Anorexia Nervosa

Anorexia Nervosa

Editors

Stephan Zipfel
Andreas Stengel
Katrin Giel

MDPI • Basel • Beijing • Wuhan • Barcelona • Belgrade • Manchester • Tokyo • Cluj • Tianjin

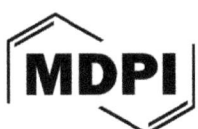

Editors

Stephan Zipfel
University Tübingen
Germany

Andreas Stengel
University Tübingen
Germany

Katrin Giel
University Tübingen
Germany

Editorial Office
MDPI
St. Alban-Anlage 66
4052 Basel, Switzerland

This is a reprint of articles from the Special Issue published online in the open access journal *Actuators* (ISSN 2076-0825) (available at: https://www.mdpi.com/journal/jcm/special_issues/anorexia_nervosa).

For citation purposes, cite each article independently as indicated on the article page online and as indicated below:

LastName, A.A.; LastName, B.B.; LastName, C.C. Article Title. *Journal Name* **Year**, *Volume Number*, Page Range.

ISBN 978-3-0365-1184-9 (Hbk)
ISBN 978-3-0365-1185-6 (PDF)

Cover image courtesy of pixabay.com user mojzagrebinfo

© 2021 by the authors. Articles in this book are Open Access and distributed under the Creative Commons Attribution (CC BY) license, which allows users to download, copy and build upon published articles, as long as the author and publisher are properly credited, which ensures maximum dissemination and a wider impact of our publications.

The book as a whole is distributed by MDPI under the terms and conditions of the Creative Commons license CC BY-NC-ND.

Contents

About the Editors vii

Preface to "Anorexia Nervosa" ix

Zaida Agüera, Georgios Paslakis, Lucero Munguía, Isabel Sánchez, Roser Granero, Jessica Sánchez-González, Trevor Steward, Susana Jiménez-Murcia and Fernando Fernández-Aranda
Gender-Related Patterns of Emotion Regulation among Patients with Eating Disorders
Reprinted from: *Journal of Clinical Medicine* 2019, 8, 161, doi:10.3390/jcm8020161 1

Gaby Resmark, Brigid Kennedy, Maria Mayer, Katrin Giel, Florian Junne, Martin Teufel, Martina de Zwaan and Stephan Zipfel
Manualised Cognitive Behaviour Therapy for Anorexia Nervosa: Use of Treatment Modules in the ANTOP Study
Reprinted from: *Journal of Clinical Medicine* 2018, 7, 398, doi:10.3390/jcm7110398 17

Celine S. Lehmann, Tobias Hofmann, Ulf Elbelt, Matthias Rose, Christoph U. Correll, Andreas Stengel and Verena Haas
The Role of Objectively Measured, Altered Physical Activity Patterns for Body Mass Index Change during Inpatient Treatment in Female Patients with Anorexia Nervosa
Reprinted from: *Journal of Clinical Medicine* 2018, 7, 289, doi:10.3390/jcm7090289 27

Katrin Ziser, Katrin E. Giel, Gaby Resmark, Christoph Nikendei, Hans-Christoph Friederich, Stephan Herpertz, Matthias Rose, Martina de Zwaan, Jörn von Wietersheim, Almut Zeeck, Andreas Dinkel, Markus Burgmer, Bernd Löwe, Carina Sprute, Stephan Zipfel and Florian Junne
Contingency Contracts for Weight Gain of Patients with Anorexia Nervosa in Inpatient Therapy: Practice Styles of Specialized Centers
Reprinted from: *Journal of Clinical Medicine* 2018, 7, 215, doi:10.3390/jcm7080215 39

Dennis Gibson and Philip S Mehler
Anorexia Nervosa and the Immune System—A Narrative Review
Reprinted from: *Journal of Clinical Medicine* 2019, 8, 1915, doi:10.3390/jcm8111915 51

Joe J. Simon, Marion A. Stopyra and Hans-Christoph Friederich
Neural Processing of Disorder-Related Stimuli in Patients with Anorexia Nervosa: A Narrative Review of Brain Imaging Studies
Reprinted from: *Journal of Clinical Medicine* 2019, 8, 1047, doi:10.3390/jcm8071047 71

Corinne Blanchet, Sébastien Guillaume, Flora Bat-Pitault, Marie-Emilie Carles, Julia Clarke, Vincent Dodin, Philibert Duriez, Priscille Gerardin, Mouna Hanachi-Guidoum, Sylvain Iceta, Juliane Leger, Bérénice Segrestin, Chantal Stheneur and Nathalie Godart
Medication in AN: A Multidisciplinary Overview of Meta-Analyses and Systematic Reviews
Reprinted from: *Journal of Clinical Medicine* 2019, 8, 278, doi:10.3390/jcm8020278 89

Gaby Resmark, Stephan Herpertz, Beate Herpertz-Dahlmann and Almut Zeeck
Treatment of Anorexia Nervosa—New Evidence-Based Guidelines
Reprinted from: *Journal of Clinical Medicine* 2019, 8, 153, doi:10.3390/jcm8020153 131

About the Editors

Professor Stephan Zipfel MD PhD; Affiliation: Internal Medicine VI, Department for Psychosomatic Medicine and Psychotherapy, University Tuebingen, Germany; E-Mail: stephan.zipfel@med.uni-tuebingen.de; Interests: anorexia nervosa; eating disorders; gut-brain axis; irritable bowel syndrome; obesity; psychotherapy.

Professor Andreas Stengel MD PhD; Affiliation: Internal Medicine VI, Department for Psychosomatic Medicine and Psychotherapy, University Tuebingen, Germany and Department for Psychosomatic Medicine, Charité University Berlin, Germany; Email: Andreas.Stengel@med.uni-tuebingen.de; Interests: anorexia nervosa; eating disorders; gut-brain axis; irritable bowel syndrome; obesity; psychogastroenterology; stress.

Professor Katrin Giel PhD; Affiliation: Department of Psychosomatic Medicine; Email: Katrin.Giel@med.uni-tuebingen.de; Interests: anorexia nervosa; eating disorders; impulsivity; obesity.

Preface to "Anorexia Nervosa"

Anorexia nervosa is a common eating disorder affecting several functions of the body. Although our knowledge of the underlying mechanism has increased, therapeutic options are still limited. This Special Issue contains 4 original and 4 review articles that discuss several aspects of anorexia nervosa and cover a broad range of topics from the bench to the bedside.

Stephan Zipfel, Andreas Stengel, Katrin Giel
Editors

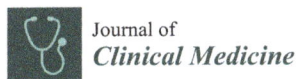 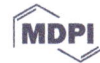

Article

Gender-Related Patterns of Emotion Regulation among Patients with Eating Disorders

Zaida Agüera [1,2,3,]*, Georgios Paslakis [2], Lucero Munguía [4], Isabel Sánchez [2], Roser Granero [1,5], Jessica Sánchez-González [2], Trevor Steward [1,2], Susana Jiménez-Murcia [1,2,4] and Fernando Fernández-Aranda [1,2,4,]*

[1] CIBER Fisiopatología Obesidad y Nutrición (CIBERobn), Instituto de Salud Carlos III, L'Hospitalet de Llobregat, 08907 Barcelona, Spain; Roser.Granero@uab.cat (R.G.); tsteward@bellvitgehospital.cat (T.S.); sjimenez@bellvitgehospital.cat (S.J.-M.)
[2] Department of Psychiatry, University Hospital of Bellvitge-IDIBELL, L'Hospitalet de Llobregat, 08907 Barcelona, Spain; paslakis@outlook.de (G.P.); isasanchez@bellvitgehospital.cat (I.S.); jsanchezg@bellvitgehospital.cat (J.S.-G.)
[3] Department of Public Health, Mental Health and Maternal-Child Nursing, School of Nursing, University of Barcelona, L'Hospitalet de Llobregat, 08907 Barcelona, Spain
[4] Department of Clinical Sciences, School of Medicine and Health Sciences, University of Barcelona, L'Hospitalet de Llobregat, 08907 Barcelona, Spain; laarcreed_lm@hotmail.com
[5] Departament de Psicobiologia i Metodologia de les Ciències de la Salut, Universitat Autònoma de Barcelona, 08193 Barcelona, Spain
* Correspondence: zaguera@bellvitgehospital.cat (Z.A.); ffernandez@bellvitgehospital.cat (F.F.-A.); Tel.: +34-93-260-72-27 (Z.A. & F.F.-A.)

Received: 2 January 2019; Accepted: 28 January 2019; Published: 1 February 2019

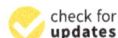

Abstract: Difficulties in emotion regulation (ER) are common in females with eating disorders (ED). However, no study to date has analyzed ER in males with ED. In the study at hand, we assessed ER in males with ED and compared results to both females with ED and healthy controls (HC). We also examined associations between ER difficulties, personality, and psychopathology. A total of 62 males with ED were compared with 656 females with ED, as well as 78 male and 286 female HC. ER was assessed by means of the Difficulties in Emotion Regulation Scale (DERS). We found that males and females with ED showed greater ER difficulties compared to HC. Pronounced general psychopathology was a shared factor associated with higher ER difficulties in both males and females with ED. However, whereas higher novelty seeking, higher cooperativeness, lower reward dependence, and lower self-directedness were related to higher ER difficulties in females with ED, lower persistence was associated with ER difficulties in males with ED. In sum, males and females with ED show similar ER difficulties, yet they are distinct in how ER deficits relate to specific personality traits. Research on strategies promoting ER in the treatment of males with ED is warranted.

Keywords: emotion regulation; males; eating disorders

1. Introduction

Emotion regulation (ER) is defined as the sum of techniques applied to manage the variety, intensity, and duration of emotions [1]. Such strategies range from the putatively less adaptive, such as dissociation, avoidance, or suppression, to the supposedly more adaptive, e.g., cognitive reappraisal or problem-solving. Difficulties in ER are a transdiagnostic feature among multiple mental disorders and may explain high comorbidity rates (e.g., with anxiety, depression, or borderline personality disorder) [2]. Accordingly, ER is proposed as a transdiagnostic target for treatment [3].

ER allows one to cope with aversive emotions, is a core feature of self-regulation, and has a profound influence on food intake behaviors [4]. Difficulties in ER are present across all types of eating disorders (ED) [5–9]. In some studies, anorexia nervosa (AN) and bulimia nervosa (BN) do not seem to significantly differ with regard to most domains of ER. Patients with binge-eating disorder (BED) show less severe ER difficulties than patients with AN or BN [5,10], although there are also studies claiming that patients with binge-eating episodes (BED, BN, and AN/binge-eating purging subtype) present more ER difficulties compared to patients with AN/restrictive subtype [11] and others have shown no differences across ED types [12]. Nevertheless, ED are associated with other behaviors linked to ER difficulties, such as substance abuse and self-harm [9,13–15].

In addition, it is unclear to which degree difficulties in ER in ED may be seen as etiopathogenetic/vulnerability or as a maintenance factor contributing to the perpetuation of the disorder. In AN, starvation and low body weight reduce the susceptibility for emotional stimuli in the short-term and are thought to serve as dysfunctional strategies to regulate aversive emotions [16,17]. Patients suffering from AN are known to have difficulties in identifying emotional states in themselves and in others (i.e., alexithymia) and may, in part, be reversed parallel to weight gain during the course of treatment [18]. This is of clinical relevance, since difficulties in identifying emotions in others are associated with difficulties in one's own ER skills [19,20]. Relatedly, the interrelation between ER and binge-eating behavior postulated in different models. According to the affect regulation theory [21], binge-eating episodes in BN are used to relieve states of negative affect. In their meta-analysis, Haedt-Matt and Keel [22] showed that negative affect immediately before an episode of binge-eating is higher than a day's average affective content and higher than the dominant affect immediately prior to an unobtrusive eating behavior. In opposition to the affect regulation theory, the aversive emotional state does not resolve immediately after the binge-eating episode, but after an apparent delay of several hours [22]. Following a binge episode, compensatory behavior in BN may prevent a further increase in negative affect. In addition, a prior study analyzing ER in female ED patients before and after treatment found that emotional dysregulation can be modified as an effect of symptomatological ED improvement [23]. With these controversial results in mind, the question of whether the emotional dysregulation is a vulnerability factor for ED, a factor that maintains and worsens with the ED or both, is still open. At present, several manualized therapies for ED focusing on ER have been published [24,25].

Nevertheless, as in the vast majority of ED studies, females are overrepresented in studies on ER in ED [7,8], and males with ED are not researched as a whole. Although females greatly outnumber males with respect to diagnosed ED, it stands to reason that ER could also play a role in eating pathology in males, as it does in females.

With regard to gender-related differences in ER, evidence is scarce and mostly derived from studies in nonclinical community samples of males and females. In the study by Hayaki and Free [26], difficulties in ER predicted disordered eating in both male and female undergraduate students. Whereas some studies have shown no global differences between genders in nonclinical cohorts [27], others have shown gender-specific affective responses to high-calorie visual cues [28]. Significantly higher levels of rumination have also been identified in females, which, as an ER strategy, mediated the relationship between gender and disordered eating [29]. Difficulties in ER were identified as important determinants of body dissatisfaction and disordered eating in a study with only undergraduate males [30].

In a recent study in a cohort suffering from ED, difficulties in ER were found to be more strongly associated with cognitively oriented ED symptoms than with behavioral symptoms, such as binge eating, purging, driven exercise, non-suicidal self-injury, or suicide attempts. However, no gender comparisons were undertaken [31]. So far, studies investigating gender-related ER differences in clinical cohorts show no relevant gender-specific differences with regard to negative affect, emotional instability, and interpersonal dysfunction in an ED cohort consisting of $n = 251$ females and $n = 137$ males [32] or with regard to emotional overeating in a BED cohort comparing $n = 172$ females and $n = 48$ males [33]. There are also divergent results showing no differences in complex emotion recognition between males with ED (*n* = 29) and healthy controls (HC) (*n* = 42) [34]. However, none of these studies in males made ER-specific instruments. Instead, the studies used subscales from a personality questionnaire as indirect measures to assess both negative affect and interpersonal dysfunction. Others have solely applied a specific measure of overeating in response to emotions, or analyzed only emotion recognition, but not ER strategies or emotion difficulties In addition, no study published to date, to our knowledge, analyzed ER in males using the different DSM-5 ED types, either because the sample size did not allow for it or because they only analyzed one ED type.

Personality traits and ER appear to be intertwined, with evidence showing links between the two in a number of studies [35,36]. For instance, difficulties in ER are implicated in the diagnostic criteria for some personality disorders (e.g., borderline personality disorder) [37]. ED are also associated with specific personality traits, including harm avoidance and low self-directedness in all ED diagnostic types, high novelty seeking in BED and BN, and high reward dependence and persistence in AN [38,39]. Males suffering from ED scored significantly lower than females with ED on harm avoidance, reward dependence, and cooperativeness, had less body image concerns, and lower general psychopathology [40]. In addition, dysfunctional personality traits are associated with higher ED severity, general psychopathology, self-harm behaviors, and worse therapy response and prognosis [41–43]. In a previous study by our group, we showed that ER difficulties mediated the relationship between personality traits (i.e., high harm avoidance and low self-directedness) and ED severity [44]. Thus, personality traits may increase vulnerability to ED pathology through ER difficulties. As these aspects were not studied in males with ED before, we incorporated an examination of the interplay between ER, personality traits, ED severity, and ED-related and general psychopathology in males with ED as further objectives of the present study.

Taking into account all the aforementioned gaps in the literature, primarily the lack of studies with clinical samples of males with ED, we aimed to examine ER in a large sample of consecutively recruited male and female patients with ED and HC, considering different DSM-5 ED types. Based on a previous research carried out at our Unit [23], which found how ER strategies improved along with improvements in eating symptoms after cognitive behavioral therapy (CBT), we analyzed the relationship between ED severity, general psychopathology, specific personality traits, and ER. In addition, assessment of the associations between ER and other behaviors commonly used to alleviate aversive emotional states, such as non-suicidal self-injury (NSSI), (reduced) interoceptive awareness, binge-eating, and purging behaviors were part of the study protocol.

2. Experimental Section

2.1. Participants

The sample consisted of 62 male participants diagnosed with ED (16-AN, 12-BN, 15-BED, 19-Other Specified Feeding or Eating Disorder (OSFED)), 656 female ED patients (140-AN, 236-BN, 100-BED, 180-OSFED), and a HC group, 286 females and 78 males, without a history of ED. The clinical groups were consecutively referred for assessment and treatment at the Eating Disorders Unit within the Department of Psychiatry at Bellvitge University Hospital in Barcelona, Spain. All patients were diagnosed according to the DSM-5 [37] criteria and assessed by senior clinicians specialized in ED. All HC came from the same catchment area as the patients. Participants were recruited between May 2013 and July 2018. In accordance with the Declaration of Helsinki, the present study was approved by the Ethics Committee of our institution (The Clinical Research Ethics Committee (CEIC) of Bellvitge University Hospital). All the participants provided signed informed consent.

2.2. Assessment

Eating Disorder Inventory-2 (EDI-2) [45]. This is a reliable and valid 91-item multidimensional self-report questionnaire that assesses different cognitive and behavioral characteristics of eating disorders: Drive for thinness, body dissatisfaction, bulimia, ineffectiveness, perfectionism, interpersonal distrust, interoceptive awareness, maturity fears, asceticism, impulse regulation, and social insecurity. This instrument was validated in a Spanish population [46]. Internal consistency was excellent in our sample ($\alpha = 0.97$ for the total scale).

Symptom Checklist-90 Items-Revised (SCL-90-R) [47]. This is a 90-item questionnaire that is widely used for assessing self-reported psychological distress and psychopathology. The test is scored on nine primary symptom dimensions: Somatization, obsessive-compulsive, interpersonal sensitivity, depression, anxiety, hostility, phobic anxiety, paranoid ideation, and psychoticism, and three global indices: Global Severity Index (GSI), Positive Symptom Total (PST), and Positive Symptom Distress Index (PSDI). This instrument was validated in a Spanish population [48]. Internal consistency was excellent in our sample (Cronbach's alpha, $\alpha = 0.98$ Cronbach's alpha).

Temperament and Character Inventory–Revised (TCI-R) [49]. The TCI-R is a 240-item questionnaire with a five-point Likert scale format. This questionnaire is a reliable and valid measure of four temperaments (harm avoidance, novelty seeking, reward dependence, and persistence) and three character dimensions (self-directedness, cooperativeness, and self-transcendence). This questionnaire was validated in a Spanish adult population [50]. Cronbach's alpha for the current sample ranged from good ($\alpha = 0.81$ for "novelty seeking") to excellent ($\alpha = 0.99$ for "persistence").

Difficulties in Emotion Regulation Scale (DERS) [51]. The DERS assesses emotion dysregulation across six subscales: (a) Nonacceptance of emotional responses, (b) difficulties in pursuing goals when having strong emotions, (c) difficulties controlling impulsive behaviors when experiencing negative emotions, (d) lack of emotional awareness, (e) limited access to emotion regulation strategies, and (f) lack of emotional clarity. Higher scores indicate more difficulties in emotion regulation. The Spanish version was validated in an adult population [44], and excellent internal consistency was found in the study sample ($\alpha = 0.96$ for the total scale).

2.3. Statistical Analysis

Statistical analysis was carried out with Stata15 for Windows. The comparison of quantitative variables between the groups was based on analysis of variance adjusted for the participants' age, education level, and civil status (ANCOVA). The estimation of the effect size of the pairwise comparisons was based on Cohen's-d coefficients ($|d| > 0.20$ was considered low, $|d| > 0.5$ was considered moderate, and $|d| > 0.8$ was considered high) [52]. In addition, Finner's procedure (a familywise error rate stepwise method which has demonstrated more powerful than Bonferroni correction) controlled the increase in Type-I error due to multiple comparisons [53].

Linear multiple regressions stratified by sex estimated the predictive capacity of clinical measures (defined as the independent variables) on ER (defined as the criterion, DERS total score). Each regression was adjusted in five blocks/steps: (a) First block-step entered and set the covariates participants' age, education, and civil status; (b) Second block added ED-related variables (EDI-2 total, onset of the ED, and duration of the ED); (c) The third block included global psychopathological state (SCL-90R GSI); (d) The fourth block entered NSSI (0 = absent; 1 = present); and (e) The fifth block included personality traits (TCI-R scale scores). The specific predictive capacity of each step/block was measured as the increase in the R^2 coefficient (ΔR^2).

Pathways analysis assessed the underlying mechanisms of the following study variables: Participants' sex and age, personality traits, EDI-2 total score, SCL-90-R GSI and DERS scale scores. This method constitutes an extension of multiple regression modeling, which aims to estimate the magnitude and significance of hypothesized associations in a set of variables with the advantage of allowing for the testing of mediational links (direct and indirect effects) [54]. Structural equation modeling (SEM) was used by defining the maximum-likelihood estimation of parameter estimation and testing goodness-of-fit through standard statistical measures: The root mean square error of approximation (RMSEA), Bentler's Comparative Fit Index (CFI), the Tucker-Lewis Index (TLI), and the standardized root mean square residual (SRMR). Adequate model fit was considered non-significant by χ^2 tests and if the following criteria were met [55]: RMSEA < 0.08, TLI > 0.9, CFI > 0.9 and SRMR < 0.1.

In this study, ER was defined as a latent variable defined by DERS scale scores, and the personality profile as a latent class defined by TCI-R scale scores.

3. Results

3.1. Sample Characteristics

Table 1 includes the description and the comparison between the four groups of the study defined by ED diagnosis and sex. Differences emerged with regards to civil status, education and age.

Table 1. Sample description.

	ED Females (n = 656)		ED Males (n = 62)		HC Females (n = 286)		HC Males (n = 78)		p-Value
	n	%	n	%	n	%	n	%	
Civil status									
Single	486	74.1%	42	67.7%	278	97.2%	77	98.7%	<0.001 *
Married-partner	114	17.4%	17	27.4%	3	1.0%	0	0.0%	
Separated-divorced	56	8.5%	3	4.8%	5	1.7%	1	1.3%	
Education									
Primary	261	39.8%	28	45.2%	6	2.1%	2	2.6%	<0.001 *
Secondary	271	41.3%	22	35.5%	276	96.5%	75	96.2%	
University	124	18.9%	12	19.4%	4	1.4%	1	1.3%	
Employed									
Student	259	39.5%	22	35.5%	120	42.0%	42	53.8%	0.077
Unemployed	397	60.5%	40	64.5%	166	58.0%	36	46.2%	
	Mean	SD	Mean	SD	Mean	SD	Mean	SD	p-Value
Age (years-old)	29.78	11.07	33.56	12.73	21.06	4.19	21.30	4.53	<0.001 *

SD: Standard deviation. * Bold: Significant comparison (0.05 level). ED: Eating disorder; HC: Healthy control.

3.2. ER and Negative Affect Measures and Comparison between Groups

The first block of Table 2 includes the results of the ANCOVA (adjusted forage, civil status, and education) comparing the four study groups (ED-women, ED-men, HC-women, and HC-men) with regard to DERS scales, EDI-2 scales, and the binge-eating/purging levels (these two last measures were only compared between ED groups). Pairwise comparisons between ED-women and ED-men reached significance in all measures (more ER difficulties for ED-women), except for DERS awareness and the EDI-2 interpersonal distrust (no differences between the two groups were obtained). ED-women registered higher mean scores in all the measures compared to HC-women. The same occurred with ED-men compared to HC-men (except for on EDI-2 perfectionism). No differences between the two HC groups (women and men) were found.

The second block of Table 2 contains the prevalence of NSSI and the comparison between the groups (comparison between the groups was based on logistic regression adjusted by the participants' age, education, and civil status). The proportion of ED-women who reported the presence of this behavior was higher than the proportion reported by ED-men (44.2% vs. 16.1%, $p < 0.001$), as well as the proportion reported by the HC-women (44.2% vs. 21.8%, $p < 0.001$). No significant differences were found comparing the HC groups (women and men) or between ED-men and HC-men.

Figure 1 includes a radar-chart for the study variables in the four groups. To allow for easy interpretation, z-standardized means were plotted.

Table 2. Comparison of DERS scales, EDI-2 scales, and negative affect between groups: ANCOVA adjusted for age, civil status, and education.

	ED Women (n = 656)		ED Men (n = 62)		HC Women (n = 286)		HC Men (n = 78)		ED Women vs. ED Men			HC Women vs. HC Men			ED Women vs. HC Women			ED Men vs. HC Men		
	Mean	SD	Mean	SD	Mean	SD	Mean	SD	p-Value	|d|		p-Value	|d|		p-Value	|d|		p-Value	|d|	
DERS scales																				
Non-acceptance	19.63	6.87	17.33	6.68	12.35	5.29	10.99	4.59	0.007 *	0.34		0.089	0.27		<0.001 *	1.19 †		<0.001 *	1.11 †	
Pursuing goals	17.64	5.03	16.07	4.89	12.98	4.12	12.47	4.31	0.013 *	0.32		0.402	0.12		<0.001 *	1.01 †		<0.001 *	0.78 †	
Impulse behaviors	17.00	6.47	14.69	6.23	10.71	4.01	9.89	3.16	0.003 *	0.36		0.267	0.23		<0.001 *	1.17 †		<0.001 *	0.97 †	
Emotional awareness	17.91	5.10	18.25	4.51	14.56	4.12	14.29	4.31	0.594	0.07		0.659	0.06		<0.001 *	0.72 †		<0.001 *	0.90 †	
Emotional regulation	25.54	8.24	22.39	8.05	15.13	5.87	14.26	5.47	0.002 *	0.39		0.370	0.15		<0.001 *	1.45 †		<0.001 *	1.18 †	
Emotional clarity	14.76	5.07	13.51	5.08	10.22	3.63	9.42	3.67	0.043 *	0.25		0.182	0.22		<0.001 *	1.03 †		<0.001 *	0.92 †	
Total score	112.46	26.94	102.25	26.02	75.95	19.27	71.31	16.95	0.002 *	0.39		0.143	0.26		<0.001 *	1.56 †		<0.001 *	1.41 †	
EDI-2 scales																				
Drive for thinness	14.23	6.02	10.51	5.60	3.74	5.04	2.75	3.45	<0.001 *	0.64 †		0.206	0.23		<0.001 *	1.89 †		<0.001 *	1.67 †	
Body dissatisfaction	17.22	7.88	11.10	8.32	6.37	6.75	4.63	4.87	<0.001 *	0.75 †		0.094	0.30		<0.001 *	1.48 †		<0.001 *	0.95 †	
Interoceptive awareness	11.83	7.06	8.32	6.43	2.83	2.89	1.94	1.99	<0.001 *	0.52 †		0.249	0.36		<0.001 *	1.67 †		<0.001 *	1.34 †	
Bulimia	7.21	5.59	3.74	4.15	1.49	1.68	1.01	0.93	<0.001 *	0.70 †		0.454	0.35		<0.001 *	1.39 †		0.001 *	0.91 †	
Interpersonal distrust	5.76	4.81	5.67	4.52	2.54	2.92	2.57	2.76	0.880	0.02		0.969	0.01		<0.001*	0.81 †		<0.001 *	0.83 †	
Ineffectiveness	11.90	7.70	8.21	7.22	2.26	3.05	2.02	2.65	<0.001 *	0.51 †		0.788	0.09		<0.001 *	1.65 †		<0.001 *	1.14 †	
Maturity fears	8.79	5.97	7.33	5.03	4.46	3.72	4.20	3.38	0.036 *	0.27		0.725	0.07		<0.001 *	0.87 †		0.001 *	0.73 †	
Perfectionism	6.18	4.36	5.05	4.00	3.99	3.55	4.08	3.34	0.037 *	0.27		0.874	0.03		<0.001 *	0.55 †		0.186	0.27	
Impulse regulation	6.84	6.03	5.55	5.21	1.28	2.27	1.47	3.06	0.047 *	0.23		0.783	0.07		<0.001 *	1.22 †		<0.001 *	0.95 †	
Ascetism	7.36	4.09	5.81	4.25	2.35	2.22	2.57	2.10	0.001 *	0.37		0.653	0.10		<0.001 *	1.52 †		<0.001 *	0.96 †	
Social insecurity	8.11	5.37	6.56	4.74	2.63	2.85	2.40	2.82	0.013 *	0.31		0.725	0.08		<0.001 *	1.28 †		<0.001 *	1.07 †	
Total score	105.43	42.63	77.88	42.60	33.89	21.52	29.50	15.65	<0.001 *	0.65 †		0.355	0.23		<0.001 *	2.12 †		<0.001 *	1.51 †	
Binge eating/purging																				
Binge episodes	3.76	6.32	1.86	2.60	—	—	—	—	0.019 *	0.39		—	—		—	—		—	—	
Purging episodes	3.96	8.75	1.29	3.60	—	—	—	—	0.018 *	0.40		—	—		—	—		—	—	
	n	%	n	%	n	%	n	%	p-Value	|d|		p-Value	|d|		p-Value	|d|		p-Value	|d|	
[1] NSSI	290	44.2%	10	16.1%	62	21.8%	19	25.0%	<0.001 *	0.64 †		0.544	0.08		<0.001 *	0.50 †		0.260	0.22	

SD: Standard deviation; NSSI: Non-suicidal self-injury; ED: Eating disorder; HC: Healthy control; EDI-2: Eating Disorder Inventory-20; DERS: Difficulties in Emotion Regulation Scale. * Bold: Significant comparison (0.05 level); † Effect size in the moderate (|d| > 0.50) to large range (|d| > 0.80); [1] Results obtained in logistic regression. — Binge and purging episodes were not registered for the HC group.

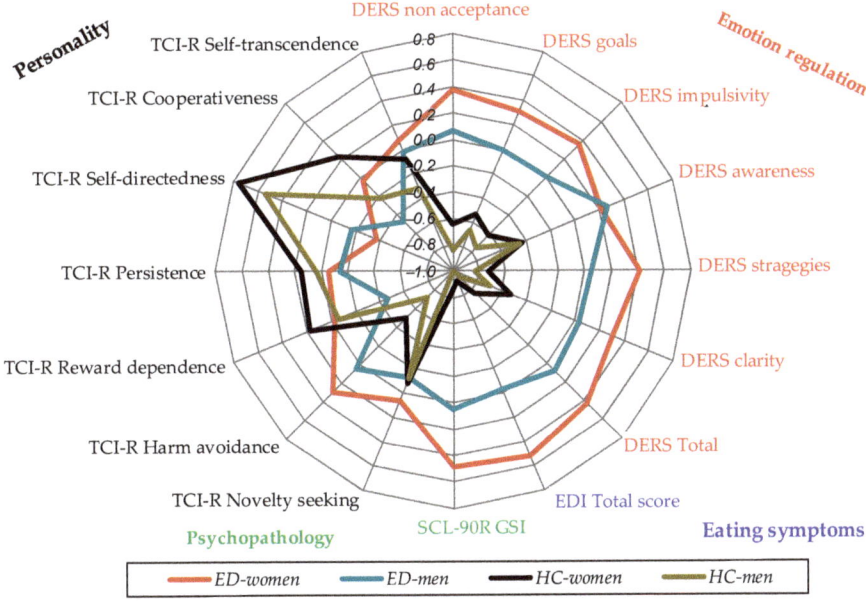

Figure 1. Radar-chart with the z-standardized means by group (*n* = 1082). DERS: Difficulties in Emotion Regulation Scale; ED: Eating disorders; EDI-2: Eating Disorders Inventory-2; HC: Healthy controls; TCI-R, SCL-90R: Symptom Checklist-90 Items-Revised; Temperament and Character Inventory revised.

3.3. Comparison of ER between ED Subtypes

Table 3 includes the ANCOVA (also adjusted for age, education, and civil status) comparing DERS scores between the ED types (AN, BN, BED, and OSFED), stratified by sex. In the female subsample as a whole, greater ER difficulties were associated with BN, followed by BED and OSFED. The lowest DERS scores were found in AN. In the male subsample, greater ER difficulties were registered in OSFED group, followed by the BN and BED groups. AN males had the lowest DERS scores. Results obtained in the men subsample must be interpreted with caution due to the low sample size of the groups.

3.4. Predictive Capacity of the Study Variables on ER

Table 4 includes the final models of the two multiple regressions measuring the predictive capacity of study variables on the DERS total score. In the ED-females model, emotion regulation difficulties were predicted by higher EDI-2 total scores, more pronounced psychopathology, higher levels in the novelty seeking and cooperativeness traits, and lower levels in the reward dependence and self-directedness traits. No significant predictive contribution of the NSSI on the DERS-total was found in the ED-females group.

For the ED-males model, DERS-total scores increased for men who reported higher scores on the EDI-2, those with higher psychopathology and lower levels in persistence.

Table 3. Comparison of DERS scales between diagnostic subtypes: ANOVA adjusted for age, civil status, and education.

Subsample	AN n = 140		BN n = 236		BED n = 100		OSFED n = 180		AN-BN		AN-BED		AN-OSFED		BN-BED		BN-OSFED		BED-OSFED	
Women	Mean	SD	Mean	SD	Mean	SD	Mean	SD	p-Value	|d|	p-Value	|d|	p-Value	|d|	p-Value	|d|	p-Value	|d|	p-Value	|d|
Nonacceptance	17.62	7.26	20.99	6.42	19.36	6.68	19.70	6.89	**<0.001** *	0.52 †	**0.046** *	0.25	**0.007** *	0.29	**0.042** *	0.25	**0.046** *	0.19	0.700	0.05
Pursuing goals	16.47	5.16	18.55	4.76	17.51	5.11	17.18	5.05	**<0.001** *	0.42	0.128	0.20	0.209	0.14	0.092	0.21	**0.006** *	0.28	0.606	0.07
Impulse behavior	15.44	6.97	18.56	6.03	16.51	6.47	16.39	6.26	**<0.001** *	0.51 †	0.225	0.16	0.186	0.14	**0.010** *	0.33	**0.001** *	0.35	0.893	0.02
Emot-awareness	17.44	5.27	18.01	4.87	18.58	5.15	17.62	5.24	0.295	0.11	0.225	0.22	0.749	0.03	0.367	0.11	0.443	0.08	0.155	0.18
Emot-regulation	23.16	8.79	27.29	7.97	25.31	7.75	24.95	7.97	**<0.001** *	0.50 †	**0.042** *	0.26	**0.049** *	0.21	**0.049** *	0.25	**0.004** *	0.29	0.739	0.05
Emot-clarity	13.77	5.50	15.22	5.00	14.49	4.53	14.77	5.02	**0.008** *	0.28	0.303	0.14	**0.042** *	0.19	0.241	0.15	0.371	0.09	0.673	0.06
Total score	103.9	29.7	118.6	24.8	111.7	25.5	110.6	26.3	**<0.001** *	0.54 †	**0.032** *	0.28	**0.025** *	0.24	**0.035** *	0.27	**0.003** *	0.31	0.752	0.04

Subsample	AN n = 16		BN n = 12		BED n = 15		OSFED n = 19		AN-BN		AN-BED		AN-OSFED		BN-BED		BN-OSFED		BED-OSFED	
Men	Mean	SD	Mean	SD	Mean	SD	Mean	SD	p-Value	|d|	p-Value	|d|	p-Value	|d|	p-Value	|d|	p-Value	|d|	p-Value	|d|
Nonacceptance	16.14	7.86	17.95	5.65	17.90	7.78	17.79	5.46	0.507	0.26	0.499	0.22	0.494	0.24	0.985	0.01	0.950	0.03	0.965	0.02
Pursuing goals	13.69	4.68	15.83	5.17	16.66	4.52	17.32	4.75	0.266	0.53 †	**0.048** *	0.65 †	**0.035** *	0.77 †	0.661	0.17	0.415	0.30	0.711	0.14
Impulse behavior	11.66	4.22	16.11	6.33	14.07	6.24	16.85	6.64	**0.043** *	0.83 †	0.286	0.51 †	**0.015** *	0.93 †	0.386	0.32	0.740	0.12	0.203	0.51 †
Emot-awareness	17.96	4.75	18.21	3.55	19.28	4.73	17.21	4.81	0.893	0.06	0.455	0.28	0.644	0.16	0.561	0.26	0.570	0.24	0.227	0.52 †
Emot-regulation	20.43	9.44	21.45	7.05	21.68	6.53	24.66	8.14	0.737	0.12	0.668	0.15	**0.049** *	0.53 †	0.942	0.03	0.275	0.52 †	0.293	0.50 †
Emot-clarity	14.31	6.38	12.20	5.19	13.75	4.63	12.71	4.27	0.315	0.36	0.777	0.10	0.387	0.29	0.458	0.31	0.798	0.11	0.591	0.23
Total score	94.2	29.3	101.7	25.1	103.3	24.1	106.5	25.0	0.466	0.28	0.356	0.34	0.180	**0.55** †	0.878	0.06	0.628	0.19	0.737	0.13

SD: Standard deviation; * Bold: Significant comparison (0.05 level). † Effect size in the moderate (|d| > 0.50) to high range (|d| > 0.80); AN: Anorexia nervosa; BN: Bulimia nervosa; BED: Binge eating disorder; OSFED: Other specified feeding or eating disorder.

Table 4. Predictive model of the DERS total score: Multiple regression stratified by sex (ED subsample, $n = 718$).

	ED Women ($n = 656$)								ED Men ($n = 62$)							
	Coefficients (Model Obtained in the Fifth Block-Step)						Change		Coefficients (Model Obtained in the Fifth Block-Step)						Change	
	B	SE	Beta	p-Value	95% CI (B)		ΔR²	p-Value	B	SE	Beta	p-Value	95% CI (B)		ΔR²	B
Covariates							0.009	0.131							0.055	0.395
Age (years-old)	−0.13	0.19	−0.054	0.497	−0.51	0.25			0.11	0.43	0.053	0.809	−0.77	0.98		
Civil status (married)	3.33	1.95	0.055	0.089	−0.50	7.15			−0.51	5.42	−0.009	0.926	−11.45	10.44		
Education level	1.51	0.94	0.041	0.107	−0.33	3.36			2.65	2.43	0.077	0.283	−2.27	7.56		
ED variables							0.533	<0.001 *							0.488	<0.001 *
EDI-2 total	0.19	0.03	0.294	<0.001 *	0.13	0.24			0.09	0.07	0.158	0.183	−0.05	0.24		
Onset of ED	−0.02	0.21	−0.005	0.934	−0.42	0.39			−0.17	0.35	−0.076	0.635	−0.88	0.54		
Duration of ED	0.05	0.20	0.017	0.798	−0.34	0.44			−0.37	0.28	−0.155	0.196	−0.94	0.20		
Psychopathology							0.073	<0.001 *							0.219	<0.001 *
SCL-90R GSI	14.61	1.55	0.397	<0.001 *	11.57	17.65			19.39	3.72	0.609	<0.001 *	11.88	26.91		
Fourth block/step							0.001	0.946							0.006	0.268
NSSI (0 = no; 1 = yes)	0.20	0.84	0.006	0.809	−1.45	1.86			−0.28	2.97	−0.007	0.924	−6.29	5.72		
TCI-R							0.025	<0.001 *							0.076	0.018 *
Novelty seeking	0.08	0.05	0.048	0.044 *	0.01	0.17			0.06	0.15	0.042	0.688	−0.24	0.35		
Harm avoidance	0.00	0.05	−0.004	0.926	−0.10	0.09			0.00	0.17	0.000	0.997	−0.34	0.34		
Reward dependence	−0.09	0.05	−0.054	0.047 *	−0.18	−0.01			−0.11	0.15	−0.060	0.470	−0.40	0.19		
Persistence	−0.05	0.04	−0.039	0.174	−0.12	0.02			−0.41	0.14	−0.256	0.005 *	−0.69	−0.13		
Self-directedness	−0.25	0.05	−0.197	<0.001 *	−0.34	−0.15			−0.21	0.16	−0.189	0.195	−0.54	0.11		
Cooperativeness	0.12	0.05	0.070	0.023 *	0.02	0.22			0.13	0.17	0.075	0.456	−0.21	0.47		
Self-transcendence	−0.04	0.05	−0.026	0.335	−0.14	0.05			0.02	0.13	0.012	0.891	−0.25	0.28		

* Bold: Significance parameter (0.05 level). DF: Degrees of freedom. ΔR²: Increase-change in R^2. ED: Eating disorders; EDI-2: Eating Disorders Inventory-2; NSSI: Non-suicidal self-injury; SCL-90R GSI: Global Severity Index of the questionnaire; Symptom Checklist-90 Items-Revised; TCI-R: Temperament and Character Inventory-Revised; B: Non-standardized B-coefficient; SE: standard error; Beta: Standardized B-coefficient; 95% CI: 95% confidence interval.

3.5. Pathways Analysis

Figure 2 includes the path-diagram with the standardized coefficients of the SEM obtained in the ED group (Table S1, supplementary material, includes the complete results valuing direct, indirect. and total effects). Goodness-of-fit was obtained (all the fit statistics were in the adequate range). The latent variable measuring ER difficulties (labeled as DERS in the figure) was directly increased for patients who presented higher ED severity (higher EDI-2 total), higher psychopathology (higher SCL-90R GSI), and who were younger. Higher scores in the latent variable measuring the personality construct (labeled as TCI-R in the figure) were also direct predictors of greater ER difficulties. ED severity and the psychopathology levels mediated the relationships between personality measures and ER, as well as between sex and ER: Higher levels in the TCI-R construct and being female increased EDI-2 interoceptive awareness and SCL-90R scores, which contributed to increases on the DERS.

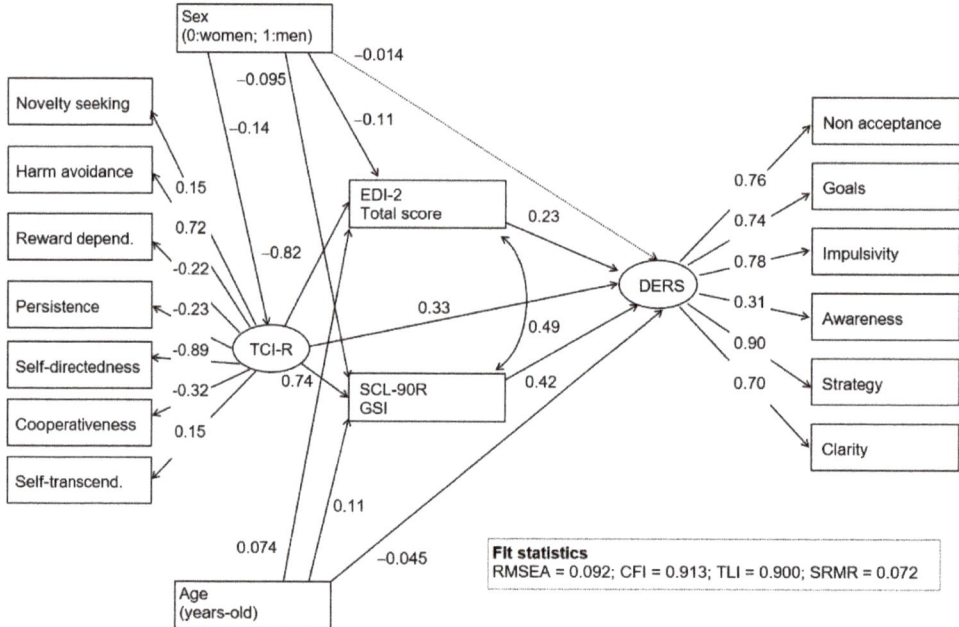

Figure 2. SEM: Standardized coefficients (ED subsample; n = 718). Continuous line: Significant parameter (0.05 level). Dash line: Nonsignificant parameter. GSI: Global Severity Index.

4. Discussion

The present study attempted to address a relevant issue in the psychopathology of male patients with ED. It aimed to provide a better knowledge regarding ER in this clinical population, analyzing and comparing ER difficulties between male and female patients with ED and HC, which was rarely studied before. Findings from this study provide new information for the treatment approach of male patients with ED, a minority in the field of ED that runs the risk of being overlooked.

Our first main finding confirmed that patients with ED, both males and females, showed greater global ER difficulties than HC. Although these results are not in accordance with prior research indicating that males with ED did not differ from HC males in emotion regulation strategies, such as emotion recognition [34], they are in line with previous studies which found that negative affect and difficulties in ER predicted disordered eating in both males and females in community samples [26,27]. These discrepancies may be due to the fact that the study by Goddard et al. [34] focused on emotional recognition and not on ER. Moreover, our results support previous findings in clinical samples that have reported decreased effective ER strategies among female patients with ED when compared with HC [10,56], suggesting that a lack of effective ER skills may prompt individuals to use disordered or abnormal eating behaviors to regulate negative affect [57], as well as contribute to body dissatisfaction and disordered eating in males [30]. Therefore, ER difficulties may act as an important etiological feature [57] or risk factor for the occurrence of EDs [23]. Although previous studies have focused primarily on females with ED, our findings also offer the possibility of generalizing these findings to males with ED.

When comparing male and female patients with ED, female patients with ED engaged in more dysfunctional ER strategies than males with ED, displaying greater scores on all DERS scales, except for DERS emotional awareness. There were no differences between male and female controls with regard to ER difficulties. First, these findings confirmed our hypothesis that both males and females with ED displayed a lack of emotional awareness. Second, the fact that female patients with ED scored higher in the most of the DERS scales, such as nonacceptance of emotional responses, limited access to emotion regulation strategies, lack of emotional clarity, and difficulties in engaging in goal-directed behavior or in controlling impulsive behaviors when experiencing negative emotions suggests that there are indeed gender-related patterns of ER in ED. However, we cannot fully exclude gender-related response bias, since males may have had a tendency to minimize or underestimate (intentionally or unintentionally) the difficulties related to their ER in order to prevent their culturally imposed, self-perceived masculinity ideals from being threatened [58]. Furthermore, males with ED appear to more often use externalizing behaviors (e.g., hetero-aggression) or to engage in drug or alcohol use/abuse to deal with emotions whereas females with ED tend to use more internalizing behaviors, such as NSSI [41]. Our results support these observations, with females with ED in the present study showing significantly more NSSI behaviors than males with ED.

Regarding ED types, our findings showed higher ER difficulties in patients with binge eating-related behaviors (BN, BED, and OSFED) compare to patients with restrictive behaviors (AN), in both males and females with ED. These results are consistent with previous studies reporting more ER difficulties among patients with binge-eating behaviors [44,59], but they are discrepant to other studies reporting less severe ER difficulties in BED patients and no significant differences between AN-R and other ED subtypes [5]. However, while females with BN showed the greatest ER deficits compared to females with other ED diagnoses, males diagnosed with OSFED were those who displayed the most ER difficulties. These differences suggest that females and males with ED engage in different disordered eating behaviors for alleviating negative affect and emotional instability. Females with ED seem to present more binge eating and purging behaviors for ER, whereas males with ED are prompt to use more heterogeneous ED-related symptomatology for alleviating emotional distress (e.g., high levels of exercise).

In terms of primary predictors, higher general psychopathology was the shared factor associated with ER difficulties in both males and females with ED. However, ED severity and different personality traits were identified as differential predictors in females and males with ED. Increased ED severity, higher novelty seeking, higher cooperativeness, lower reward dependence, and lower self-directedness were related to higher ER difficulties in females with ED, while lower persistence was associated with ER difficulties in males with ED. Thus, in females with ED, difficulties in ER were associated with a tendency to be more impulsive and intolerant of routine, and which are linked with seeking little emotional support, the unwillingness to be sociable, and having difficulty in expressing feelings and thoughts [60]. On the other hand, in males with ED, difficulties with ER were associated with low persistence, that is, a tendency to be less perseverant in situations of frustration and fatigue [60]. In light of our results, our findings suggest that personality differences may impact ER difficulties, therefore, it would be important to assess for personality traits and consider potential gender-related differences [61,62]. In this regard, it may also be useful to apply ER-based adjuvant treatments focused on reducing impulsivity and increasing self-directedness and reward dependence for females with ED, and specific treatment approaches for males with ED where increased persistence management are specifically addressed.

Finally, another emergent finding was that both ED severity and general psychopathology mediated the relationships between personality and ER difficulties. This may open a new line of research that allows for knowing if the improvement in the ED symptomatology could establish changes in emotion dysregulation. In this sense, a previous study in females with ED found ER improvements after CBT (treatment as usual, without any specific module addressing ER), especially in patients with BN. This study found that improvements in ER were the largest in those with a better treatment outcome [23]. In this line, our results reinforce this concept, suggesting that ED severity and psychopathology may be associated with ER difficulties. In addition, although our study is transversal and does not allow us to analyze the causality, we suggest the existence of a bidirectional pathological process that has ER difficulties acting as a maintenance factors for the ED. However, these findings do not exclude the possibility that ER is also a vulnerability factor for ED. The lack of longitudinal studies analyzing individuals before developing the ED does not allow us to identify if the ER is an etiopathogenic factor of the disorder or if, on the contrary, difficulties in ER are aggravated with the ED. It is most likely that ER is probably acting in both directions, both as a vulnerability factor and as a maintenance factor for the disorder (which is aggravated by psychopathology). With this in mind, we hypothesize that treatment enhanced with a module aimed at improving ER skills could benefit the treatment outcome of ED patients. Further studies should address this point.

Also, the results suggest that, a more dysfunctional personality profile and being female increased the risk of higher ED severity and general psychopathology, which contributed to an increase in ER difficulties in patients with ED. In this vein, a recent study found that depression moderated the association between ER difficulties and binge eating in patients with BED, suggesting that individuals who experience more intense emotions are more affected by difficulties in ER [8]. Again, the above is consistent with the need for treatment based on addressing the difficulties of ER in ED patients, since, although being aware of one's own emotions is not sufficient for an adaptive emotional regulation [44], it is the first step to improving it.

Limitations and Strengths

The present study should be evaluated within the context of its limitations. First, as we only assessed patients with ED that were seeking treatment in a clinical setting, the patient cohorts may not be representative of all patients with ED. In addition, ER difficulties were assessed by means of the DERS. Although this is a validated instrument for the assessment of ER, it may not capture other relevant aspects of ER, such as ER strategies or skills (e.g., reappraisal, stimulus control, etc.). Finally, due to the study's cross-sectional design, no conclusions can be drawn with regard to response to treatment between genders.

Notwithstanding these limitations, the current study has also several strengths that should be noted. One of the strengths of our study includes the relatively large number of males with ED in our sample and our comparison with females with ED, as well as with male and female healthy controls. For the first time, we addressed ER in a large sample of males with ED, including different DSM-5 types. As far as we know, this is the first study assessing predictors of difficulties in ER in females and males with ED.

5. Conclusions

There is a growing interest in addressing difficulties in ER in the treatment of patients with ED. However, most ER-based studies were performed in females with ED and, to date, no study was carried out in males with all DSM-5 ED diagnoses. Our findings suggest that treatments focusing on enhancing ER abilities are likely to be beneficial to both female and male patients with ED. Our findings also suggest a bidirectional relationship, that is, if we improve eating symptomatology and general psychopathology, we could improve ER in these patients. However, our results also provide evidence for the need to design specific treatments for males and females with ED that address shared and differential gender-related features associated to emotion dysregulation, such as impulsivity and reward dependence in females, and persistence in males with ED. Taking into account all of the aforementioned factors, further research should be addressed to validate and complement our results, including other measures of ER. Likewise, longitudinal designs may offer insight into gender-related responses of ER difficulties to ED treatments. Findings of this kind may, in fact, provide further evidence for the need of gender-specific, ER-centered treatments as a further step toward individualized psychotherapy.

Supplementary Materials: The following are available online at http://www.mdpi.com/2077-0383/8/2/161/s1, Table S1: SEM: tests of direct, indirect and total effects (ED subsample, n = 718).

Author Contributions: Conceptualization: Z.A., I.S., J.S.-G., S.J.-M., and F.F.-A.; Methodology: Z.A. and R.G.; Formal Analysis: R.G.; Investigation: Z.A. and G.P.; Data Curation: Z.A. and R.G.; Writing-Original Draft Preparation: G.P., R.G., and Z.A.; Writing-Review & Editing: L.M., I.S., J.G.-S., Z.A., T.S., S.J.-M., and F.F.-A.; Supervision: Z.A., F.F.-A., and S.J.-M.; Funding Acquisition: F.F.-A. and S.J.-M.

Funding: We thank CERCA Programme / Generalitat de Catalunya for institutional support. This research was funded by Instituto de Salud Carlos III (ISCIII) (grant numbers: PI14/00290 and PI17/01167), by Ministerio de Economía y Competitividad (grant number PSI2015-68701-R), by Ministerio de Sanidad, Servicios Sociales e Igualdad (grant number PR338/17), PERIS (Generalitat de Catalunya, SLT006/17/00077), and co-funded by FEDER funds /European Regional Development Fund (ERDF), a way to build Europe. CIBERObn is an initiative of ISCIII.

Conflicts of Interest: The authors declare no conflict of interest. The funders had no role in the design of the study; in the collection, analyses, or interpretation of data; in the writing of the manuscript, and in the decision to publish the results.

References

1. Gratz, K.L.; Weiss, N.H.; Tull, M.T. Examining emotion regulation as an outcome, mechanism, or target of psychological treatments. *Curr. Opin. Psychol.* **2015**, *3*, 85–90. [CrossRef] [PubMed]
2. Neacsiu, A.D.; Herr, N.R.; Fang, C.M.; Rodriguez, M.A.; Rosenthal, M.Z. Identity disturbance and problems with emotion regulation are related constructs across diagnoses. *J. Clin. Psychol.* **2015**, *71*, 346–361. [CrossRef]
3. Sloan, E.; Hall, K.; Moulding, R.; Bryce, S.; Mildred, H.; Staiger, P.K. Emotion regulation as a transdiagnostic treatment construct across anxiety, depression, substance, eating and borderline personality disorders: A systematic review. *Clin. Psychol. Rev.* **2017**, *57*, 141–163. [CrossRef]
4. Macht, M. How emotions affect eating: A five-way model. *Appetite* **2008**, *50*, 1–11. [CrossRef]
5. Brockmeyer, T.; Skunde, M.; Wu, M.; Bresslein, E.; Rudofsky, G.; Herzog, W.; Friederich, H.C. Difficulties in emotion regulation across the spectrum of eating disorders. *Compr. Psychiatry* **2014**, *55*, 565–571. [CrossRef]
6. Kittel, R.; Brauhardt, A.; Hilbert, A. Cognitive and emotional functioning in binge-eating disorder: A systematic review. *Int. J. Eat. Disord.* **2015**, *48*, 535–554. [CrossRef] [PubMed]
7. Haynos, A.F.; Roberto, C.A.; Attia, E. Examining the associations between emotion regulation difficulties, anxiety, and eating disorder severity among inpatients with anorexia nervosa. *Compr. Psychiatry* **2015**, *60*, 93–98. [CrossRef] [PubMed]
8. Kenny, T.E.; Singleton, C.; Carter, J.C. Testing predictions of the emotion regulation model of binge-eating disorder. *Int. J. Eat. Disord.* **2017**, *50*, 1297–1305. [CrossRef]
9. Schaumberg, K.; Welch, E.; Breithaupt, L.; Hübel, C.; Baker, J.H.; Munn-Chernoff, M.A.; Yilmaz, Z.; Ehrlich, S.; Mustelin, L.; Ghaderi, A.; et al. The science behind the academy for eating disorders' nine truths about eating disorders. *Eur. Eat. Disord. Rev.* **2017**, *25*, 432–450. [CrossRef]
10. Svaldi, J.; Caffier, D.; Tuschen-Caffier, B. Emotion suppression but not reappraisal increases desire to binge in women with binge eating disorder. *Psychother. Psychosom.* **2010**, *79*, 188–190. [CrossRef]
11. Danner, U.N.; Sternheim, L.; Evers, C. The importance of distinguishing between the different eating disorders (sub)types when assessing emotion regulation strategies. *Psychiatry Res.* **2014**, *215*, 727–732. [CrossRef] [PubMed]
12. Svaldi, J.; Griepenstroh, J.; Tuschen-Caffier, B.; Ehring, T. Emotion regulation deficits in eating disorders: A marker of eating pathology or general psychopathology? *Psychiatry Res.* **2012**, *197*, 103–111. [CrossRef] [PubMed]

13. Cucchi, A.; Ryan, D.; Konstantakopoulos, G.; Stroumpa, S.; Kaçar, A.S.; Renshaw, S.; Landau, S.; Kravariti, E. Lifetime prevalence of non-suicidal self-injury in patients with eating disorders: A systematic review and meta-analysis. *Psychol. Med.* **2016**, *46*, 1345–1358. [CrossRef] [PubMed]
14. Dingemans, A.; Danner, U.N.; Parks, M. Emotion regulation in binge eating disorder: A review. *Nutrients* **2017**, *9*, 1274. [CrossRef] [PubMed]
15. Carlson, L.; Steward, T.; Agüera, Z.; Mestre-Bach, G.; Magaña, P.; Granero, R.; Jiménez-Murcia, S.; Claes, L.; Gearhardt, A.N.; Menchón, J.M.; et al. Associations of food addiction and nonsuicidal self-injury among women with an eating disorder: A common strategy for regulating emotions? *Eur. Eat. Disord. Rev.* **2018**, *26*, 629–637. [CrossRef] [PubMed]
16. Brockmeyer, T.; Holtforth, M.G.; Bents, H.; Kämmerer, A.; Herzog, W.; Friederich, H.C. Starvation and emotion regulation in anorexia nervosa. *Compr. Psychiatry* **2012**, *53*, 496–501. [CrossRef] [PubMed]
17. Hatch, A.; Madden, S.; Kohn, M.; Clarke, S.; Touyz, S.; Williams, L.M. Anorexia nervosa: Towards an integrative neuroscience model. *Eur. Eat. Disord. Rev.* **2010**, *18*, 165–179. [CrossRef] [PubMed]
18. Oldershaw, A.; Lavender, T.; Sallis, H.; Stahl, D.; Schmidt, U. Emotion generation and regulation in anorexia nervosa: A systematic review and meta-analysis of self-report data. *Clin. Psychol. Rev.* **2015**, *39*, 83–95. [CrossRef] [PubMed]
19. Harrison, A.; Sullivan, S.; Tchanturia, K.; Treasure, J. Emotional functioning in eating disorders: Attentional bias, emotion recognition and emotion regulation. *Psychol. Med.* **2010**, *40*, 1887–1889. [CrossRef]
20. Brown, T.A.; Avery, J.C.; Jones, M.D.; Anderson, L.K.; Wierenga, C.E.; Kaye, W.H. The impact of alexithymia on emotion dysregulation in anorexia nervosa and bulimia nervosa over time. *Eur. Eat. Disord. Rev.* **2018**, *26*, 150–155. [CrossRef] [PubMed]
21. Polivy, J.; Herman, C.P. Etiology of binge eating: Psychological mechanisms. In *Binge Eating: Nature, Assessment and Treatment*; Fairburn, C.G., Wilso, G.T., Eds.; Guilford Press: New York, NY, USA, 1993; pp. 173–205.
22. Haedt-Matt, A.A.; Keel, P.K. Revisiting the affect regulation model of binge eating: A meta-analysis of studies using ecological momentary assessment. *Psychol. Bull.* **2011**, *137*, 660–681. [CrossRef] [PubMed]
23. Mallorquí-Bagué, N.; Vintró-Alcaraz, C.; Sánchez, I.; Riesco, N.; Agüera, Z.; Granero, R.; Jiménez-Múrcia, S.; Menchón, J.M.; Treasure, J.; Fernández-Aranda, F. Emotion regulation as a transdiagnostic feature among eating disorders: Cross-sectional and longitudinal approach. *Eur. Eat. Disord. Rev.* **2018**, *26*, 53–61. [CrossRef] [PubMed]
24. Safer, D.L.; Telch, C.F.; Chen, E.Y. *Dialectical Behavior Therapy for Binge Eating and Bulimia*; Guilford Press: New York, NY, USA, 2009.
25. Sipos, V.; Schweiger, U.; Jauch-Chara, K.; Faßbinder, E. Treatment of eating disorders by emotion regulation. *Psychother. Psychosom. Med. Psychol.* **2017**, *67*, 431–435. [PubMed]
26. Hayaki, J.; Free, S. Positive and negative eating expectancies in disordered eating among women and men. *Eat. Behav.* **2016**, *22*, 22–26. [CrossRef] [PubMed]
27. Ambwani, S.; Slane, J.D.; Thomas, K.M.; Hopwood, C.J.; Grilo, C.M. Interpersonal dysfunction and affect-regulation difficulties in disordered eating among men and women. *Eat. Behav.* **2014**, *15*, 550–554. [CrossRef] [PubMed]
28. Anderson, L.M.; Reilly, E.E.; Thomas, J.J.; Eddy, K.T.; Franko, D.L.; Hormes, J.M.; Anderson, D.A. Associations among fear, disgust, and eating pathology in undergraduate men and women. *Appetite* **2018**, *125*, 445–453. [CrossRef] [PubMed]
29. Opwis, M.; Schmidt, J.; Martin, A.; Salewski, C. Gender differences in eating behavior and eating pathology: The mediating role of rumination. *Appetite* **2017**, *110*, 103–107. [CrossRef] [PubMed]
30. Lavender, J.M.; Anderson, D.A. Contribution of emotion regulation difficulties to disordered eating and body dissatisfaction in college men. *Int. J. Eat. Disord.* **2010**, *43*, 352–357. [CrossRef] [PubMed]
31. Pisetsky, E.M.; Haynos, A.F.; Lavender, J.M.; Crow, S.J.; Peterson, C.B. Associations between emotion regulation difficulties, eating disorder symptoms, non-suicidal self-injury, and suicide attempts in a heterogeneous eating disorder sample. *Compr. Psychiatry* **2017**, *73*, 143–150. [CrossRef] [PubMed]
32. Ivanova, I.V.; Tasca, G.A.; Proulx, G.; Bissasda, H. Contribution of interpersonal problems to eating disorder psychopathology via negative affect in treatment-seeking men and women: Testing the validity of the interpersonal model in an understudied population. *Clin. Psychol. Psychother.* **2017**, *24*, 952–964. [CrossRef] [PubMed]

33. Masheb, R.M.; Grilo, C.M. Emotional overeating and its associations with eating disorder psychopathology among overweight patients with Binge eating disorder. *Int. J. Eat. Disord.* **2006**, *39*, 141–146. [CrossRef] [PubMed]
34. Goddard, E.; Carral-Fernández, L.; Denneny, E.; Campbell, I.C.; Treasure, J. Cognitive flexibility, central coherence and social emotional processing in males with an eating disorder. *World J. Biol. Psychiatry* **2014**, *15*, 317–326. [CrossRef] [PubMed]
35. Pollock, N.C.; McCabe, G.A.; Southard, A.C.; Zeigler-Hill, V. Pathological personality traits and emotion regulation difficulties. *Personal. Individ. Differ.* **2016**, *95*, 168–177. [CrossRef]
36. Borges, L.M.; Naugle, A.E. The role of emotion regulation in predicting personality dimensions. *Personal. Ment. Health* **2017**, *11*, 314–334. [CrossRef] [PubMed]
37. American Psychiatric Association. *Diagnostic and Statistical Manual of Mental Disorders: DSM-5*; American Psychiatric Association: Washington, DC, USA, 2013.
38. Agüera, Z.; Krug, I.; Sanchez, I.; Granero, R.; Penelo, E.; Penas-Lledo, E.; Jimenez-Murcia, S.; Menchon, J.M.; Fernández-Aranda, F. Personality changes in bulimia nervosa after a cognitive behaviour therapy. *Eur. Eat. Disord. Rev.* **2012**, *20*, 379–385. [CrossRef] [PubMed]
39. Atiye, M.; Miettunen, J.; Raevuori-Helkamaa, A. A meta-analysis of temperament in eating disorders. *Eur. Eat. Disord. Rev.* **2015**, *23*, 89–99. [CrossRef] [PubMed]
40. Núñez-Navarro, A.; Agüera, Z.; Krug, I.; Jiménez-Murcia, S.; Sánchez, I.; Araguz, N.; Gorwood, P.; Granero, R.; Penelo, E.; Karwautz, A.; et al. Do men with eating disorders differ from women in clinics, psychopathology and personality? *Eur. Eat. Disord. Rev.* **2012**, *20*, 23–31. [CrossRef]
41. Claes, L.; Jiménez-Murcia, S.; Agüera, Z.; Castro, R.; Sánchez, I.; Menchón, J.M.; Fernández-Aranda, F. Male eating disorder patients with and without non-suicidal self-injury: A comparison of psychopathological and personality features. *Eur. Eat. Disord. Rev.* **2012**, *20*, 335–338. [CrossRef]
42. Hintsanen, M.; Jokela, M.; Cloninger, C.R.; Pulkki-Råback, L.; Hintsa, T.; Elovainio, M.; Josefsson, K.; Rosenström, T.; Mullola, S.; Raitakari, O.T.; et al. Temperament and character predict body-mass index: A population-based prospective cohort study. *J. Psychosom. Res.* **2012**, *73*, 391–397. [CrossRef]
43. Rodríguez-Cano, T.; Beato-Fernandez, L.; Rojo-Moreno, L.; Vaz-Leal, F.J. The role of temperament and character in the outcome of depressive mood in eating disorders. *Compr. Psychiatry* **2014**, *55*, 1130–1136. [CrossRef]
44. Wolz, I.; Agüera, Z.; Granero, R.; Jiménez-Murcia, S.; Gratz, K.L.; Menchón, J.M.; Fernández-Aranda, F. Emotion regulation in disordered eating: Psychometric properties of the Difficulties in Emotion Regulation Scale among Spanish adults and its interrelations with personality and clinical severity. *Front. Psychol.* **2015**, *6*, 907. [CrossRef] [PubMed]
45. Garner, D.M. *Eating Disorder Inventory-2*; Psychological Assessment Resources: Odessa, Ukraine, 1991.
46. Garner, D.M. *Inventario de Trastornos de la Conducta Alimentaria (EDI-2)—Manual*; TEA: Madrid, Spain, 1998.
47. Derogatis, L.R. *SCL-90-R: Symptom Checklist-90-R. Administration, Scoring and Procedures Manuall—II for the Revised Version*; Clinical Psychometric Research: Towson, MD, USA, 1994.
48. Derogatis, L.R. *SCL-90-R. Cuestionario de 90 Síntomas-Manual*; TEA: Madrid, Spain, 2002.
49. Cloninger, C.R. *The Temperament and Character Inventory—Revised*; Center for Psychobiology of Personality, Washington University: St Louis, MO, USA, 1999.
50. Gutiérrez-Zotes, J.A.; Bayón, C.; Montserrat, C.; Valero, J.; Labad, A.; Cloninger, C.R. Temperament and Character Inventory-Revised (TCI-R). Standardization and normative data in a general population sample. *Actas Esp. Psiquiatr.* **2004**, *32*, 8–15.
51. Gratz, K.L.; Roemer, L. multidimensional assessment of emotion regulation and dysregulation: development, factor structure, and initial validation of the difficulties in emotion regulation scale. *J. Psychopathol. Behav. Assess.* **2004**, *26*, 41–54. [CrossRef]
52. Kelley, K.; Preacher, K.J. On effect size. *Psychol. Methods* **2012**, *17*, 137–152. [CrossRef] [PubMed]
53. Finner, H. On a monotonicity problem in step-down multiple test procedures. *J. Am. Stat. Assoc.* **1993**, *88*, 920–923. [CrossRef]
54. Kline, R.B. *Principles and Practice of Structural Equation Modeling*, 2nd ed.; Gilford Press: New York, NY, USA, 2005.
55. Barrett, P. Structural equation modelling: Adjudging model fit. *Personal. Individ. Differ.* **2007**, *42*, 815–824. [CrossRef]

56. Lavender, J.M.; Wonderlich, S.A.; Engel, S.G.; Gordon, K.H.; Kaye, W.H.; Mitchell, J.E. Dimensions of emotion dysregulation in anorexia nervosa and bulimia nervosa: A conceptual review of the empirical literature. *Clin. Psychol. Rev.* **2015**, *40*, 111–122. [CrossRef]
57. Donahue, J.M.; Reilly, E.E.; Anderson, L.M.; Scharmer, C.; Anderson, D.A. Evaluating associations between perfectionism, emotion regulation, and eating disorder symptoms in a mixed-gender sample. *J. Nerv. Ment. Dis.* **2018**, *206*, 900–904. [CrossRef]
58. Kinnaird, E.; Norton, C.; Tchanturia, K. Clinicians' views on treatment adaptations for men with eating disorders: A qualitative study. *BMJ Open* **2018**, *8*, e021934. [CrossRef]
59. Aloi, M.; Rania, M.; Caroleo, M.; De Fazio, P.; Segura-García, C. Social cognition and emotional functioning in patients with binge eating disorder. *Eur. Eat. Disord. Rev.* **2017**, *25*, 172–178. [CrossRef]
60. Cloninger, C.R.; Svrakic, D.M.; Przybeck, T.R. A psychobiological model of temperament and character. *Arch. Gen. Psychiatry* **1993**, *50*, 975–990. [CrossRef] [PubMed]
61. Greenberg, S.T.; Schoen, E.G. Males and eating disorders: Gender-based therapy for eating disorder recovery. *Prof. Psychol. Res. Pract.* **2008**, *39*, 464–471. [CrossRef]
62. Agüera, Z.; Sánchez, I.; Granero, R.; Riesco, N.; Steward, T.; Martín-Romera, V.; Jiménez-Murcia, S.; Romero, X.; Caroleo, M.; Segura-García, C.; et al. Short-Term Treatment Outcomes and Dropout Risk in Men and Women with Eating Disorders. *Eur. Eat. Disord. Rev.* **2017**, *25*, 293–301. [CrossRef] [PubMed]

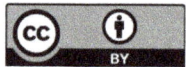 © 2019 by the authors. Licensee MDPI, Basel, Switzerland. This article is an open access article distributed under the terms and conditions of the Creative Commons Attribution (CC BY) license (http://creativecommons.org/licenses/by/4.0/).

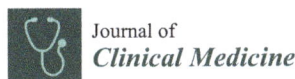

Article

Manualised Cognitive Behaviour Therapy for Anorexia Nervosa: Use of Treatment Modules in the ANTOP Study

Gaby Resmark [1,*], Brigid Kennedy [1,2], Maria Mayer [1], Katrin Giel [1], Florian Junne [1], Martin Teufel [3], Martina de Zwaan [4] and Stephan Zipfel [1]

1. Department of Psychosomatic Medicine and Psychotherapy, University Hospital Tübingen, 72076 Tübingen, Germany; brigid.kennedy@med.uni-tuebingen.de (B.K.); maria.mayer@med.uni-tuebingen.de (M.M.); katrin.giel@med.uni-tuebingen.de (K.G.); florian.junne@med.uni-tuebingen.de (F.J.); stephan.zipfel@med.uni-tuebingen.de (S.Z.)
2. School of Psychology, The University of Sydney, Camperdown 2006, Australia
3. Department of Psychosomatic Medicine and Psychotherapy, University of Duisburg-Essen, 45147 Essen, Germany; martin.teufel@lvr.de
4. Department of Psychosomatic Medicine and Psychotherapy, Hannover Medical School, 30625 Hannover, Germany; dezwaan.martina@mh-hannover.de
* Correspondence: gaby.resmark@med.uni-tuebingen.de; Tel.: +49-(0)7071-29-86719

Received: 16 October 2018; Accepted: 26 October 2018; Published: 29 October 2018

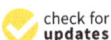

Abstract: Standardised treatment manuals facilitate therapy planning and enhance comparability for research purposes. Within the Anorexia Nervosa Treatment of Out Patients (ANTOP) study, the largest multisite outpatient intervention trial in anorexia nervosa (AN) to date, manualised enhanced cognitive-behavioural therapy (CBT-E) was offered as one treatment modality. The manual consisted of 9 modules, of which *Motivation, Nutrition, Formulation and Relapse Prevention* were compulsory. Homework worksheets were provided, to ensure the transfer of therapeutic improvements to daily life. This study investigated the use of modules and worksheets in order to explore practice styles of trained therapists in the treatment of AN. This secondary analysis was based on log-sheets (n = 2604) CBT-E therapists completed after each session. Frequencies of modules and worksheets used across all sessions were calculated. Relationships, such as that between use of module and duration of illness, were examined. The most commonly used module was *Motivation*. In patients with longer illness duration, the module *Self Esteem* seemed to be particularly important. The worksheet *Scales*, balancing the pros and cons of AN, was prioritised by therapists. The results underline the importance of motivational work in the treatment of AN, including validating the ambivalence experienced by most AN patients. With increasing duration of illness, resource-oriented elements, such as self esteem stabilisation, should be of focus.

Keywords: anorexia nervosa; cognitive behaviour therapy; manualised treatment; modules; worksheets

1. Introduction

Treatment manuals for psychotherapeutic interventions guarantee that the path of treatment remains relatively focused, ensuring a standardised quality of therapy [1]. The clear structure associated with manualised treatment also increases transparency associated with the treatment, and with that, patient motivation [2]. Yet, the use of treatment manuals continues to be a controversial discussion point in the psychotherapy field [2]. Critics argue that use of manuals leads to rigid treatment, which neglects individual components of the patient's disorder, and reduces scope for therapist innovation [1,2].

Manuals exist for a vast array of treatments, including cognitive behaviour therapy (CBT) [3–5]. A convincing bank of evidence suggests that manualised CBT is effective in treating eating disorders [6–8]. Studies have shown that CBT can produce weight gain in anorexia nervosa (AN) patients [9], as well as improvements in eating disorder pathology for patients with AN [9], bulimia nervosa and eating disorders not otherwise specified [10]. A recently developed modified version of CBT, called enhanced cognitive behaviour therapy (CBT-E) [3], employs a transdiagnostic approach addressing all eating disorders. CBT-E has been shown to produce lasting improvements in body-mass index and eating disorder pathology in AN patients [11], and to be equally as effective as other "standard" treatment options [11,12].

One aspect which warrants consideration is the inclusion of modules in CBT treatment manuals. Modules are a form of building block for the treatment [4]; they outline the focal points of the planned treatment and seek to guide the therapy. Several modular CBT manuals have been developed to treat eating disorders; often, these manuals provide a wide selection of modules for therapists and patients to choose from [3–5,13]. Worksheets are another element often included as a supplementary resource to accompany modules; for example, in Wilhelm et al.'s CBT manual for body dysmorphic disorder [5] and in Legenbauer and Vocks' manual for anorexia and bulimia treatment [4]. Legenbauer and Vocks' manual [4], only available in German, is a practical manual designed for the cognitive behavioural treatment of eating disorders. The manual contains chapters addressing specific concepts related to eating disorders, such as motivation. Each chapter is accompanied by specific activities and detailed worksheets to assist the therapy. Worksheets can be used in-session and administered as homework, and facilitate the transfer of therapeutic progress into daily life. Similarly, Fairburn's CBT-E manual considers "Next Steps", an alternative term for homework, to be an integral component of treatment [3]. Most CBT manuals provide a rather clear structure, but should be seen as a guide, rather than an inflexible, predetermined protocol [14].

While past research has demonstrated that modular treatment manuals can produce positive treatment effects in eating disorder patients, to the authors' knowledge, no research has investigated the actual *implementation* of such manuals. Hence, there is an absence of research investigating the ways in which therapists execute manualised treatment. This study aimed to tackle this research gap, by investigating the practice styles of therapists administering a manualised CBT-E treatment to outpatients with AN. The manual of focus, written in German, was developed in 2007, prior to the publication of Fairburn's CBT-E manual [3]. It was written based on a 2-day workshop delivered by Fairburn. The manual was designed specifically for the ANTOP (Anorexia Nervosa Treatment of Out Patients) study, a German multisite randomised control trial in outpatients with AN [15,16]. The design and main outcome of the ANTOP study have been published elsewhere [15,16]. The present study sought to answer the following research questions:

- What were the most commonly used modules?
- What were the most commonly used worksheets?
- Was there a relationship between stage of therapy and module used?
- Was there a relationship between duration of illness and module used?

2. Methods

2.1. CBT-E in the ANTOP Study

This study was conducted as a secondary analysis of data from the ANTOP study. In one arm of this study, AN patients received 40 individual sessions of CBT-E over 10 months. Therapy was categorised into three stages: stage 1 (sessions 1–16) involved therapy twice a week for 2 months, stage 2 (sessions 17–32) involved therapy once a week for 4 months, and stage 3 (sessions 33-40) involved therapy once every 2 weeks for 4 months. Twenty-four CBT therapists, trained initially by Fairburn, used the specifically designed CBT-E ANTOP manual to guide treatment. The manual contained 9 modules, 4 of which were compulsory (Table 1). Worksheets were also provided for optional use during sessions and as homework. At the time of the ANTOP manual development, Fairburn's available material did not contain any worksheets, and hence, worksheets were taken from Legenbauer and Vocks' German CBT manual [4]. At the end of each therapy session, therapists were required to fill out a log-sheet, documenting detailed information regarding the content of the session. Although several modules could be used per session, therapists were required to record the single module which was the main focus throughout that session. Therapists could also record up to 2 worksheets given to the patient in the session, or as homework. This information provided the data for the current analysis.

Table 1. Modules in the Anorexia Nervosa Treatment of Out Patients (ANTOP) study CBT-E manual.

Module	Module Content
Compulsory Modules	
Motivation (Starting Well)	Building a therapeutic relationship, reflecting on pros and cons of anorexia nervosa (AN), and discussing healthy eating behaviours
Nutrition	Establishing and maintaining a regular healthy eating pattern
Formulation	Understanding what causes and maintains the individual's eating disorder
Relapse Prevention (Ending Well)	Maintaining positive behavioural changes learnt throughout the course of therapy and preparing to cope with setbacks
Optional Modules	
Cognitive Restructuring	Learning to challenge dysfunctional beliefs concerning eating, weight and the body
Mood Regulation	Recognising and coping with negative emotions
Social Skills	Improving communication and conflict resolutions skills
Body Image	Addressing the negative attitudes towards patients' own bodies, and the influence of perceived figure/weight on self-worth
Self Esteem and Resources	Increasing self-worth: Identifying strengths, establishing new hobbies and interests, reflecting on what brings happiness

2.2. Sample

Of the eighty AN patients assigned to the CBT-E arm in the ANTOP study, 78 commenced treatment and 65 completed treatment (that is, they attended at least 27 of the 40 sessions). Only female, adult patients (aged $\geq$ 18 years) were included in the ANTOP study. When the study commenced, patients' mean age was 27.4 years and mean body-mass index (kg/m^2) was 16.82. Forty-nine patients (61%) had an illness duration of less than or equal to 6 years, and 31 (39%) had AN for longer than 6 years [16]. The data used for this secondary analysis comprised of 2604 session logs; this number was less than the total possible number of session logs (3120) as not all patients completed all 40 treatment sessions. Only logs which contained relevant information regarding the component of interest were included in each analysis.

The ANTOP study was approved by the ethics board of the faculty of medicine, University Hospital Tübingen, on the 21/02/2006 (ref: 440/2006). Additionally, the study was approved by the ethics committees at each of the participating treatment centres. All procedures performed in studies involving human participants were in accordance with the ethical standards of the institutional and/or national research committee and with the 1975 Helsinki declaration and its later amendments or comparable ethical standards.

2.3. Statistics

All statistical analyses were conducted using IBM SPSS Statistics version 25 (IBM, Armonk, NY, USA). Frequency tests were conducted in order to identify the most commonly used modules and worksheets across all CBT-E sessions. Crosstabs were displayed in order to investigate the relationship between choice of module and stage of therapy. An overall chi square test of independence was conducted to determine the relationship between module and duration of illness, followed by post hoc standardised residuals testing (absolute value greater than 2.00 indicated significance [17]). Patients were classified into two groups: those with an illness duration of equal to or less than 6 years, and those with an illness longer than 6 years. Duration of illness was classified in this way, because in the ANTOP study the randomisation had been stratified according to this dichotomised variable.

3. Results

3.1. Modules

Across all 2604 CBT-E sessions, the focus module was recorded a total of 2411 times. Figure 1 depicts frequencies of module use.

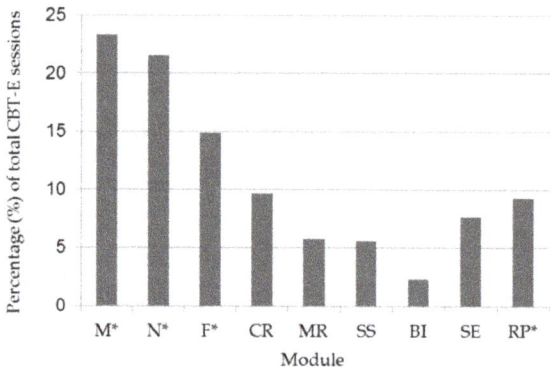

Figure 1. Frequency (percentage) of focus modules (n = 2411) used throughout treatment. M = Motivation, N = Nutrition, F = Formulation, CR = Cognitive Restructuring, MR = Mood Regulation, SS = Social Skills, BI = Body Image, SE = Self Esteem, RP = Relapse Prevention. Asterisks represent compulsory modules.

3.2. Relationship between Module and Stage of Therapy

As can be seen in Figure 2, stage of therapy appeared to influence choice of module. While Stage 1 sessions focused on modules such as *Motivation* and *Nutrition* most frequently, over 50% of Stage 3 sessions focused on *Relapse Prevention*.

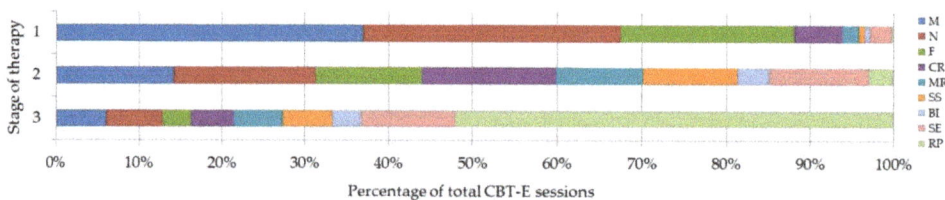

Figure 2. Relationship between frequency (percentage) of applied modules (n = 2411) and stage of therapy. M = Motivation, N = Nutrition, F = Formulation, CR = Cognitive Restructuring, MR = Mood Regulation, SS = Social Skills, BI = Body Image, SE =Self Esteem, RP =Relapse Prevention. Stage 1: sessions 1–16, Stage 2: sessions 17–32, Stage 3: sessions 33–40.

3.3. Relationship between Module and Duration of Illness

There was a statistically significant relationship between choice of module and duration of illness, X^2 (8, n = 2411) = 15.937, p = 0.043. Post-hoc tests analysing standardised residuals revealed that differences between the duration of illness groups lay in the use of the *Self Esteem and Resources* module; this module was used significantly more often with patients who had a duration of illness longer than 6 years, compared to those who had an illness duration of 6 years or less.

3.4. Worksheets

The use of worksheets was recorded 888 times across all session logs. 590 additional records of worksheet use were excluded from analysis, as they did not refer to any of the 55 worksheets made available to the therapists. A list of the top ten most commonly used worksheets was generated using frequency analysis (Table 2).

Table 2. Top ten distributed worksheets, listed in descending order according to frequency used (*n* = 888).

Name of Worksheet (Module)	Number of Times Distributed (%)
The Scales (Motivation)	107 (12)
Family relationships (Formulation)	56 (6.3)
Two letters to the eating disorder (Motivation)	53 (6.0)
How I'd like to change my eating behaviour (Nutrition)	43 (4.8)
Cognitive distortions (Cognitive Restructuring)	37 (4.2)
What have I learnt (Formulation)	34 (3.8)
Analysis of a monitoring record (Nutrition)	29 (3.3)
Paths to change (Nutrition)	27 (3.0)
Toolbox for emergencies (Relapse Prevention)	26 (2.9)
What I need to be content (Self Esteem)	26 (2.9)

The Scales was the most commonly used worksheet, distributed 107 times (12%). This worksheet involved patients recording the short- and long-term pros and cons of their eating disorder on either side of a balance scale. Next to each pro or con, they were instructed to write a number from 1 to 100, indicating how important they considered this factor to be. After completing their list, patients were asked to consider both the pros and cons lists in their entireties and to assign each side of the scale a number. This number was to be used as a measure of whether the eating disorder is more friend or foe.

Family relationships was the second most commonly used worksheet, distributed 56 times (6.3%). This worksheet involved patients reflecting on the relationships within their family, specifically throughout their pubescent years, or whichever period they feel was most important for the development of their eating disorder. Patients were instructed to draw or write the names of their family members (including themselves) within a rectangle. They were told to use lines to connect the family members; normal lines represented positive and stable relationships, and dotted lines represented relationships characterised by conflict. On the left of the page, in the smaller boxes, patients listed the distinctive traits they believe characterise each of their family members. The general aim of this worksheet was to encourage reflection on family relationships, and also to identify factors potentially influencing the emergence and persistence of the disorder. For information on further worksheets, see Legenbauer and Vocks' Manual.

4. Discussion

This secondary analysis of data from the ANTOP study provides insight into the practice styles of experienced therapists administering manualised CBT-E to outpatients with AN. It sheds light on which modules and corresponding worksheets were most commonly used. Additionally, it considers the use of modules in more depth, in particular in relation to stage of therapy and duration of illness.

The four most commonly used modules overall were *Motivation, Nutrition, Formulation* and *Cognitive Restructuring,* suggesting that they are arguably the most important modules of focus during CBT-E for AN patients. It is, however, important to acknowledge that three of these four modules were indeed compulsory modules, meaning they were required to be used for at least 5 of the 40 sessions. The fact that focus was given more often to the optional module *Cognitive Restructuring* than to the compulsory module *Relapse Prevention* can be interpreted in two ways. On the one hand, cognitive restructuring represents an essential strategy within CBT. On the other hand, just over a quarter of the ANTOP sample still had full syndrome AN at the end of treatment [16]; this might have resulted in less use of *Relapse Prevention*, as use of this module often assumes absence of symptoms. It should also be acknowledged that although module choice was oriented around patient needs, choice of module would have also been influenced by the therapists' practice styles and beliefs.

The *Motivation* and *Nutrition* modules were of the greatest focus, both being distributed in over 20% of sessions. These findings coincide with the extensive bank of literature suggesting that these aspects should be of pivotal focus throughout AN treatment. The ego syntonic nature of the illness often contributes to an ambivalence to change in AN patients [18]; the symptoms which characterise the illness, such as dangerously low body weight, are unfortunately characteristics which patients value, and hence often wish to maintain. Indeed, patients with AN rarely seek treatment on an entirely voluntary basis [18]. There is evidence that a patient's motivation to change is arguably one of the strongest predictors of treatment success [19,20]. Nutrition is another pivotal aspect to successful CBT-E treatment of AN as patients need to normalise their eating behaviour and restore weight in order to overcome the illness [21,22]. Additionally, evidence suggests that with better nutrition, cognitive functioning can be improved, and subsequently, responsiveness to interventions [23].

The limited use of the *Body Image* module also warrants consideration. Disturbed body image is one of the characterising features of AN [24–27]. Indeed, body image distortion is not only a predictor of the development of AN [25], but also for the longevity of the diagnosis, and likelihood of relapse [24]. Perceptions of body image have also been found to be significantly related to depression and anxiety symptoms in AN patients [26]. It is, therefore, clear that body image is intimately intertwined with AN, and should accordingly be of pivotal focus in treatment. Yet, the current data analysis revealed that the *Body Image* module was surprisingly the least frequently used module among the ANTOP therapists; specifically, it was used in less than 3% of sessions. The current findings provide evidential support for the concern that body image disturbances are somewhat neglected in eating disorder therapy [4,28]. Accordingly, treatment outcomes might be improved by placing more focus on body image disturbances [25]. Research comparing two versions of CBT for eating disorder patients revealed that treatment which specifically addressed body image disturbance produced greater improvements at end of treatment and one year follow up, than CBT treatment which did not [29]. When considered in conjunction with this research, the current findings highlight a potential limitation in current treatment practice; that therapists are perhaps not placing enough emphasis on the concept of body image in their treatment of AN patients.

Data analysis found that during stage 1 (sessions 1–16) therapy sessions, the *Motivation* and *Nutrition* modules were of predominant focus. These findings are in line with existing literature [3,30], which suggests that in order for therapy to be successful, initial stages of therapy should address aspects such as patient's motivation to engage in therapy, healthy eating habits, and weight gain. Analysis also revealed that over 50% of stage 3 sessions focused on the *Relapse Prevention* module. This again coincides with the literature, which suggests that in order to ensure long-term results, final stages of treatment should address how progress can be maintained upon cessation of therapy, and how relapse can be prevented [3,30]. Overall, these results suggest that therapists administering CBT-E in the ANTOP study were administering therapy in a manner that is in accordance with the suggested progression of AN treatment.

There was a significant relationship between duration of illness and choice of modules, specifically in the use of the *Self Esteem and Resources* module. This module was significantly more likely to be used for patients who had an illness duration of longer than 6 years. Current research suggests that although some patients do recover fully from AN, approximately 20% of patients go on to develop a severe and enduring form of the disorder that is resistant to treatment [31]. Touyz and colleagues argue that this subset of patients have a unique set of needs, different to those of other AN patients, and hence suggest that a different approach should be taken in their treatment [32,33]. This approach, closely linked to the Recovery Model [32], does not view recovery simply as an absence of symptoms. Instead, focus is shifted away from weight gain towards aspects such as improving quality of life and hope for the future [33]. The findings from the current study seem to compliment this alternative approach. In their treatment of longer suffering AN, CBT-E therapists of the ANTOP study seemed to deem it necessary to place greater focus on resource-oriented aspects outside of the AN symptomatology, such as the *Self Esteem and Resources* module.

The data analysis also revealed which of the available 55 worksheets were used most frequently. In accordance with the priority given to the *Motivation* module, the worksheet *The Scales*, addressing the pros and cons of the eating disorder, was used almost double the amount of times than any other worksheet. *Family Relationships*, which required patients to construct a family diagram, was the second most frequently used worksheet. The frequent use of these worksheets highlights the importance of these specific topics of motivation and relationships throughout the treatment process.

Limitations and Future Research

While the design and conduct of the ANTOP study followed the highest aspirations of international standards in clinical research, this subproject was limited due to its nature as a secondary analysis. Consequently, the results must be considered as hypotheses to be tested in future studies. It was a completer analysis, meaning only data provided by patients currently in treatment could be considered. Additionally, the categorical nature of the data limited the scientific quality of the analysis; mainly descriptive analysis was provided. Finally, although this study included an in-depth analysis of the practice styles of experienced therapists, it did not assess the effectiveness of these practice styles. Future research would therefore benefit from investigating whether use of certain modules, or combinations of modules, results in better treatment outcomes for AN patients. Furthermore, it could be useful to investigate whether certain worksheets were more commonly used in younger patients, as many of them were designed in a "girlish" way (e.g., the worksheet *My Strengths* in the *Self Esteem* module was pink and decorated with flowers), and so therapists may have chosen not to give them to older patients.

5. Conclusions

To the authors' knowledge this is the first scientific analysis which explores the practical application of a modular therapy manual in the treatment of eating disorders. Analysing individual outpatient therapy administered by experienced therapists involved in the ANTOP study, this paper provides other therapists with practical recommendations regarding the use of modules and corresponding worksheets within manualised CBT-E for AN. Analysis revealed that *Motivation*, *Nutrition*, *Formulation* and *Cognitive Restructuring* were the most common modules of focus. In particular, *Motivation* and *Nutrition* seemed to be most relevant during the initial stages of treatment, whereas *Relapse Prevention* was more relevant in the final treatment stage. The module *Self Esteem* appeared to be particularly relevant for patients who had a duration of illness longer than 6 years, a finding which complements recent research advocating a so-called recovery model for long-term sufferers of AN. *Body Image* was often neglected; a concerning finding, in light of recent research highlighting the importance of addressing body image disturbances in AN patients. The most commonly used worksheet was *The Scales* within the module *Motivation*. These findings underline the importance of actively addressing the ambivalence often present in patients with AN in order to facilitate readiness for change. Furthermore, the findings show clearly that modern manualised CBT is much more than teaching strategies and techniques. It should leave room to address themes that might maintain the individual's eating disorder and therefore need to be solved in order to allow for recovery.

Author Contributions: Conceptualisation, G.R., K.G., F.J. and S.Z.; methodology, G.R., B.K., M.M., K.G. and F.J.; formal analysis, B.K., M.M. and K.G.; investigation, G.R., B.K., M.M., K.G., F.J., M.T., M.d.Z. and S.Z.; resources, G.R., K.G., F.J. and S.Z.; data curation, G.R., B.K., M.M., and K.G.; writing—original draft preparation, G.R., B.K. and M.M.; writing—review and editing, G.R., B.K., M.M., K.G., F.J. and S.Z.; visualisation, G.R., B.K., and M.M.; supervision, G.R., K.G., F.J., and S.Z.; project administration, G.R.

Funding: This study was a secondary analysis of the ANTOP study data. The ANTOP study was funded by The German Federal Ministry of Education and Research (Bundesministerium für Bildung und Forschung (BMBF)), project number 01GV0624. The ANTOP study was part of the BMBF research programme Research Networks on Psychotherapy.

Acknowledgments: Worksheets in the ANTOP study were taken from Legenbauer T, Vocks S (2006). Manual der kognitiven Verhaltenstherapie bei Anorexie und Bulimie. Springer, Heidelberg. The contribution the authors have made to the ANTOP study is greatly appreciated. We thank all members of the ANTOP study group for their contributions to the original ANTOP paper.

Conflicts of Interest: The authors declare no conflict of interest.

References

1. Lang, P. Einstellung von Psychotherapeuten zu Therapieleitlinien und Manualisierter Therapie bei Anorexia Nervosa und Bulimia Nervosa. Ph.D. Thesis, Universität Ulm, Ulm, Gremany, 2010. [CrossRef]
2. Addis, M.; Cardemil, E.; Duncan, B.; Miller, S. Does Manualization Improve Therapy Outcomes? In *Evidence-Based Practices in Mental Health: Debate and Dialogue on the Fundamental Questions*; Norcross, J., Beutler, L., Levant, R., Eds.; American Psychological Association: Washington, DC, USA, 2006; pp. 131–160.
3. Fairburn, C.G. *Cognitive Behavior Therapy and Eating Disorders*; Guilford Press: New York, NY, USA, 2008.
4. Legenbauer, T.; Vocks, S. *Manual der kognitiven Verhaltenstherapie bei Anorexie und Bulimie*; Springer: Heidelberg, Germany, 2006.
5. Wilhelm, S.; Phillips, K.; Steketee, G. *Cognitive-Behavioral Therapy for Body Dysmorphic Disorder: A Treatment Manual*; Guilford Press: New York, NY, USA, 2013.
6. Cooper, Z.; Doll, H.; Hawker, D. Testing a new cognitive behavioral treatment for obesity: A randomized controlled trial with three-year follow-up. *Behav. Res. Ther.* **2010**, *48*, 706–713. [CrossRef] [PubMed]
7. Fairburn, C.G.; Cooper, Z.; Doll, H.A.; O'Connor, M.E.; Bohn, K.; Hawker, D.M.; Wales, J.A.; Palmer, R.L. Transdiagnostic cognitive-behavioral therapy for patients with eating disorders: A two-site trial with 60-week follow-up. *Am. J. Psychiatry* **2009**, *166*, 311–319. [CrossRef] [PubMed]
8. Wilhelm, S.; Phillips, K.; Didie, E. Modular cognitive-behavioral therapy for body dysmorphic disorder: A randomized controlled trial. *Behav. Ther.* **2014**, *45*, 314–327. [CrossRef] [PubMed]
9. Dalle Grave, R.; Calugi, S.; Conti, M. Inpatient cognitive behavior therapy for anorexia nervosa: A randomized controlled trial. *Psychother. Psychosom.* **2013**, *82*, 390–398. [CrossRef] [PubMed]
10. Knott, S.; Woodward, D.; Hoefkens, A.; Limbert, C. Cognitive behavior therapy for bulimia nervosa and eating disorders not otherwise specified: Translation from randomized controlled trial to clinical setting. *Behav. Cognit. Psychother.* **2015**, *43*, 641–654. [CrossRef] [PubMed]
11. Byrne, S.; Wade, T.; Hay, P.; Touyz, S.; Fairburn, C.; Treasure, J.; Schmidt, U.; McIntosh, V.; Allen, K.; Fursland, A.; et al. A randomised controlled trial of three psychological treatments for anorexia nervosa. *Psychol. Med.* **2017**, *47*, 2823–2833. [CrossRef] [PubMed]
12. Zeeck, A.; Herpertz-Dahlmann, B.; Friederich, H.-C.; Brockmeyer, T.; Resmark, G.; Hagenah, U.; Ehrlich, S.; Cuntz, U.; Zipfel, S.; Hartmann, A. Psychotherapeutic treatment for anorexia nervosa: A systematic review and network meta-analysis. *Front. Psychiatry* **2018**, *9*, 158. [CrossRef] [PubMed]
13. Cooper, Z.; Fairburn, C.; Hawker, D. *Cognitive–Behavioral Treatment of Obesity: A Clinician's Guide*; Guilford Press: New York, NY, USA, 2003.
14. Rießen, I.; Zipfel, S.; Groß, G. Ambulante manualisierte Verhaltenstherapie bei Anorexia nervosa—Erfahrungsbericht aus der Supervision. *Psychotherapeut* **2010**, *55*, 496–502. [CrossRef]
15. Wild, B.; Friederich, H.-C.; Gross, G.; Teufel, M.; Herzog, W.; Giel, K.E.; de Zwaan, M.; Schauenburg, H.; Schade-Brittinger, C.; Schäfer, H.; et al. The ANTOP study: Focal psychodynamic psychotherapy, cognitive-behavioural therapy, and treatment-as-usual in outpatients with anorexia nervosa—A randomized controlled trial. *Trials* **2009**, *10*, 23. [CrossRef] [PubMed]
16. Zipfel, S.; Wild, B.; Friederich, H.-C.; Teufel, M.; Schellberg, D.; Giel, K.E.; de Zwaan, M.; Dinkel, A.; Herpertz, S.; Burgmer, M.; et al. Focal psychodynamic therapy, cognitive behaviour therapy, and optimised treatment as usual in outpatients with anorexia nervosa (ANTOP study): Randomised controlled trial. *Lancet* **2014**, *383*, 127–137. [CrossRef]
17. Beasley, T.; Schumacker, R. Multiple regression approach to analyzing contingency tables: Post hoc and planned comparison procedures. *J. Exp. Educ.* **1995**, *64*, 79–93. [CrossRef]

18. Vitousek, K.; Watson, S.; Wilson, G. Enhancing motivation for change in treatment-resistant eating disorders. *Clin. Psychol. Rev.* **1998**, *18*, 391–420. [CrossRef]
19. Dagmar, O.; Aebi, M.; Winkler Metzke, C.; Steinhausen, H.-C. Motivation to change, coping, and self-esteem in adolescent anorexia nervosa: A validation study of the Anorexia Nervosa Stages of Change Questionnaire. *J. Eat Disord.* **2017**, *5*, 11. [CrossRef]
20. Neugebauer, Q. *Motivation in the Treatment of Anorexia Nervosa: A Systematic Review of Theoretical and Empirical Literature*; Pepperdine University: California, CA, USA, 2013.
21. Yager, J.; Devlin, M.; Halmi, K.; Herzog, D.; Mitchell, J.; Powers, P.; Zerbe, K. Treatment of patients with eating disorders, third edition. *Am. J. Psychiatry* **2006**, *163*, 4–54.
22. Bruch, H. Anorexia nervosa: Therapy and theory. *Am. J. Psychiatry* **1982**, *139*, 1531–1538. [CrossRef] [PubMed]
23. Marzola, E.; Nasser, J.; Hashim, S. Nutritional rehabilitation in anorexia nervosa: Review of the literature and implications for treatment. *BMC Psychiatry* **2013**, *13*, 290. [CrossRef] [PubMed]
24. Caspi, A.; Amiaz, R.; Davidson, N.; Czerniak, E.; Gur, E.; Kiryati, N.; Harari, D.; Furst, M.; Stein, D. Computerized assessment of body image in anorexia nervosa and bulimia nervosa: Comparison with standardized body image assessment tool. *Arch. Womens Ment. Health* **2017**, *20*, 139–147. [CrossRef] [PubMed]
25. Delinsky, S. *Body Image and Anorexia Nervosa*; Cash, T., Smolak, L., Eds.; Guilford Press: New York, NY, USA, 2011; pp. 279–287.
26. Junne, F.; Zipfel, S.; Wild, B.; Martus, P.; Giel, K.; Resmark, G.; Friederich, H.-C.; Teufel, M.; de Zwaan, M.; Dinkel, A.; et al. The relationship of body image with symptoms of depression and anxiety in patients with anorexia nervosa during outpatient psychotherapy: Results of the ANTOP study. *Psychotherapy* **2016**, *53*, 141–151. [CrossRef] [PubMed]
27. Zipfel, S.; Giel, K.; Bulik, C. Anorexia nervosa: Aetiology, assessment, and treatment. *Lancet Psychiatry* **2015**, *2*, 1099–1111. [CrossRef]
28. Junne, F.; Wild, B.; Resmark, G.; Giel, K.E.; Teufel, M.; Martus, P.; Ziser, K.; Friederich, H.-C.; de Zwaan, M.; Löwe, B.; et al. The importance of body image disturbances for the outcome of outpatient psychotherapy in patients with anorexia nervosa: Results of the ANTOP-study. *Eur. Eat. Disord. Rev.* **2018**. [CrossRef] [PubMed]
29. Marco, J.; Perpina, C.; Botella, C. Effectiveness of cognitive behavioral therapy supported by virtual reality in the treatment of body image in eating disorders: One year follow-up. *Psychiatry Res.* **2013**, *209*, 619–625. [CrossRef] [PubMed]
30. Pike, K.; Carter, J.; Olmsted, M. Cognitive-behavioral therapy for anorexia nervosa. In *the Treatment of Eating Disorders: A Clinical Handbook*; Grilo, C., Mitchell, J., Eds.; The Guilford Press: New York, NY, USA, 2010; pp. 83–107.
31. Steinhausen, H.-C. The outcomes of anorexia nervosa in the 20th century. *Am. J. Psychiatry* **2002**, *159*, 1284–1293. [CrossRef] [PubMed]
32. Dawson, L.; Rhodes, P.; Touyz, S. The recovery model and anorexia nervosa. *Aust. N. Z. J. Psychiatry* **2014**, *48*, 1009–1016. [CrossRef] [PubMed]
33. Touyz, S.; Le Grange, D.; Lacey, J.; Hay, P. *Managing Severe and Enduring Anorexia Nervosa: A Clinician's Guide*; Routledge: New York, NY, USA, 2016.

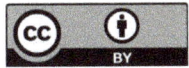

© 2018 by the authors. Licensee MDPI, Basel, Switzerland. This article is an open access article distributed under the terms and conditions of the Creative Commons Attribution (CC BY) license (http://creativecommons.org/licenses/by/4.0/).

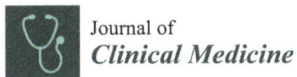 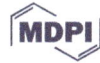

Article

The Role of Objectively Measured, Altered Physical Activity Patterns for Body Mass Index Change during Inpatient Treatment in Female Patients with Anorexia Nervosa

Celine S. Lehmann [1,2], Tobias Hofmann [1], Ulf Elbelt [1,3], Matthias Rose [1], Christoph U. Correll [2,4,5], Andreas Stengel [1,6,*,†] and Verena Haas [2,*,†]

1. Center for Internal Medicine and Dermatology, Department of Psychosomatic Medicine, Charité-Universitätsmedizin Berlin, 12200 Berlin, Germany; celine-sina.lehmann@charite.de (C.S.L.); Tobias.Hofmann@charite.de (T.H.); Ulf.Elbelt@charite.de (U.E.); Matthias.Rose@charite.de (M.R.)
2. Department of Child and Adolescent Psychiatry, Charité-Universitätsmedizin Berlin, 13353 Berlin, Germany; ccorrell@northwell.edu
3. Center for Internal Medicine with Gastroenterology and Nephrology, Division for Endocrinology, Diabetes and Nutrition, Charité-Universitätsmedizin Berlin, 12200 Berlin, Germany
4. Donald and Barbara Zucker School of Medicine at Hofstra/Northwell, Hempstead, NY 11549, USA
5. Department of Psychiatry, The Zucker Hillside Hospital, Glen Oaks, NY 11004, USA
6. Department of Psychosomatic Medicine and Psychotherapy, Medical University Hospital Tübingen, 72076 Tübingen, Germany
* Correspondence: Andreas.Stengel@charite.de (A.S.); verena.haas@charite.de (V.H.); Tel.: +49-30-450-653-588 (A.S.); +49-30-450-566-399 (V.H.)
† These authors contributed equally to the manuscript.

Received: 23 August 2018; Accepted: 12 September 2018; Published: 18 September 2018

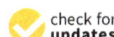

Abstract: Increased physical activity (PA) affects outcomes in patients with anorexia nervosa (AN). To objectively assess PA patterns of hospitalized AN patients in comparison with healthy, outpatient controls (HC), and to analyze the effect of PA on Body Mass Index (BMI) change in patients with AN, we measured PA in 50 female patients with AN (median age = 25 years, range = 18–52 years; mean BMI = 14.4 ± 2.0 kg/m^2) at the initiation of inpatient treatment and in 30 female healthy controls (median age = 26 years, range = 19–53 years; mean BMI = 21.3 ± 1.7 kg/m^2) using the SenseWear™ armband. Duration of inpatient stay and weight at discharge were abstracted from medical records. Compared with controls, AN patients spent more time in very light-intensity physical activity (VLPA) (median VLPA = 647 vs. 566 min/day, $p = 0.004$) and light-intensity physical activity (LPA) (median LPA = 126 vs. 84 min/day, $p < 0.001$) and less time in moderate-intensity physical activity (MPA) (median MPA = 82 vs. 114 min/day, $p = 0.022$) and vigorous physical activity (VPA) (median VPA = 0 vs. 16 min/day, $p < 0.001$). PA and BMI increase were not associated in a linear model, and BMI increase was mostly explained by lower admission BMI and longer inpatient stay. In a non-linear model, an influence of PA on BMI increase seemed probable (jack knife validation, $r^2 = 0.203$; $p < 0.001$). No direct association was observed between physical inactivity and BMI increase in AN. An altered PA pattern exists in AN patients compared to controls, yet the origin and consequences thereof deserve further investigation.

Keywords: accelerometry; eating disorders; motor restlessness; physical inactivity

1. Introduction

The role of increased physical activity (PA) for the onset and maintenance of anorexia nervosa (AN) is increasingly recognized. Being associated with a longer duration of inpatient treatment [1] and higher rates of a chronic outcome [2] as well as drop-out from treatment [3], increased PA can be regarded as a significant factor in the persistence of the disease [4]. However, high level PA is addressed insufficiently by current research [5]. As a consequence, a deeper understanding of the mechanisms underlying altered PA in AN as well as for the development of suitable therapeutic strategies to manage PA during weight restoration efforts are urgently warranted to improve outcomes for patients with AN.

Elevated levels of physical activity have been observed in 30–80% of patients suffering from AN [6,7], with this high range probably resulting from varying methods of PA measurement [8]. When assessed with subjective measurement tools including exercise questionnaires, patients reported higher total PA in comparison with a control group, yet simultaneous objective PA assessment using actigraphy yielded similar PA levels [9], suggesting that self-report overestimated PA in patients with AN and that objective assessments are needed to obtain accurate results. In addition, PA behavior is complex and has multiple dimensions; therefore, objective quantification of PA targets different components. Previous studies on objectively assessed PA in AN have yielded mixed results, with some reporting no differences in time spent in moderate to vigorous and daytime PA [10], or fidgeting [8], while others reported increased moderate to vigorous PA duration [3] and seated non-exercise PA [11] between AN inpatients and controls.

In a previous study [12], we focused on a potential link between high PA in AN and hypoleptinemia using a multisensor body monitor (Sensewear™ armband) for objective PA detection in hospitalized adults with AN. Results indicated that the use and interpretation of accelerometry, employed to objectively assess PA in AN patients, needs to be developed further and should also include parameters of physical inactivity. Building on the previous findings based on simple step count, the present study focused on a more detailed analysis of an expanded set of objectively measured PA patterns and intensities in adult females with AN, including inactivity parameters and adding a comparison to normal weight controls. We aimed to investigate the relationship between different PA patterns and BMI increase during inpatient treatment. We hypothesized that during inpatient treatment (I), hospitalized adult AN patients show increased low intensity PA in comparison with healthy controls, (II) increased low-level PA and BMI increase are inversely related, and (III) physical inactivity and BMI increase are directly related.

2. Subjects and Methods

2.1. Study Population

We enrolled 50 female adults with AN who were admitted to the Department of Psychosomatic Medicine at Charité—Universitätsmedizin Berlin for inpatient treatment of AN between 2011 and 2016. Patient inclusion criteria were: A diagnosis of AN according to ICD-10 (International Statistical Classification of Diseases and Related Health Problems, 10th Revision), restrictive, purging or atypical type, as well as a BMI < 17.5 kg/m^2. Exclusion criteria were: age <18 years, current pregnancy or a diagnosed psychotic episode. Information about the duration of the illness, comorbidities as well as medication at the beginning and end of the treatment program were retrieved from anamnestic data and medical reports. Between 2015 and 2016, we also recruited 30 sex-matched and similar aged normal weight healthy controls (HC), consisting mostly of clinical staff and relatives thereof. A BMI between 18.5 and 25 kg/m^2 served as inclusion criteria. Exclusion criteria were: Any known major medical or psychiatric disease and any condition with significant influence on PA. All participants gave written informed consent, and the study was approved by the institutional ethics committee of the Charité—Universitätsmedizin Berlin.

2.2. Anthropometry

Weight of all patients was measured to the nearest 0.1 kg via a digital scale (Seca 771, Vogel & Halke, Hamburg, Germany) and height to the nearest 0.5 cm via a stadiometer (Seca 220 Stadiometer, Vogel & Halke, Hamburg, Germany) [13]. Measurements took place in the morning between 7 and 8 a.m. after overnight fasting and in underwear. Weight of the controls was measured after a 2-h fast using a chair scale (MCB300K100M, KERN & Sohn GmbH, Balingen, Germany) and height was measured using a stadiometer (Vogel & Halke). BMI was calculated as kg/m^2.

2.3. Bioelectrical Impedance Analysis

Whole-body bioimpedance was measured by Nutriguard-M (Data Input, Darmstadt, Germany; electrodes: Bianostic-AT, Data Input) as part of the patients' clinical measurements. For bioimpedance analysis (BIA) of the normal-weight controls Biacorpus RX 4004 (MEDICAL HealthCare GmbH, Karlsruhe, Germany; Electrodes: BIA Classictabs, Medical HealthCare GmbH, Karlsruhe, Germany) was used. Patients and controls were weighed after fasting for at least 2 h, voiding and an equilibration period in a supine position. The equilibration period of both AN patients and controls lasted at least 10 min. BIA was carried out in accordance to the manufacturer's instructions, and body composition was calculated with Body Comp software (Version 9.0, Professional Scientific, Medical Health Care GmbH, Karlsruhe, Germany).

2.4. PA Assessment

PA was measured in AN patients after inpatient admission and inclusion into the study. Using a portable armband device (SenseWear™ PRO3 armband; BodyMedia, Inc., Pittsburgh, PA, USA), PA was continuously detected over a 3-day period (Friday to Sunday). During the time of PA detection, the study population was not restricted regarding their daily physical activity [13]. A day was included into data analysis if the armband had been worn for at least 20.5 h [13]. Measurements of controls took place while they stayed in their usual environment and by using the SenseWear™ PRO3 or the SenseWear™ MF armband. According to a statement of the manufacturer from 15 March 2011, the Sensewear Pro 3 and MF models were shown to be functionally equivalent in terms of sensor technology and data analysis (manufacturers statement on equivalency available on request).

The Sensewear armband is a multi-sensor device worn on the upper dominant arm which enables a continuous physiological PA detection [14] by measuring parameters such as heat flow, galvanic skin response (GSR), body temperature and near-body temperature [15]. An integrated two-axial accelerometer captures the movement of the upper arm as well as the position of the body [14]. The information captured by the five sensors and participant characteristics (age, sex, weight, height, smoker or non-smoker and handedness) [16] are integrated and analyzed by a proprietary software (SenseWear™ Software, Version 8.0, BodyMedia, Inc., Pittsburgh, PA, USA). This program is based upon algorithms of the manufacturer and able to analyze the collected raw data at different metabolic equivalent (MET) values. The latter represents a standardized indicator which is independent of time, body weight and sex [15]. One MET is equivalent to 1 kcal/h/kg body weight and serves as useful parameter to describe the energy expenditure [17] and intensity [15] of a specific activity. The MET value ranges from 1 MET while at rest [17] and 1.1 METs when driving in a car to 2–4 METs when doing housework [15], and can reach maximum values of 20 METs when doing excessive sports [15]. According to previous studies, we used six different MET categories to classify different activity intensities of PA within our AN and control group:

- A MET-value ≤ 1.0 was defined as the rate of energy expenditure while at rest [17].
- Activities with a MET-value ≤ 1.8 were considered as sedentary behavior [18].
- Thus, we concluded to form a new category ranging from ≥ 1.1 to ≤ 1.8 METs to describe very light-intensity physical activities (VLPA).
- Light-intensity physical activities (LPA) were defined as MET-values >1.8 and <3 [18].

- Moderate-intensity activities (MPA) were defined as ≥3 METs to <6 METs [17,18].
- Vigorous-intensity activities (VPA) were divided firstly into MET-values ranging from ≥6 to ≤9, and secondly into values >9 METs [3].

2.5. Statistical Analysis

Based on a prior study of 11 AN patients and 10 HCs whose activity was measured with a shoe-based accelerometer at three time points: (I) while eating lunch, (II) filling out questionnaires, and (III) watching television for 1 h, power was sufficient with 19 analyzed individuals to demonstrate a significant difference in total PA levels (df = 1.19, f = 5.68, $p = 0.03$) [11]. However, we aimed to assess activity continuously for 3 days and parse the analyses into six different PA intensity levels, i.e., (I) at rest, (II) very light, (III) light, (IV) moderate, (V) vigorous and (VI) vigorous >9 METs. Therefore, we assumed that at least four times more patients (i.e., $n = 44$) would be required to have sufficient power. For organizational purposes we capped HCs at $n = 30$ (assuming less heterogeneity among HCs); we increased the sample size of AN patients to $n = 50$.

A p-value of <0.05 was set as the significance threshold. All variables were tested in a two-sided fashion. All data are presented as mean ± standard deviation (SD) if following a normal distribution, otherwise as median (25th/75th percentile), or absolute frequency (relative frequency %). Quartiles were computed using R type 8 so that the resulting quantile estimates were approximately median-unbiased, regardless of the distribution. Data following a Gaussian distribution were analyzed by t-tests. Wilcoxon tests were applied for group differences for quantitative response variables not following a Gaussian distribution. Analyses for categories were performed by Fisher's exact test. To test the relationship between BMI change and various potential predictors, univariate and multivariate linear models were computed. A regression tree was computed, as this approach does not make assumptions on distributions or linearity. This machine learning technique computes a series of prediction thresholds to split a data set. Given our relatively small sample, splitting the data set into learning and test sets was not feasible; therefore, we applied a jack-knife procedure, classifying each subject based on a tree build from the remaining patients. Statistical analyses were computed using R version 3.4.2, R Core Team 2017.

3. Results

3.1. Characterization of the Study Population Including Medical Details, Comorbidities, Medications, and Body Composition

Table 1 shows the patients' demographic characteristics and body composition data upon hospital admission compared to the healthy control group. The two study groups did not significantly differ in age ($p = 0.057$). Body weight, BMI, body fat, and lean mass were significantly lower in patients with AN compared to controls (all: $p < 0.001$; Table 1). Regarding phase angle, i.e., the ratio of body cell mass to fat-free mass as an indicator of cellular health and integrity, AN patients had significantly lower values than controls ($p < 0.001$; Table 1).

Medical details, comorbidities, and current medications of the study populations are summarized in a supplemental table (Supplementary Table S1). Forty-eight percent of the patients were diagnosed with restrictive AN, 26% with purging AN, and 26% with atypical AN. In terms of comorbidities, AN patients had significantly more pericardial effusion ($p < 0.001$), episodes of depression ($p < 0.001$), and at least one comorbidity (AN = 96% vs. C = 33%, $p < 0.001$). No statistically significant differences existed for other medical disorders. In terms of medication, a significant difference between both groups existed only for psychopharmacological treatment, with none of the controls (C) but 16% of the AN patients receiving medication on admission ($p = 0.021$). No significant difference existed for oral contraceptives ($p = 0.052$), L-thyroxine ($p = 0.632$), or taking no medication (AN, 35% vs. C, 37%; $p = 1.000$).

Table 1. Demographic characteristics and bioimpedance data in patients with anorexia nervosa on admission and in the healthy control group.

Measurement Parameters	Anorexia Nervosa Baseline (n = 50)	Controls (n = 30)	p
Demographic parameters			
Age (years)	25 (21/30)	26 (23/35)	0.057
Weight (kg)	39.9 ± 6.6 (28.4–58.8)	60.5 ± 5.8 (51.2–71.9)	<0.001
Height (cm)	166 ± 7 (152–185)	169 ± 6 (159–180)	0.128
BMI (kg/m^2)	14.4 ± 2.0 (8.9–17.7)	21.3 ± 1.7 (18.8–25.0)	<0.001
Duration of illness (months)	72 (15/134)	N/A	
Body composition			
Phase angle (°)	4.5 (3.8/5.1)	5.9 (5.5/6.4)	<0.001
Fat mass (kg)	2.9 ± 2.7 (1–12.5)	16.0 ± 3.1 (11.3–22.5)	<0.001
Fat mass (%)	6.7 ± 5.2 (2.1–21.6)	26 ± 3 (21–32)	<0.001
Fat-free mass (kg)	37 ± 4 (27–46)	44 ± 3 (39–53)	<0.001
Fat-free mass (%)	93 ± 5 (78–98)	74 ± 3 (68–79)	<0.001

Data are expressed as mean ± SD (range) or as median (25th/75th percentile). BMI, Body Mass Index; N/A, not applicable; AN, anorexia nervosa.

3.2. Comparison of Physical Activity and MET Intensities

PA data and time spent in different levels of physical activity of 50 hospitalized AN patients compared to 30 ambulatory healthy controls are outlined in Table 2. Both groups engaged in similar levels of activity in terms of average steps and total distance per day. However, patients with AN had a greater range regarding the step count; 2479–31876 vs. 6507–22948 steps (Table 2). Significant differences were observed in daily average METs with patients presenting lower median values than controls. Patients with AN spent significantly more time in very low ($p = 0.004$) and low ($p < 0.001$) levels of PA than controls. Conversely, AN patients spent significantly less time in PA below the very low PA level ($p < 0.001$), in moderate ($p = 0.022$) as well as in 6–9 MET vigorous activity level ($p < 0.001$; Table 2). However, no significant differences were found for markers of physical inactivity: Both groups spent nearly the same duration of time on recumbency and sleep.

Table 2. Physical activity and the division into different MET cut-offs in patients with anorexia nervosa on admission and in the healthy control group.

Measurement Parameters	Anorexia Nervosa Baseline (n = 50)	Controls (n = 30)	p
Physical activity			
Number of steps per day	11,305 ± 6064 (2479–31,876)	11,098 ± 3973 (6507–22,948)	0.854
Total distance (km/day)	10.2 ± 5.5 (2.3–25.2)	9.8 ± 4.0 (4.6–19.2)	0.769
Metabolic equivalents (METs per day)	1.40 (1.40/1.60)	1.70 (1.50/1.80)	<0.001
Duration of recumbency (min/day)	483 (443/527)	500 (440/560)	0.348
Duration of sleep (min/day)	427 (375/457)	408 (363/484)	0.842
PA ≤ 1 METs duration (min/day)	496 (448/536)	588 (502/643)	<0.001
VLPA 1.1–1.8 METs duration (min/day)	647 (569/703)	566 (499/631)	0.004
LPA 1.8–3 METs duration (min/day)	126 (92/188)	84 (71/108)	<0.001
MPA 3–6 METs duration (min/day)	82 (44/130)	114 (79/165)	0.022
VPA 6–9 METs duration (min/day)	0 (0/3)	16 (8/35)	<0.001
VPA > 9 METs duration (min/day)	0.0 (0.0/0.0)	0.0 (0.0/3.2)	0.063

Data are expressed as mean ± SD (range) or as median (25th/75th percentile). LPA, light-intensity physical activity; MET, metabolic equivalent; MPA, moderate-intensity physical activity; PA, physical activity; VLPA, very light-intensity physical activity; VPA, vigorous-intensity physical activity.

3.3. BMI Change

Table 3 summarizes clinical outcome parameters of AN patients on admission and at discharge from inpatient treatment. On average, AN patients achieved a weight gain of 2.1 ± 2.3 kg during the 32-day (25th percentile: 26 days; 75th percentile: 63 days) inpatient treatment program. The BMI increased by 0.7 ± 0.8 kg/m², which is equivalent to a BMI increase of 4%. The mean rate of weight gain in AN was 0.29 kg/week and ranged from −0.44 kg/week up to 1.35 kg/week. Seven (14%) out of the 50 AN patients lost weight during their inpatient stay.

Table 3. Clinical outcome parameters of patients with anorexia nervosa.

Measurement Parameters	Anorexia Nervosa Baseline (n = 50)	Anorexia Nervosa Discharge (n = 50)	p
Clinical outcome			
Weight (kg)	39.9 ± 6.6 (28.4–58.8)	42.0 ± 6.2 (31.4–59.7)	<0.001
Total weight gain (kg)	-	2.1 ± 2.3 (−1.4–9.6)	
BMI (kg/m²)	14.4 ± 2.0 (8.9–17.7)	15.2 ± 1.8 (11.7–18.3)	<0.001
BMI increase (kg/m²)	-	0.7 ± 0.8 (−0.5–2.8)	
BMI increase (%)	-	4 (1/10)	

Data are expressed as mean ± SD (range) or as median (25th/75th percentile); BMI, Body Mass Index.

3.4. Association between Physical Activity and Clinical Outcome

In an univariate regression analysis with BMI increase in % as the dependent variable and a range of potential predictive factors as independent variables (length of inpatient stay, phase angle, BMI on admission, steps, total distance, PA at different MET intensities, duration of sleep and recumbency), only length of inpatient stay ($r = 0.154$; $p < 0.001$), phase angle ($r = -2.95$; $p = 0.002$) and BMI on admission ($r = -1.99$; $p < 0.001$) were significant predictors (presented in Figure 1 with Spearman rank correlation). In a multivariable model, length of inpatient stay ($p < 0.001$) and BMI on admission ($p = 0.029$) remained significant predictors and duration of sleep became significant ($r = -0.0107$; $p = 0.019$) as well. In addition, for MPA a trend ($r = 0.0111$; $p = 0.089$) towards becoming a significant positive predictor of BMI increase was observed.

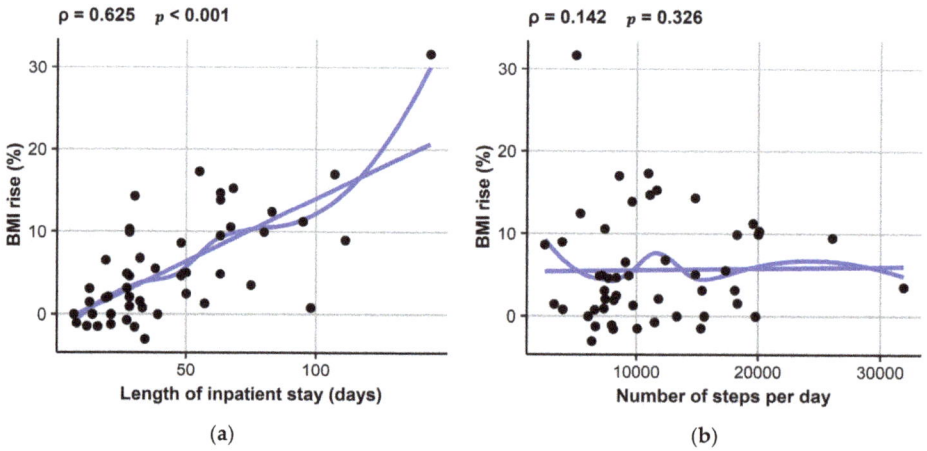

Figure 1. Associations between BMI increase in % and (a) length of inpatient stay and (b) number of steps per day applying Spearman rank correlation. BMI, Body Mass Index.

In an exploratory regression tree model (Figure 2), the following parameters were relevant predictors of percent BMI change: length of inpatient stay, BMI on admission, and number of steps.

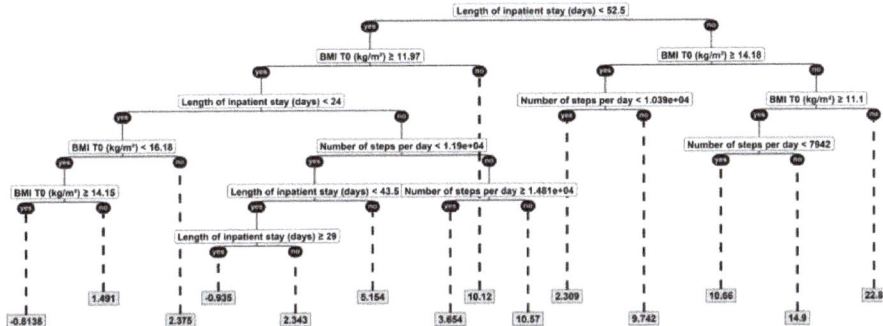

Figure 2. Regression tree for non-linear modelling to test the relation between BMI percent change and further parameters. BMI, Body Mass Index.

With this non-linear model, the association between actual and predicted BMI percent change could be predicted with an $r^2 = 0.81$ (Figure 3).

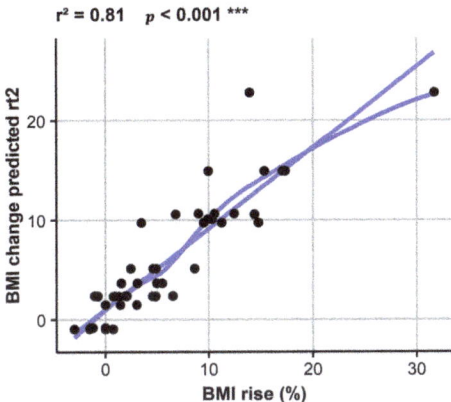

Figure 3. Non-linear model on predicted vs. measured BMI change. BMI, Body Mass Index.

Furthermore, validation of this prediction model by jack-knife analysis was successful ($r^2 = 0.203$; $p < 0.001$). The importance score for length of inpatient stay was 1026, for admission BMI 822, and for number of steps 453, potentially suggesting at least a small effect of PA measured as steps on % BMI increase. Applying these statistical procedures also for LPA as a parameter for low level activity, data yielded a similar value for r^2 for steps as well as an importance score of 562 for LPA, indicating also a slight effect of LPA on BMI change comparable in strength to that of steps.

4. Discussion

In our study, the following main results emerged: (1) Compared with healthy controls, AN patients spent more time engaging in light and less time engaging in vigorous intensity PA; (2) the patient's BMI increase during inpatient treatment was largely predicted by low BMI on admission and longer duration of inpatient stay; (3) high step count and time in light-intensity PA only emerged as potential predictors of lower BMI increase in an exploratory and non-linear model; and (4) contrary to our assumption, the duration of sleep as a marker of physical inactivity was inversely associated with BMI increase.

Few studies have objectively measured low intensity PA in AN inpatients compared with healthy controls. Our findings demonstrating increased low intensity PA are consistent with a previous study using a shoe-based monitor [11]. Using the SenseWear armband, El Ghoch et al. [3] also observed that AN patients spent less time in high intensity PA, yet contrary to our findings time spent in light-intensity PA did not differ between groups and the patients showed a significantly higher moderate and vigorous PA duration. The division into two low intensity MET categories (1.1–1.8 and 1.8–3) in the present study as opposed to one category (1.1–3 METs) in the study by El Ghoch [3] may explain the different and more detailed results. Differences in time spent with moderate to vigorous PA might relate to varying approaches with respect to the restriction of PA on the wards or to practical opportunities to exercise in the environment outside the ward. The choice of different PA assessment tools should also be taken into account: When assessing PA with movement sensors, there was no difference in time spent on "fidgeting" (operationalized as "body position change counts") between AN patients and controls [8]. Yet, the authors of that study mentioned problems with measurement technology consisting of several leads and wires, which might have affected compliance and PA behavior of the study participants.

A better understanding of the origin of distinct PA patterns in AN patients is warranted. Increased light PA in AN might be a consequence of negative energy balance resulting in a foraging response to increase PA to find food [19,20] or linked with a distinct phenotype characterized by disturbed energy homeostasis specifically associated with increased PA despite severe weight loss [6,21]. Further origins for increased light PA in AN might be an attempt of emotion regulation [6,22] or the desire to lose weight [4,23]. Interestingly, when interviewed 57 years after participating in the Minnesota starvation experiment in 1944/1945, the volunteer men did not report an increased drive for PA while starving [23]. To add to the complexity of altered PA in AN, the surrounding conditions during the time of PA assessment might play a considerable role. When obese volunteers were subjected to 24-h measurements of energy turnover within a metabolic chamber [24] for analysis of spontaneous PA, with exercise being prohibited within the chamber, the authors hypothesized that such forced reduction of voluntary exercise may have resulted in the partially observed increased engagement in spontaneous PA [25]. Similarly, in 16 healthy, male volunteers who underwent 8 weeks of experimental overfeeding, two-thirds of the increase in total daily energy expenditure was due to increased non-exercise activity thermogenesis (NEAT) [26]. Individual variation in NEAT accounted for the 10-fold differences in fat storage that occurred with overfeeding, suggesting that during positive energy balance, high activation of NEAT results in difficulties to gain weight for some individuals. The phenomenon of high NEAT and concomitantly energy needs of 4000 kcal/day to gain weight was recently documented in a case report of a young woman with AN at the end of therapy [27]. We believe that it is important for the tailoring of suitable PA interventions for AN patients to find an answer to the question whether increased low-level PA is an AN-specific phenotype that is linked with physiological processes during starvation and refeeding, or whether such PA behavior is related to restrictive treatment setting characteristics irrespective of AN, which may also be observable in other populations. Therefore, the current restrictive handling of PA during AN treatment may need to be reconsidered since an increase in low-level PA could provoke higher daily energy expenditure and might hinder weight recovery. Increased voluntary exercise could be accompanied by a decrease in spontaneous PA [25]. Concomitantly, Calogero et al. [28] investigated the effectiveness of an exercise program in patients with eating disorders, reporting on weight improvements through this intervention and concluding that patients in the exercise program may have been less likely to exercise secretly, whereas patients in the control group may have exercised unsupervised.

A low admission BMI was identified as a major determinant for BMI increase in AN. Resting energy expenditure proportionally declines with BMI [29], physiologically leading to a more rapid weight regain at the beginning of treatment. Longer inpatient stay also predicted BMI increase which may be at least in part explained by the rules in our adult treatment setting where patients were discharged if they continuously failed to meet the expected weight targets. On the other hand, patients who stayed in treatment longer also had more time to gain weight. Since only a slight effect of PA on BMI increase was observed and only by conducting an exploratory analysis, the admission BMI and duration of stay had an overall much greater, independent and overriding predictive power on BMI increase in AN. Whether an association between PA and weight trajectory in AN can be detected may depend on certain study characteristics, i.e., measurement technique and time point of PA assessment. There was no association between (I) PA duration at different MET intensities and daily steps at inpatient discharge and BMI at 1-year follow up [30]; (II) PA level operationalized as the average acceleration in m/s^2/min from both feet and BMI or rate of weight gain in AN patients admitted to an inpatient unit [11], and (III) time spent on feet at low-weight within 2 weeks of hospital admission or 1-month post-treatment discharge and 12 months BMI trajectory [8]. However, a longer on-feet duration at the inpatient weight restored time point was associated with a more rapid decrease in BMI over the 12 months following discharge [8]. Interestingly, a retrospective study applying questionnaires for PA assessment 6 months and 1 week prior to inpatient admission in 20 adolescents with AN found that an increase in PA—and not a decrease in food intake—was associated with the need for inpatient treatment [31]. These findings give rise to at least some effect of PA on the weight and illness trajectory of AN, and stress the need for further, systematic studies on this topic.

In the present study, no linear and direct associations between sleep duration and recumbency, conceptualized as physical inactivity parameters, and weight gain during AN treatment existed. Similarly, others could not find associations between sleep patterns and BMI [32], or between changes in sleep patterns and changes in BMI [33]. In the latter study, there was a significant direct association between baseline sleep time and BMI. In the present study, the contribution of sleep duration to variance of BMI increase was only of minor effect size. However, unexpectedly, in a multivariable model, the duration of sleep was inversely associated with BMI increase. In obesity, short sleep duration is known to be associated with increased food intake and excess body weight [34,35]. Whether this link also applies to patients with AN needs further investigation.

While we used objective PA assessments at standardized time points close to hospital admission, which are different from other studies that assessed PA across various stages of AN treatment [11], our findings also need to be interpreted within their limitations. Firstly, the validity of the SenseWear armband in severely underweight AN patients is unknown, and raw data and algorithms within the armband software are not accessible to researchers. Nonetheless, we consider this technology suitable for PA detection due to its easy handling compared to other devices [8] and the fact that multiple sensors enable the distinction between various types of PA, the recording of actual on-body time as well as time spent on sleep [14]. Second, whether our controls were of comparable socioeconomic background, and whether the wearing of the armband motivated them to work out more than usual remains unclear. Given that PA analysis was conducted between hospitalized AN patients and healthy controls within their everyday environment and thus in two very different settings, comparability of data may be argued. As a consequence, PA patterns of the patients in the present study may not be representative of other patients with AN under other types of care. However, finding a suitable control group for hospitalized patients is difficult, as healthy people are not hospitalized, and hospitalized patients for other reasons than AN are likely to suffer from a medical condition which affects PA patterns.

In conclusion, we found that AN patients spent more time engaging in light, and less time engaging in vigorous intensity PA than controls, and that the BMI increase during inpatient treatment was predicted by low admission BMI and longer inpatient treatment. Furthermore, high step count and time in light-intensity PA only emerged as potential predictors of lower BMI increase in an exploratory and non-linear model. This latter finding indicates that the effect of PA on the disease course of AN should be quantified and clarified further and that more complex models may need to be employed in future research on this topic. Since PA behavior is likely influenced by multiple factors including age, psychological and nutritional parameters, assessment of these potential modifiers in future studies may contribute to a better understanding of PA variability in AN.

Supplementary Materials: The following are available online at http://www.mdpi.com/2077-0383/7/9/289/s1, Table S1: Medical details, comorbidities, and medication of study patients and the healthy controls.

Author Contributions: Data curation, C.S.L., T.H. and A.S.; Project administration, T.H., U.E., A.S. and V.H.; Writing—original draft, C.S.L.; Writing—review & editing, T.H., U.E., M.R., C.U.C., A.S. and V.H.

Funding: This work was supported by funding of the Swiss Anorexia Nervosa Foundation (Project Number 23-13) and Charité University Funding (UFF 89/441-176, A.S.).

Acknowledgments: We thank Andreas Busjahn for his support with the statistical analysis; Magdalena Brinkmann, Karin Johansson and Christina Hentzschel for their assistance with the organization of clinical assessments. We acknowledge support by Deutsche Forschungsgemeinschaft and Open Access Publishing Fund of Charité University Berlin.

Conflicts of Interest: Correll has been a consultant and/or advisor to or has received honoraria from: Alkermes, Allergan, Angelini, Gerson Lehrman Group, IntraCellular Therapies, Janssen/J&J, LB Pharma, Lundbeck, Medavante, Medscape, Merck, Neurocrine, Otsuka, Pfizer, ROVI, Servier, Sunovion, Takeda, and Teva. He has provided expert testimony for Bristol-Myers Squibb, Janssen, and Otsuka. He served on a Data Safety Monitoring Board for Lundbeck, ROVI and Teva. He received royalties from UpToDate and grant support from Janssen and Takeda. He is also a shareholder of LB Pharma.

References

1. Solenberger, S.E. Exercise and eating disorders: A 3-year inpatient hospital record analysis. *Eat. Behav.* **2001**, *2*, 151–168. [CrossRef]
2. Strober, M.; Freeman, R.; Morrell, W. The long-term course of severe anorexia nervosa in adolescents: Survival analysis of recovery, relapse, and outcome predictors over 10–15 years in a prospective study. *Int. J. Eat. Disord.* **1997**, *22*, 339–360. [CrossRef]
3. El Ghoch, M.; Calugi, S.; Pellegrini, M.; Milanese, C.; Busacchi, M.; Battistini, N.C.; Bernabè, J.; Dalle Grave, R. Measured physical activity in anorexia nervosa: Features and treatment outcome. *Int. J. Eat. Disord.* **2013**, *46*, 709–712. [CrossRef] [PubMed]
4. Carrera, O.; Adan, R.A.; Gutierrez, E.; Danner, U.N.; Hoek, H.W.; van Elburg, A.A.; Kas, M.J. Hyperactivity in anorexia nervosa: Warming up not just burning-off calories. *PLoS ONE* **2012**, *7*, e41851. [CrossRef] [PubMed]
5. Gümmer, R.; Giel, K.E.; Schag, K.; Resmark, G.; Junne, F.P.; Becker, S.; Zipfel, S.; Teufel, M. High levels of physical activity in anorexia nervosa: A systematic review. *Eur. Eat. Disord. Rev.* **2015**, *23*, 333–344. [CrossRef] [PubMed]
6. Kostrzewa, E.; van Elburg, A.A.; Sanders, N.; Sternheim, L.; Adan, R.A.; Kas, M.J. Longitudinal changes in the physical activity of adolescents with anorexia nervosa and their influence on body composition and leptin serum levels after recovery. *PLoS ONE* **2013**, *8*, e78251. [CrossRef] [PubMed]
7. Rizk, M.; Lalanne, C.; Berthoz, S.; Kern, L.; EVHAN Group; Godart, N. Problematic exercise in anorexia nervosa: Testing potential risk factors against different definitions. *PLoS ONE* **2015**, *10*, e0143352. [CrossRef] [PubMed]
8. Gianini, L.M.; Klein, D.A.; Call, C.; Walsh, B.T.; Wang, Y.; Wu, P.; Attia, E. Physical activity and post-treatment weight trajectory in anorexia nervosa. *Int. J. Eat. Disord.* **2016**, *49*, 482–489. [CrossRef] [PubMed]
9. Keyes, A.; Woerwag-Mehta, S.; Bartholdy, S.; Koskina, A.; Middleton, F.; Connan, F.; Webster, P.; Schmidt, U.; Campbell, I.C. Physical activity and the drive to exercise in anorexia nervosa. *Int. J. Eat. Disord.* **2015**, *48*, 46–54. [CrossRef] [PubMed]
10. Sauchelli, S.; Arcelus, J.; Sánchez, I.; Riesco, N.; Jiménez-Murcia, S.; Granero, R.; Gunnard, K.; Baños, R.; Botella, C.; de la Torre, R.; et al. Physical activity in anorexia nervosa: How relevant is it to therapy response? *Eur. Psychiatry* **2015**, *30*, 924–931. [CrossRef] [PubMed]
11. Belak, L.; Gianini, L.; Klein, D.A.; Sazonov, E.; Keegan, K.; Neustadt, E.; Walsh, B.T.; Attia, E. Measurement of fidgeting in patients with anorexia nervosa using a novel shoe-based monitor. *Eat. Behav.* **2017**, *24*, 45–48. [CrossRef] [PubMed]
12. Stengel, A.; Haas, V.; Elbelt, U.; Correll, C.U.; Rose, M.; Hofmann, T. Leptin and physical activity in adult patients with anorexia nervosa: Failure to demonstrate a simple linear association. *Nutrients* **2017**, *9*, 1210. [CrossRef] [PubMed]
13. Hofmann, T.; Elbelt, U.; Ahnis, A.; Kobelt, P.; Rose, M.; Stengel, A. Irisin levels are not affected by physical activity in patients with anorexia nervosa. *Front. Endocrinol. (Lausanne)* **2014**, *4*, 202. [CrossRef] [PubMed]

14. Andre, D.; Pelletier, R.; Farringdon, J.; Safier, S.; Talbott, W.; Stone, R.; Vyas, N.; Trimble, J.; Wolf, D.; Vishnubhatla, S.; et al. The Development of the SenseWear® Armband, a Revolutionary Energy Assessment Device to Assess Physical Activity and Lifestyle. BodyMedia Inc., 2006. Available online: http://1fw.dotfit.com/sites/63/templates/categories/images/1783/Dev_SenseWear_article.pdf (accessed on 23 August 2018).
15. Das Armband Kompendium. Available online: http://www.body-coaches.de/wp-content/uploads/Armband_Anleitung.pdf (accessed on 23 August 2018).
16. Gastin, P.B.; Cayzer, C.; Dwyer, D.; Robertson, S. Validity of the ActiGraph GT3X+ and BodyMedia SenseWear Armband to estimate energy expenditure during physical activity and sport. *J. Sci. Med. Sport* **2018**, *21*, 291–295. [CrossRef] [PubMed]
17. Physical Activity Guidelines Advisory Committee. *Physical Activity Guidelines for Americans*; US Department of Health and Human Services: Washington, DC, USA, 2008; pp. 15–34.
18. Scheers, T.; Philippaerts, R.; Lefevre, J. Patterns of physical activity and sedentary behavior in normal-weight, overweight and obese adults, as measured with a portable armband device and an electronic diary. *Clin. Nutr.* **2012**, *31*, 756–764. [CrossRef] [PubMed]
19. Sternheim, L.; Danner, U.; Adan, R.; van Elburg, A. Drive for activity in patients with anorexia nervosa. *Int. J. Eat. Disord.* **2015**, *48*, 42–45. [CrossRef] [PubMed]
20. Adan, R.A.; Hillebrand, J.J.; Danner, U.N.; Cardona Cano, S.; Kas, M.J.; Verhagen, L.A. Neurobiology driving hyperactivity in activity-based anorexia. *Curr. Top. Behav. Neurosci.* **2011**, *6*, 229–250. [PubMed]
21. Casper, R.C. Restless activation and drive for activity in anorexia nervosa may reflect a disorder of energy homeostasis. *Int. J. Eat. Disord.* **2016**, *49*, 750–752. [CrossRef] [PubMed]
22. Bratland-Sanda, S.; Sundgot-Borgen, J.; Rø, Ø.; Rosenvinge, J.H.; Hoffart, A.; Martinsen, E.W. Physical activity and exercise dependence during inpatient treatment of longstanding eating disorders: An exploratory study of excessive and non-excessive exercisers. *Int. J. Eat. Disord.* **2010**, *43*, 266–273. [CrossRef] [PubMed]
23. Eckert, E.D.; Gottesman, I.I.; Swigart, S.E.; Casper, R.C. A 57-year follow-up investigation and review of the Minnesota study on human starvation and its relevance to eating disorders. *Arch. Psychol.* **2018**, *2*, 3.
24. Ravussin, E.; Lillioja, S.; Anderson, T.E.; Christin, L.; Bogardus, C. Determinants of 24-hour energy expenditure in man. Methods and results using a respiratory chamber. *J. Clin. Investig.* **1986**, *78*, 1568–1578. [CrossRef] [PubMed]
25. Garland, T., Jr.; Schutz, H.; Chappell, M.A.; Keeney, B.K.; Meek, T.H.; Copes, L.E.; Acosta, W.; Drenowatz, C.; Maciel, R.C.; van Dijk, G.; et al. The biological control of voluntary exercise, spontaneous physical activity and daily energy expenditure in relation to obesity: Human and rodent perspectives. *J. Exp. Biol.* **2011**, *214*, 206–229. [CrossRef] [PubMed]
26. Levine, J.A.; Eberhardt, N.L.; Jensen, M.D. Role of nonexercise activity thermogenesis in resistance to fat gain in humans. *Science* **1999**, *283*, 212–214. [CrossRef] [PubMed]
27. Haas, V.; Stengel, A.; Mähler, A.; Gerlach, G.; Lehmann, C.; Boschmann, M.; de Zwaan, M.; Herpertz, S. Metabolic barriers to weight gain in patients with anorexia nervosa: A young adult case report. *Front. Psychiatry* **2018**, *9*. [CrossRef] [PubMed]
28. Calogero, R.M.; Pedrotty, K.N. The practice and process of healthy exercise: An investigation of the treatment of exercise abuse in women with eating disorders. *Eat. Disord.* **2004**, *12*, 273–291. [CrossRef] [PubMed]
29. Haas, V.K.; Gaskin, K.J.; Kohn, M.R.; Clarke, S.D.; Müller, M.J. Different thermic effects of leptin in adolescent females with varying body fat content. *Clin. Nutr.* **2010**, *29*, 639–645. [CrossRef] [PubMed]
30. El Ghoch, M.; Calugi, S.; Pellegrini, M.; Chignola, E.; Dalle Grave, R. Physical activity, body weight, and resumption of menses in anorexia nervosa. *Psychiatry Res.* **2016**, *246*, 507–511. [CrossRef] [PubMed]
31. Higgins, J.; Hagman, J.; Pan, Z.; MacLean, P. Increased physical activity not decreased energy intake is associated with inpatient medical treatment for anorexia nervosa in adolescent females. *PLoS ONE* **2013**, *8*, e61559. [CrossRef] [PubMed]
32. Delvenne, V.; Kerkhofs, M.; Appelboom-Fondu, J.; Lucas, F.; Mendlewicz, J. Sleep polygraphic variables in anorexia nervosa and depression: A comparative study in adolescents. *J. Affect. Disord.* **1992**, *25*, 167–172. [CrossRef]
33. El Ghoch, M.; Calugi, S.; Bernabè, J.; Pellegrini, M.; Milanese, C.; Chignola, E.; Dalle Grave, R. Sleep patterns before and after weight restoration in females with anorexia nervosa: A longitudinal controlled study. *Eur. Eat. Disord. Rev.* **2016**, *24*, 425–429. [CrossRef] [PubMed]

34. Wu, Y.; Zhai, L.; Zhang, D. Sleep duration and obesity among adults: A meta-analysis of prospective studies. *Sleep Med.* **2014**, *15*, 1456–1462. [CrossRef] [PubMed]
35. Cappuccio, F.P.; Taggart, F.M.; Kandala, N.B.; Currie, A.; Peile, E.; Stranges, S.; Miller, M.A. Meta-analysis of short sleep duration and obesity in children and adults. *Sleep* **2008**, *31*, 619–626. [CrossRef] [PubMed]

© 2018 by the authors. Licensee MDPI, Basel, Switzerland. This article is an open access article distributed under the terms and conditions of the Creative Commons Attribution (CC BY) license (http://creativecommons.org/licenses/by/4.0/).

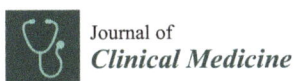 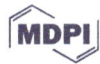

Article

Contingency Contracts for Weight Gain of Patients with Anorexia Nervosa in Inpatient Therapy: Practice Styles of Specialized Centers

Katrin Ziser [1,*], Katrin E. Giel [1], Gaby Resmark [1], Christoph Nikendei [2], Hans-Christoph Friederich [3], Stephan Herpertz [4], Matthias Rose [5], Martina de Zwaan [6], Jörn von Wietersheim [7], Almut Zeeck [8], Andreas Dinkel [9], Markus Burgmer [10], Bernd Löwe [11], Carina Sprute [12], Stephan Zipfel [1] and Florian Junne [1]

1. Department of Psychosomatic Medicine and Psychotherapy, Medical University Hospital Tuebingen, Osianderstr. 5, 72076 Tuebingen, Baden-Wuerttemberg, Germany; katrin.giel@med.uni-tuebingen.de (K.E.G.); gaby.resmark@med.uni-tuebingen.de (G.R.); stephan.zipfel@med.uni-tuebingen.de (S.Z.); florian.junne@med.uni-tuebingen.de (F.J.)
2. Department of General Internal and Psychosomatic Medicine, Heidelberg University Hospital, Im Neuenheimer Feld 410, 69120 Heidelberg, Baden-Wuerttemberg, Germany; christoph.nikendei@med.uni-heidelberg.de
3. Clinical Institute of Psychosomatic Medicine and Psychotherapy, University Hospital Duesseldorf, Moorenstraße 5, 40225 Duesseldorf, Nordrhein-Westfalen, Germany; hans-christoph.friederich@med.uni-duesseldorf.de
4. Department of Psychosomatic Medicine and Psychotherapy, LWL University Hospital, Ruhr-University Bochum, Alexandrinenstr. 1-3, 44791 Bochum, Nordrhein-Westfalen, Germany; stephan.herpertz@rub.de
5. Division of Psychosomatic Medicine, Charité University Hospital Berlin, Hindenburgdamm 30, 12200 Berlin, Berlin, Germany; rose@charite.de
6. Department of Psychosomatic Medicine and Psychotherapy, Hannover Medical School, Carl-Neuberg-Straße 1, 30625 Hannover, Niedersachsen, Germany; dezwaan.martina@mh-hannover.de
7. Department of Psychosomatic Medicine and Psychotherapy, University Hospital Ulm, Albert-Einstein-Allee 23, 89081 Ulm, Baden-Wuerttemberg, Germany; joern.vonwietersheim@uniklinik-ulm.de
8. Department of Psychosomatic Medicine and Psychotherapy, University Hospital Freiburg, Hauptstr. 8, 79104 Freiburg, Baden-Wuerttemberg, Germany; almut.zeeck@uniklinik-freiburg.de
9. Department of Psychosomatic Medicine and Psychotherapy, Klinikum rechts der Isar, Technical University of Munich, Langerstr. 3, 81675 Munich, Bayern, Germany; a.dinkel@tum.de
10. Department of Psychosomatic Medicine and Psychotherapy, University Hospital Muenster, Domagkstr. 22, 48149 Muenster, Nordrhein-Westfalen, Germany; markus.burgmer@ukmuenster.de
11. Institute and Outpatient Clinic for Psychosomatic Medicine and Psychotherapy, University Hospital Hamburg-Eppendorf, Martinistraße 52, 20246 Hamburg-Eppendorf, Hamburg, Germany; b.loewe@uke.de
12. Department of Psychosomatic Medicine and Psychotherapy, LVR-University Hospital, University Duisburg-Essen, Virchowstr. 174, 45147 Essen, Nordrhein-Westfalen, Germany; carina.sprute@lvr.de
* Correspondence: katrin.ziser@med.uni-tuebingen.de; Tel.: +49-7071-29-83610

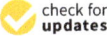

Received: 1 August 2018; Accepted: 11 August 2018; Published: 14 August 2018

Abstract: The treatment of patients with anorexia nervosa (AN) is often challenging, due to a high degree of ambivalence towards recovery and weight gain these patients often express. One part of the multimodal treatment is the utilization of treatment contracts (i.e., contingency contracts) that aim to motivate patients to gain weight by applying positive and negative consequences for the (non-)achievement of weight goals. The main aim of this study is to assess and analyze current standards of contingency contracts' utilization in German eating disorder centers. $n = 76$ mental health professionals of twelve specialized university centers in Germany that are currently or were formerly treating patients with AN in an inpatient setting participated. Most experts use contingency contracts in their clinic with weekly weight goals ranging between 500 and 700 g. Overall effectiveness and significance of contingency contracts for the inpatient treatment of patients with AN was rated high. Typical characteristics of a contingency contract in specialized German university hospital centers, such as the most frequent consequences, are described. The survey results assist the planning of further studies aiming to improve the multimodal treatment of patients with AN. For clinical practice, using external motivators such as contingency contracts as well as targeting internal motivation (e.g., by using motivational interviewing) is proposed.

Keywords: Anorexia nervosa; treatment contracts; weight gain; inpatient treatment; survey

1. Introduction

According to the Diagnostic and Statistical Manual of Mental Disorders (DSM-5), anorexia nervosa (AN) is a mental disorder characterized by an intense fear of gaining weight and body image disturbances that lead to restricted food intake relative to the required food intake (restrictive subtype) or other behaviors promoting weight loss such as excessive exercising or purging behavior (binge-purge subtype) [1]. Despite a twelve-month prevalence rate of 0.8% within the German population, AN is one of the mental disorders with the highest mortality [2–4]. In the long term, only approximately half of patients completely recover, whereas roughly 20 percent develop a chronic form of the disorder [5,6]. It takes an average of five to six years to achieve complete recovery [2]. This reflects the challenges associated with treatment, resulting from a high degree of ambivalence towards recovery and weight gain patients with AN often express [7,8].

According to German treatment recommendations, patients with severe AN (Body Mass Index (BMI) < 15) are treated in inpatient settings that regard weight restoration as one of the focal points for recovery [9]. Initial weight gain and symptom-orientation have been shown to predict good outcomes [10,11]. Nonetheless, a study by Schlegl and colleagues suggests that about one third of patients with AN do not show a significant response to intensive inpatient treatment [12]. Thus, there is still room for improvement in inpatient treatment approaches for patients with AN [13].

One indispensable part of the multimodal treatment approach for patients with AN is the utilization of a treatment contract, which is implemented to induce motivation for weight gain. Treatment contracts are currently routinely used in the inpatient treatment of patients with AN in Germany [14–17]. They are verbal or written agreements with the patient that contain mostly, but not exclusively, weight goals. Frequently, they outline the amount of weight that should be gained in a defined period of time during the inpatient stay (e.g., each week). Positive consequences for reaching these weight goals and negative consequences for not fulfilling weight goals are determined. Treatment contracts to induce weight gain in patients with AN can also be called weight contracts or contingency contracts for weight gain.

A recent systematic review by our group showed that despite their routine usage in inpatient treatment, contingency contracts for weight gain are an understudied topic and the empirical evidence base is scarce [18]. The majority of publications included in our review were of rather historical nature with few current contributions. We could, however, identify a development from restrictive applications of treatment contracts, e.g., in the form of bed rest to more collaborative approaches. These collaborative approaches try to actively involve patients into the contingency contracting process, e.g., by negotiating terms of the contract or letting patients choose consequences.

In terms of clinical application, there is some guidance in available treatment manuals for AN [15,19] with written examples of contracts. However, this guidance seems to stem from clinical expertise which is valuable but not sufficient to ensure high treatment standards. Currently, it is unclear whether treatment manuals are used and if done so, how the contingency contract process is organized in German eating disorder centers.

The main aim of the present study is to assess and analyze the utilization of contingency contracts for weight gain in German university hospitals specializing in eating disorders by means of a survey. Current approaches used by these specialized centers for collaboration with the patient are investigated, as well as strategies to enhance the patients' autonomy and motivation in the treatment contract process. Experiences of mental health professionals during the treatment contract process are also described. Finally, as an exploratory question, the role of professional characteristics in the contingency contract process is examined.

2. Experimental Section

2.1. Study Centers

Twelve specialized university hospital centers in Germany were invited and participated in this multicenter study. Mental health professionals who are currently or were formerly treating patients with AN in an inpatient setting were eligible for participation.

2.2. Sample

The study sample consists of $n = 76$ medical doctors and clinical psychologists between the ages of 24 and 60 ($M = 37.95$, $SD = 8.28$). For a detailed sample description, see Table 1.

Table 1. Demographic characteristics of the study sample ($n = 76$).

Variables	M (SD)	%
Gender: female		71.1
Clinical experience in psychotherapy/psychosomatic medicine/psychiatry in years	7.75 (7.20)	
Occupational group		
Medical doctor		61.8
Clinical psychologist		36.8
Both		1.3
Estimated number of treated patients with anorexia nervosa		
<20		34.2
20–40		23.7
41–60		14.5
61–80		6.6
81–100		9.2
>100		11.8
Main therapeutic orientation		
Cognitive-behavior psychotherapy		29.7
Psychodynamic psychotherapy		70.3

2.3. Measures

The online survey contained questions concerning the following topics: (1) demographic characteristics (including e.g., therapeutic orientation and clinical work experience); (2) questions about the utilization of and criteria for implementing contingency contracts into the inpatient treatment routine (e.g., percentage of patients that receive a contingency contract, timepoint of conclusion, duration, standardization of the procedure); (3) precise form of the contingency contract (e.g., verbal, written, freely formulated); (4) weight goals, control days and consequences for achieving or not achieving the weight goals; (5) circumstances that lead to a termination of contingency contracts; (6) experienced emotions of experts during the contingency contract process and appraisal of effectiveness. Items were either dichotomous (applicable–not applicable) or measured on a seven-point Likert scale (e.g., 1 never–7 always). All items relating to the contingency contract were newly developed for this survey.

After the demographic questions, a definition of contingency contracts in the context of inpatient treatment of patients with AN was given for clarification. Contingency contracts in the form of a weight contract were defined as follows: "A weight contract is a verbal or written agreement with a patient that determines weight changes and/or behavioral changes (e.g., eating behavior) that are linked to consequences for the patient."

2.4. Procedure

Invitational links were sent to representatives of all of the study centers, who then forwarded the invitation to eligible expert staff. Upon clicking on the survey link, experts were informed about the survey and protection of data privacy. They had to give consent in order to start the survey. Upon reaching the final page, experts were informed that the survey is finished and thanked for their participation.

2.5. Statistical Analyses

Means, standard deviations and percentages are reported for sample descriptions. Since variables were mostly not normally distributed, Mann–Whitney U tests for the analyses of single differences of means were used. To analyze potential associations between variables, Spearman rho correlations are reported. All statistical analyses were performed using IBM SPSS Statistics version 24 (IBM Corporation, Armonk, NY, USA). The level of significance for all analyses was set at $\alpha = 0.05$.

3. Results

3.1. Utilization

All of the experts reported that contingency contracts are utilized in their institution for inpatients with AN. They estimated that 87.6 percent of patients with AN in their department and 87.9 percent of their own patients with AN receive a contingency contract (annualized rate). The majority of experts (90.8%) reported using a standardized procedure to put contingency contracts in place. Of those, almost all reported having a guideline/manual provided within the department (98.6%) versus e.g., a published manual.

3.2. Preparation and Conclusion

About two thirds of experts (65.8%) reported preparing contingency contracts before inpatient treatment, for example at a preliminary (outpatient) consultation. 14.5 percent of the experts reported on giving written information about contingency contracts to the patient before admission to the ward. The majority of experts (78.4%) reported that contingency contracts are finalized in the first week of the inpatient stay. Only 5.2 percent of experts reported finalizing contingency contracts in the second week of inpatient treatment and 5.3 percent reported on not having a set time point for concluding contingency contracts.

3.3. Weight Contingencies and Weight Goals

Most experts (88.2%) reported setting standardized weekly contingents for weight gain, ranging between 300 g and 800 g per week. The most frequent weight gain goals are 700 g per week (44.8%), 500 g per week (37.3%) and 800 g per week (10.4%). The determination of the designated weight goal differs between the institutions: 46.1 percent of experts indicated individually negotiating the weight goal with the patients, and 39.5 percent of experts indicated that the weight goal is orientated at normal or close to normal weight with BMIs ranging between 17 and 19 kg/m^2. One expert indicated using different BMIs according to the age group of the patient for determining normal weight. For 15.8 percent of experts, weight goals were adapted to the planned duration of treatment. Only 6.6 percent of experts reported on not having a determined weight goal.

3.4. Revisiting, Changing and Terminating Contingency Contracts

Experts reported on revisiting the contingency contract with the patients at determined time points (47.4%), predominantly during ward rounds. Some other cases, e.g., if weight loss occurred, also made it necessary to revisit contingency contracts. For a smaller proportion of experts, revisiting the contingency contract occurred routinely after weighing the patient (28.9%), in the event of negative consequences (28.9%) or in the event of positive consequences (25.0%). Only 27.6 percent of experts reported on revisiting the contingency contract in each session.

Changing contingency contracts in the course of the inpatient treatment seemed to be handled quite differently: About one third of the experts (32.9%) reported on changing contingency contracts when patients lost weight and/or dropped below a certain BMI or when patients could not catch up to the required amount of weight gain anymore (31.6%). Some experts (7.8%) reported that changes/adaptions of the contingency contract were not intended whereas other experts reported on individually adapting contingency contracts over the course of treatment. Individually adapting might for instance take the form of temporarily changing from weight gain to weight maintenance. Some experts also reported on discharging patients from the ward for motivational reasons if weight goals were repeatedly not achieved. Patients were then offered the possibility of a re-admission after one or two weeks if they achieved some weight gain on their own.

About half of the experts (48.6%) reported that terminating contingency contracts did not happen in their institution, whereas 39.2 percent indicated that contingency contracts were terminated in special cases. These include the achievement of normal weight, somatic reasons (e.g., refeeding syndrome, infections) or if other symptoms gain priority (e.g., impulsive behavior).

3.5. Consequences

Consequences mostly depended on weight loss (90.8%) and weight gain (86.8%). One quarter of experts also reported that consequences could depend on symptoms like vomiting/purging, exercising/physical activity and eating behavior. Consequences were routinely applied after checking weight, either after every weighing (31.6%) or every second weighing (47.4%). Experts reported on choosing positive consequences themselves (23.7%) or letting the patient choose positive consequences from a list (17.1%) or freely (26.3%). In about a quarter of cases (24.7%), consequences were already determined in the contingency contract or were negotiated with the patient (13.0%). In regards to negative consequences, 36.8% experts reported determining the consequences themselves, as opposed to letting patients choose from a list (21.1%) or freely (11.8%).

Most frequently used positive consequences were the cessation of ward restriction (84.2%), being able to temporarily leave the hospital (82.9%) and the cessation of a liquid diet. Other mentioned positive consequences were: extension of treatment opportunities (e.g., patients could also participate in art or music therapy), cessation of accompanied eating, cessation of nasogastric feeding, and opportunities to temporarily leave the ward. When patients could choose their own positive consequences, chosen consequences included: buying themselves something nice, having their hair done, having a meal outside of the hospital, meeting friends, taking a bath, watching a movie/going to the cinema, bringing one's musical instrument to the ward and using the music room.

The most frequently used negative consequences were restriction to the ward (86.8%) and additional high caloric nutrients (69.7%). Further mentioned negative consequences were movement bans, nasogastric feeding, closely accompanied eating, and restrictions on using the phone or having visitors. The ultimate negative consequence was discharge from the hospital.

3.6. Overall Effectiveness and Factors of Success from the Experts' Points of View

Overall effectiveness of contingency contracts in the inpatient treatment of patients with AN was rated as 'effective for the most part' ($M = 5.72$, $SD = 0.74$). Greater clinical work experience was associated with a higher appraisal of the relevance of contingency contracts for the inpatient treatment of patients with AN ($r_s = 0.328$, $p = 0.006$).

Among the factors experts rated as important for the success of a contingency contract were general factors such as therapeutic alliance ($M = 6.67$, $SD = 0.53$), empathy of the therapist ($M = 6.58$, $SD = 0.62$) and motivation of the patient ($M = 6.53$, $SD = 0.67$). Factors such as having a written record of the contingency contract ($M = 6.56$, $SD = 0.67$) and having a copy of the contingency contract available for the patient ($M = 6.47$, $SD = 0.71$) were also rated as important. For a detailed rating of factors of success, see Figure 1.

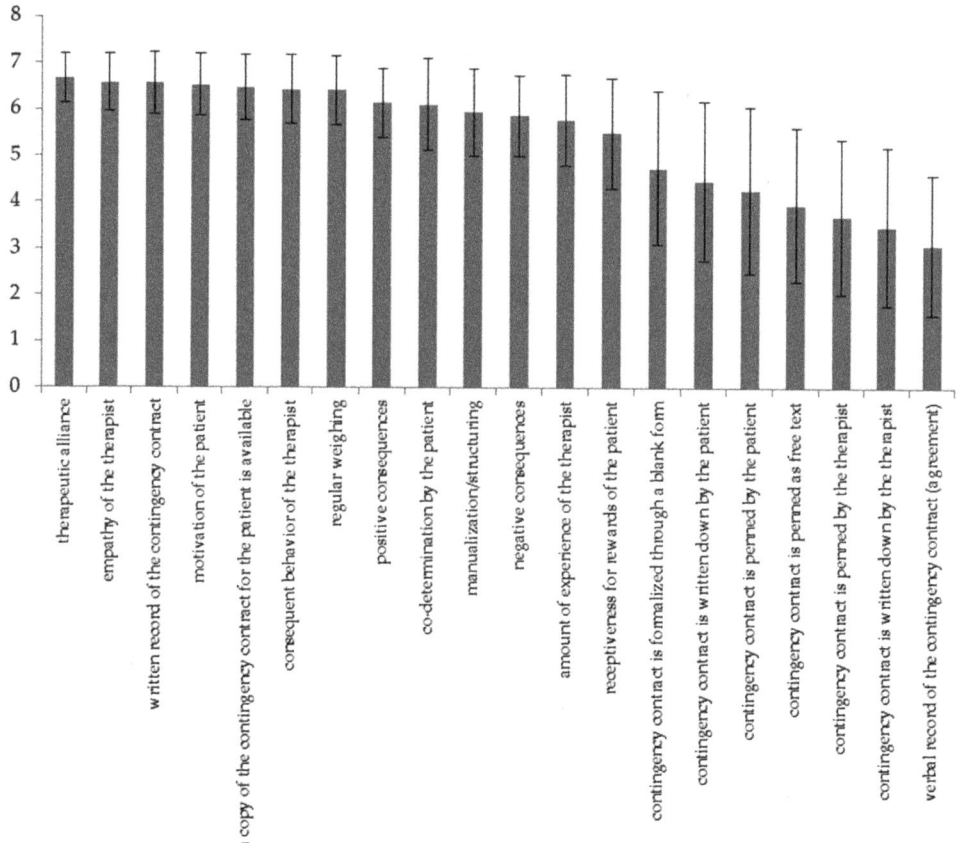

Figure 1. Factors of success of contingency contracts for anorexia nervosa (AN) by expert ratings. Factors of success were rated on a 7-point Likert scale from 1 'not important at all' to 7 'very important'.

3.7. Emotions Experienced by the Experts during the Contingency Contract Negotiation and Emotional Burden

On average, experts rated the overall significance of contingency contracts for the inpatient treatment of patients with AN as 'significant for the most part' to 'very significant' ($M = 6.27$, $SD = 1.00$). They reported on not experiencing the contingency contract process (preparation, negotiation and conclusion) as emotionally straining ($M = 3.95$, $SD = 1.65$), however there was a significant correlation between experiencing emotional strain and the amount of clinical work experience in years of $r_s = -0.355$, $p = 0.002$. This indicates that when clinical work experience increases, emotional strain during the contingency contract process decreases.

Experts reported mainly experiencing a sense of responsibility ($M = 5.20$, $SD = 1.09$), compassion ($M = 4.80$, $SD = 1.09$) and strain ($M = 4.54$, $SD = 1.20$) during the negotiation of contingency contracts. Other emotions (tension, relaxation, ambivalence, frustration, anger and rejection) were reported as being experienced 'rarely' to 'occasionally'.

3.8. Group Differences

Potential differences in appraising contingency contracts in the inpatient treatment of patients with AN were tested between occupational groups (medical doctors vs. psychologists) and between therapeutic orientations (behavior therapy vs. psychodynamic therapy). Regarding differences between occupational groups, there were no significant differences in emotions experienced during the negotiation of contingency contracts (all $Us > 406.50$, all $ps > 0.171$). However, medical doctors rated the ethical tenability of contingency contracts, especially regarding the application of negative consequences such as restriction to the ward, higher than psychologists ($U = 373.50$, $p = 0.008$).

Regarding the emotions experienced during the contingency contract process, differences in how ambivalence was experienced were found between therapeutic orientations ($U = 314.00$, $p = 0.060$). Specifically, psychodynamic therapists experienced more ambivalence while negotiating a contingency contract. There were no group differences for the other listed emotions (all $Us > 362.00$, all $ps > 0.302$). For the ratings of factors of success, there was only one significant difference between the therapeutic orientations: Behavioral therapists rated recording the contingency contract in a written form as more important compared to psychodynamic therapists ($U = 359.00$, $p = 0.019$).

4. Discussion

This study analyzed characteristics, utilization and appraisal of contingency contracts for weight gain in AN in German university hospitals specializing in the treatment of eating disorders. Experts were asked about their preparation, negotiation, conclusion and revisions of contingency contracts for patients with AN, their overall rating of effectiveness, as well as experienced emotions and possible emotional strain during this process.

4.1. Similarities of Contingency Contracts in Specialized Eating Disorder Centers

As expected, the majority of patients with AN receive a contingency contract in the participating institutions. Although not following a published manual, utilization in all centers follows internal guidelines or manuals. The most commonly used weight goals range between 500 and 800 g per week and are therefore in line with current recommendations of treatment guidelines for eating disorders [9,20].

Consequences are usually dependent on weight gain and/or weight loss. Only a few experts reported also putting consequences on other eating disorder related behaviors such as excessive exercising or vomiting. Having weight gain or weight loss as a sole focus of contingency contracts for patients with AN presumably originates from early behavioristic approaches of contingency management [18]. In light of a holistic treatment approach however, it seems advisable to consider other eating disorder related behaviors such as excessive exercising or vomiting as part of the contingency contract as well.

In sum, the present study uncovered basic characteristics of contingency contracts shared by the majority of experts. A typical contingency contract in specialized eating disorder centers in Germany can therefore be described as presented in Figure 2.

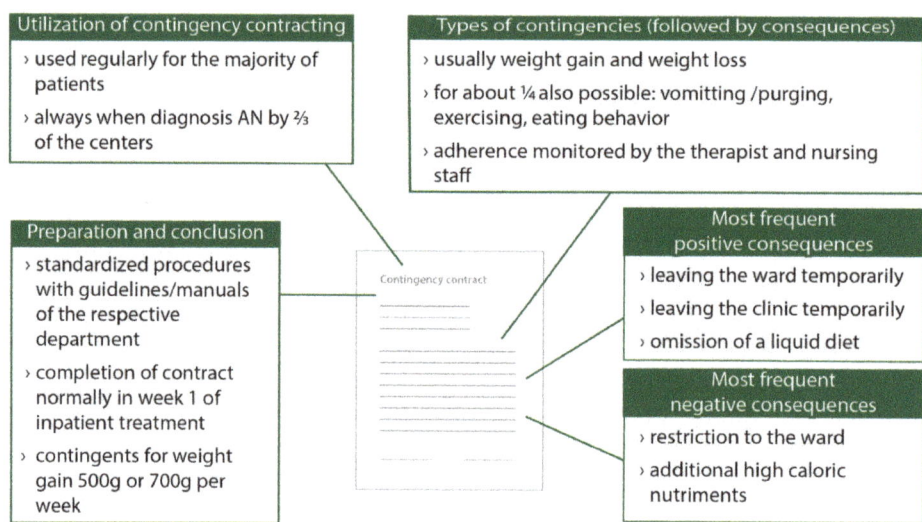

Figure 2. Characteristics of typical contingency contracts in specialized German university centers; AN = anorexia nervosa.

4.2. Differences of Contingency Contracts in Specialized Eating Disorder Centers

The three major aspects, in which participating institutions differ, are their definitions of weight goals, when and how contingency contracts are revisited and the choice of consequences. The definition of weight goals and the revisiting of contingency contracts possibly reflect the different self-developed manuals of the eating disorder centers. One half of experts negotiate weight goals with the patient, also taking aspects such as planned duration of stay into consideration. Another 40% orientate themselves toward a BMI value that should be achieved (low normal). One possible explanation for different BMI goals, ranging between 17 and 19 kg/m^2, is the continued discussion surrounding which BMI cut-off should be used to indicate non-anorectic weight for patients with AN [1,21].

Herzog and colleagues [22] showed that lower weekly weight goals (500 g) led to a higher achieved weight at the end of treatment, compared to higher weekly weight goals (750 g). In contrast, there are studies showing that higher weekly caloric intake led to higher overall weight gain (e.g., [23]). A recent systematic review [24] demonstrated that higher calorie refeeding is not associated with increased risk of the refeeding syndrome, at least for mildly and moderately affected patients. However, inpatient therapy is mainly indicated for severely ill patients and caution regarding caloric intake in the first days of treatment should be applied. Hence, for severely malnourished patients, there is no evidence to change current approaches. However, the long-term impact of different approaches is unknown [24], therefore no clear recommendation can be made from the literature concerning what (weekly) weight goals or BMI goals should be set [9].

4.3. Collaborative Approaches within the Contingency Contract Process

One of the aims of the current study was to identify approaches to incorporate patients into the contingency contract process in order to motivate them and enhance compliance and autonomy. In concrete terms, patients (and parents for younger patients) can for example co-determine weight goals, choose consequences and write down the contingency contract in their own words. We found that about 30% of experts let their patients choose consequences or negotiate consequences with the patient and almost half of the experts negotiate weight goals with their patients. This seems promising especially considering that patients are often ambivalent to restore weight [25]. However, letting patients co-determine weight goals can bare the risk of setting weight goals that are too small. Additionally, negotiating weight goals and weight contingencies with the patient instead of setting them oneself can be a wearisome task for the therapist.

In the literature covering the topic of collaboration in the field of AN, there is a clear preference for collaborative approaches by patients as well as therapists [26]. Furthermore, Williams and Reid [25] showed in their qualitative study that patients with AN feel low self-efficacy about changing behaviors. On one side, AN gives them a sense of control, but the disorder also causes strong feelings of loss of control. The authors conclude that this ambivalence patients experience should be targeted in a collaborative manner [25]. In line with this evidence and the systematic review, which shows an overall movement from the utilization of (directive) contingency management towards more collaborative contingency contracts [18], contingency contracts in Germany should intensify their focus on collaboration within the weight contract process.

4.4. Implications for Clinical Practice

Motivational aspects are one of the main considerations for the improvement of treatment and care for patients with AN [27] and are taken into consideration for example by integrating motivation-based therapeutic styles into treatment [28,29]. Motivation of patients has been shown to play an essential role concerning dropout rates and treatment compliance [30]. Furthermore, internal motivation to change was identified as one of the positive predictors of clinically significant changes in eating disorder psychopathology in patients with AN quantitatively [12] as well as qualitatively in patients' reports [31]. It is therefore worth considering a shift in the treatment approach, from motivating the patients externally through a contingency contract, to enhancing internal motivation for example by incorporating a motivations-based treatment style. Indeed, some of the authors are currently developing a motivation-based intervention, incorporating motivational aspects into the inpatient treatment of patients with AN, which they plan to soon test against existing treatment options.

4.5. Experiences of Experts with the Contingency Contract Process

Although there was great variation in emotions experienced by the participating experts during the contingency contract process, on average there was no extremely negative or positive emotions which evidently accompanied this process. Additionally, it could be shown that the emotional burden for experts decreased with the years of experience, which coincides with clinical impressions. We found no significant differences between occupational groups (physician versus psychologist) or therapeutic orientation (behavioral versus psychodynamic psychotherapy). It would be interesting, however, to also investigate the emotional experiences of nurses and other caregivers in the inpatient environment.

4.6. Limitations and Prospects

The main limitation of the study is its descriptive nature; as no causal conclusions about the reported associations and group differences can be drawn. Furthermore, only specialized university centers were included which heightened the risk of a selection/recruitment bias. Although a fair amount of specialized university centers in Germany participated, not all could be included, raising the question of representativeness. However, given that this is the first study attempting to describe the contingency contract process in specialized centers in Germany, this account provides a valuable contribution to the evidence base.

The usefulness of contingency contracting practice styles for patients with AN in other countries would also be of high interest. Taking into account that patients in other countries might be treated in outpatient or day-patient settings more frequently, it might be more difficult to track positive and negative consequences. However, this would also entail the chance for greater collaboration between patients and therapists, potentially lessening the chance of patients fearing 'to be controlled' and enabling them to gain more autonomy. There are some reports about the utilization of contingency contracts around the world [18], however to the best of our knowledge, studies about practice styles that go beyond the treatment program of one specific clinic, are missing.

5. Conclusions

The majority of experts use contingency contracts for their patients with AN. Most contracts involve weekly weight goals and there is strong consensus regarding the most frequent positive and negative consequences following weight gain or loss. This knowledge can help define and implement best practices concerning contingency contracting in the treatment of patients with AN. It also gives insight into current practice, and is therefore useful for the planning of further studies aiming to improve the efficacy of treatments procedures for patients with AN. For clinical practice, using external motivators such as contingency contracts as well as targeting internal motivation (e.g., by using motivational interviewing) is proposed.

Author Contributions: Conceptualization, K.Z., F.J., S.Z., K.E.G. and G.R.; Methodology, K.Z., F.J., S.Z., K.E.G. and G.R.; Formal Analysis, K.Z.; Investigation, K.Z., F.J., S.Z., K.E.G., G.R., C.N., H.-C.F., S.H., M.R., M.d.Z., J.v.W., A.Z., A.D., M.B., B.L. and C.S.; Resources, F.J., K.E.G. and S.Z.; Data Curation, K.Z.; Writing-Original Draft Preparation, K.Z.; Writing-Review & Editing, K.Z., F.J., S.Z., K.E.G., G.R., C.N., H.-C.F., S.H., M.R., M.d.Z., J.v.W., A.Z., A.D., M.B., B.L. and C.S.; Visualization, K.Z.; Supervision, F.J. and S.Z.; Project Administration, K.Z.

Acknowledgments: K.Z. is supported by the "Konrad Adenauer Stiftung" (Konrad Adenauer Foundation).

Conflicts of Interest: The authors declare no conflict of interest.

References

1. American Psychiatric Association. *Diagnostic and Statistical Manual of Mental Disorders*, 5th ed.; American Psychiatric Association: Washington, DC, USA, 2013.
2. Jacobi, F.; Höfler, M.; Strehle, J.; Mack, S.; Gerschler, A.; Scholl, L.; Busch, M.A.; Hapke, U.; Maske, U.; Seiffert, I. Twelve-months prevalence of mental disorders in the German health interview and examination survey for adults–Mental health module (DEGS1-MH): A methodological addendum and correction. *Int. J. Methods Psychiatr. Res.* **2015**, *24*, 305–313. [CrossRef] [PubMed]
3. Zipfel, S.; Giel, K.E.; Bulik, C.M.; Hay, P.; Schmidt, U. Anorexia nervosa: Aetiology, assessment, and treatment. *Lancet Psychiatry* **2015**, *2*, 1099–1111. [CrossRef]
4. Arcelus, J.; Mitchell, A.J.; Wales, J.; Nielsen, S. Mortality rates in patients with anorexia nervosa and other eating disorders: A meta-analysis of 36 studies. *Arch. Gen. Psychiatry* **2011**, *68*, 724–731. [CrossRef] [PubMed]
5. Miller, C.A.; Golden, N.H. An introduction to eating disorders: Clinical presentation, epidemiology, and prognosis. *Nutr. Clin. Pract.* **2010**, *25*, 110–115. [CrossRef] [PubMed]
6. Zipfel, S.; Löwe, B.; Reas, D.L.; Deter, H.-C.; Herzog, W. Long-term prognosis in anorexia nervosa: Lessons from a 21-year follow-up study. *Lancet* **2000**, *355*, 721–722. [CrossRef]
7. Cockell, S.J.; Geller, J.; Linden, W. Decisional balance in anorexia nervosa: Capitalizing on ambivalence. *Eur. Eating Disord. Rev.* **2003**, *11*, 75–89. [CrossRef]
8. Abbate-Daga, G.; Amianto, F.; Delsedime, N.; De-Bacco, C.; Fassino, S. Resistance to treatment and change in anorexia nervosa: A clinical overview. *BMC Psychiatry* **2013**, *13*, 294–311. [CrossRef] [PubMed]
9. Herpertz, S.; Herpertz-Dahlmann, B.; Fichter, M.; Tuschen-Caffier, B.; Zeeck, A. *S3-Leitlinie Diagnostik und Behandlung der Essstörungen*; Springer: Berlin/Heidelberg, Germany, 2011.
10. Sly, R.; Morgan, J.F.; Mountford, V.A.; Lacey, J.H. Predicting premature termination of hospitalised treatment for anorexia nervosa: The roles of therapeutic alliance, motivation, and behaviour change. *Eating Behav.* **2013**, *14*, 119–123. [CrossRef] [PubMed]
11. Zeeck, A.; Hartmann, A. Relating therapeutic process to outcome: Are there predictors for the short-term course in anorexic patients? *Eur. Eating Disord. Rev.* **2005**, *13*, 245–254. [CrossRef]
12. Schlegl, S.; Quadflieg, N.; Löwe, B.; Cuntz, U.; Voderholzer, U. Specialized inpatient treatment of adult anorexia nervosa: Effectiveness and clinical significance of changes. *BMC Psychiatry* **2014**, *14*, 258. [CrossRef] [PubMed]
13. Keel, P.K.; Brown, T.A. Update on course and outcome in eating disorders. *Int. J. Eating Disord.* **2010**, *43*, 195–204. [CrossRef] [PubMed]

14. Hartmann, A.; Zeeck, A.; Barrett, M.S. Interpersonal problems in eating disorders. *Int. J. Eating Disord.* **2010**, *43*, 619–627. [CrossRef] [PubMed]
15. Legenbauer, T.; Vocks, S. *Manual der kognitiven Verhaltenstherapie bei Anorexie und Bulimie*; Springer: Berlin, Germany, 2014.
16. Schauenburg, H.; Friederich, H.-C.; Wild, B.; Zipfel, S.; Herzog, W. Fokale psychodynamische psychotherapie der anorexia nervosa. *Psychotherapeut* **2009**, *54*, 270–280. [CrossRef]
17. Herzog, W.; Friederich, H.-C.; Wild, B.; Löwe, B.; Zipfel, S. Magersucht. *Therapeutische Umschau* **2006**, *63*, 539–544. [CrossRef] [PubMed]
18. Ziser, K.; Resmark, G.; Giel, K.E.; Becker, S.; Stuber, F.; Zipfel, S.; Junne, F. The effectiveness of contingency management in the treatment of patients with anorexia nervosa: A systematic review. *Eur. Eating Disord. Rev.* **2018**, 1–15. [CrossRef] [PubMed]
19. Borgart, E.-J.; Meermann, R. *Essstörungen*; Huber: Bern, Switzerland, 2004.
20. National Guideline Alliance UK. *Eating Disorders: Recognition and Treatment*; National Institute for Health and Care Excellence (NICE): London, UK, 2017.
21. Hebebrand, J.; Bulik, C.M. Critical appraisal of the provisional DSM-5 criteria for anorexia nervosa and an alternative proposal. *Int. J. Eating Disord.* **2011**, *44*, 665–678. [CrossRef] [PubMed]
22. Herzog, T.; Zeeck, A.; Hartmann, A.; Nickel, T. Lower targets for weekly weight gain lead to better results in inpatient treatment of anorexia nervosa: A pilot study. *Eur. Eating Disord. Rev.* **2004**, *12*, 164–168. [CrossRef]
23. Solanto, M.V.; Jacobson, M.S.; Heller, L.; Golden, N.H.; Hertz, S. Rate of weight gain of inpatients with anorexia nervosa under two behavioral contracts. *Pediatrics* **1994**, *93*, 989–991. [PubMed]
24. Garber, A.K.; Sawyer, S.M.; Golden, N.H.; Guarda, A.S.; Katzman, D.K.; Kohn, M.R.; Le Grange, D.; Madden, S.; Whitelaw, M.; Redgrave, G.W. A systematic review of approaches to refeeding in patients with anorexia nervosa. *Int. J. Eating Disord.* **2016**, *49*, 293–310. [CrossRef] [PubMed]
25. Williams, S.; Reid, M. Understanding the experience of ambivalence in anorexia nervosa: The maintainer's perspective. *Psychol. Health* **2010**, *25*, 551–567. [CrossRef] [PubMed]
26. Geller, J.; Brown, K.E.; Zaitsoff, S.L.; Goodrich, S.; Hastings, F. Collaborative versus directive interventions in the treatment of eating disorders: Implications for care providers. *Prof. Psychol. Res. Pract.* **2003**, *34*, 406–413. [CrossRef]
27. Anderson, L.K.; Reilly, E.E.; Berner, L.; Wierenga, C.E.; Jones, M.D.; Brown, T.A.; Kaye, W.H.; Cusack, A. Treating eating disorders at higher levels of care: Overview and challenges. *Curr. Psychiatry Rep.* **2017**, *19*, 48. [CrossRef] [PubMed]
28. Geller, J.; Dunn, E.C. Integrating motivational interviewing and cognitive behavioral therapy in the treatment of eating disorders: Tailoring interventions to patient readiness for change. *Cogn. Behav. Pract.* **2011**, *18*, 5–15. [CrossRef]
29. Bunyan, M.; Crowley, J.; Smedley, N.; Mutti, M.F.; Cashen, A.; Thompson, T.; Foster, J. Feasibility of training nurses in motivational interviewing to improve patient experience in mental health inpatient rehabilitation: A pilot study. *J. Psychiatr. Ment. Health Nursing* **2017**, *24*, 221–231. [CrossRef] [PubMed]
30. Mander, J.; Teufel, M.; Keifenheim, K.; Zipfel, S.; Giel, K.E. Stages of change, treatment outcome and therapeutic alliance in adult inpatients with chronic anorexia nervosa. *BMC Psychiatry* **2013**, *13*, 111. [CrossRef] [PubMed]
31. Federici, A.; Kaplan, A.S. The patient's account of relapse and recovery in anorexia nervosa: A qualitative study. *Eur. Eating Disord. Rev.* **2008**, *16*, 1–10. [CrossRef] [PubMed]

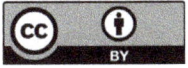

© 2018 by the authors. Licensee MDPI, Basel, Switzerland. This article is an open access article distributed under the terms and conditions of the Creative Commons Attribution (CC BY) license (http://creativecommons.org/licenses/by/4.0/).

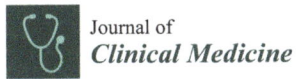

Review

Anorexia Nervosa and the Immune System—A Narrative Review

Dennis Gibson [1],* and Philip S Mehler [2]

[1] Assistant Medical Director, ACUTE Center for Eating Disorders @ Denver Health; Assistant Professor of Medicine, University of Colorado School of Medicine; 777 Bannock St., Denver, CO 80204, USA

[2] President, Eating Recovery Center; Founder and Executive Medical Director, ACUTE Center for Eating Disorders @ Denver Health; Glassman Professor of Medicine, University of Colorado School of Medicine; 7351 E Lowry Blvd, Suite 200, Denver, CO 80230, USA; Philip.mehler@dhha.org

* Correspondence: dennis.gibson@dhha.org; Tel.: +303-602-5067; Fax: +303-602-3811

Received: 13 September 2019; Accepted: 4 November 2019; Published: 8 November 2019

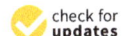

Abstract: The pathogenesis of an increasing number of chronic diseases is being attributed to effects of the immune system. However, its role in the development and maintenance of anorexia nervosa is seemingly under-appreciated. Yet, in examining the available research on the immune system and genetic studies in anorexia nervosa, one becomes increasingly suspicious of the immune system's potential role in the pathophysiology of anorexia nervosa. Specifically, research is suggestive of increased levels of various pro-inflammatory cytokines as well as the spontaneous production of tumor necrosis factor in anorexia nervosa; genetic studies further support a dysregulated immune system in this disorder. Potential contributors to this dysregulated immune system are discussed including increased oxidative stress, chronic physiological/psychological stress, changes in the intestinal microbiota, and an abnormal bone marrow microenvironment, all of which are present in anorexia nervosa.

Keywords: anorexia nervosa; eating disorders; immune system; inflammation; cytokines

---

1. Introduction

The importance of the immune system in the pathogenesis of a large number of diseases is being increasingly accepted. Although its contribution toward organic disease is easily appreciated, the realization that the immune system is also capable of contributing to the pathogenesis of mental health disorders has only recently become more recognized as the effects of inflammation on the central nervous system function have been discovered [1]. Furthermore, research has identified significant pleiotropy between the immune system and mental health disorders [2]. However, the impact of inflammation toward the development and maintenance of anorexia nervosa has not been elucidated at this time. Anorexia nervosa, a mental illness characterized by extreme weight loss due to restricted intake resulting from an extreme fear of weight gain, ultimately impacts every organ system and has a very high recidivism rate due to the lack of efficacious treatment options. If indeed anorexia nervosa is associated with a pro-inflammatory state, as this paper will attempt to argue, weight restoration, an essential component of treatment, then becomes that much more difficult due to the hunger suppressing and weight loss effects associated with the pro-inflammatory cytokines. This paper will attempt to argue for this pro-inflammatory state by summarizing the research findings of the immune system in anorexia nervosa and how they compare to the findings in primary malnutrition. However, much of the current research on this topic is of lower quality, and this paper is not meant to serve as a systematic review. With that said, a review of the majority of the publications on the immune system in anorexia nervosa has been attempted.

One first becomes intrigued by the possibility of a dysregulated immune system in anorexia nervosa when examining the frequency of infection in patients with anorexia nervosa. Although anorexia nervosa is a subtype of malnutrition, individuals with anorexia nervosa curiously may not suffer the same increased incidence of infection as found in other types of malnutrition [3]. A pro-inflammatory state is suggested when comparing the immunologic findings in anorexia nervosa, a state of starvation secondary to a primary mental health disease, to those present in primary malnutrition (that are related to inadequate energy intake and not secondary to another condition such as cancer, infection, malabsorption, etc.).

Genome wide association studies, which are non-biased studies examining the entire genome for genetic variations occurring more frequently in a certain population, provide additional evidence for a dysregulated immune system that is potentially involved in the pathogenesis of anorexia nervosa. One locus found to be significantly affiliated with anorexia nervosa is associated with multiple autoimmune disorders [4]. Research has indeed found an increased association between anorexia nervosa and various autoimmune diseases, with a bidirectional relationship [5–7]. In addition, individuals with auto-inflammatory disease (when the innate immune system attacks various host tissues) are at a higher risk for the development of an eating disorder [6]. Curiously, there is a case report of an individual with long-standing juvenile idiopathic arthritis and anorexia nervosa who exhibited improvement in body weight and appetite after treatment with infliximab (anti-TNF therapy) [8]. There is another case report of an individual with a 12-year history of anorexia nervosa pre-dating by many years a diagnosis of Crohn's disease, who experienced significant weight gain and no further relapse in psychopathology several months after beginning immunosuppressive therapy [9].

Another genetic finding approaching significance in anorexia nervosa involves a locus containing early B cell factor 1, which encodes a transcription factor important for immune system development, regulation of adipocyte/osteoblast differentiation and possible interaction with leptin signaling [10]. A region on chromosome 7, which includes various taste receptor genes, but also a gene important for cell–cell adhesion, apoptosis, and the immune response to pathogens, was also found to approach significance in the anorexia nervosa population [11].

After comparing the immunologic findings in primary malnutrition to those found in anorexia nervosa, suspicion arises as to why these differences exist. Potential contributors to these immunologic differences between primary malnutrition and anorexia nervosa will then briefly be discussed. First, a brief review of the immune system is warranted [12,13].

2. The Innate Immune System Overview

The innate immune system is largely composed of dendritic cells (DC), monocytes, macrophages, neutrophils, natural killer cells (NK), and the complement factors. These cells serve as the first line of nonspecific defense against potential pathogens, and are constantly surveilling the human body, recognizing highly conserved molecules on pathogens. Identification of these structural motifs by pathogen recognition receptors (i.e., Toll-like receptors) on immune system cells stimulates phagocytosis or activates other aspects of the immune system, with the ultimate goal being pathogen destruction. Complement is also capable of binding these non-host molecules, thereby marking the pathogen for destruction by phagocytes and initiating the inflammatory cascade. In addition, NK cells are capable of pathogen recognition via Toll-like receptors, and they destroy pathogens through apoptosis. However, these NK cells differ from other immune cells in that their cell killing must first be downregulated through binding to host antigens.

Macrophages and neutrophils are both capable of phagocytosis. Activation of these cells leads to upregulation of various transcription factors that, in turn, leads to the production of various pro-inflammatory genes. Cytokines, substances that induce an inflammatory response through communication with various immune cells, aid in the recruitment of other immune cells through chemotaxis, increase vascular permeability, and perform multiple other actions on the immune system are released from the activated immune cells and largely serve to alter cell behavior.

3. The Adaptive Immune System Overview

The adaptive immune system is composed of cell-mediated immunity, which involves the T cell response, and humoral immunity, which involves the B cell response. The adaptive immune system is more specific for pathogens, can take days to weeks to mount a response given use of immunologic memory, and comes into significant play when the innate immune system is incapable of controlling the reproduction of pathogens. The adaptive immune system becomes activated in lymph nodes when B cells, DCs, and macrophages present proteins derived from pathogens to cells of the adaptive immune system.

The cell-mediated immune response is highly dependent upon T cells. T lymphocytes are produced in the marrow and mature in the thymus gland. T cells can be divided into cytotoxic T cells (CD8) and helper T cells (CD4), which can be further divided into Th1 and Th2 type cells. Naïve T cells become activated when their receptors, which are highly specific for a particular protein, bind to antigen presenting cells such as DCs and macrophages. Activated cytotoxic T cells are then capable of pathogen killing by recognizing very specific proteins located on the pathogen. CD4 cells will differentiate into Th1 cells or Th2 cells depending upon the local cytokine milieu. Naïve T helper cells favor Th1 differentiation in the presence of interleukin (IL)-12 and interferon (IFN)-γ and Th2 differentiation in the presence of IL-4. The Th1 helper cells then produce increased amounts of IL-2 and IFN-γ, favoring cell-mediated immunity, while the Th2 helper cells produce increased amounts of the cytokines IL-4, IL-5, IL-10, and IL-13, favoring humoral immunity. In general, the Th1 response is more pro-inflammatory than the Th2 response. Naïve helper T cells can also differentiate into T regulatory cells, which serve to downregulate the immune response.

Cell-mediated immunity is largely tested through delayed cutaneous hypersensitivity (macrophage interaction with CD4 helper T cells causes the release of Th1 cytokines, which then recruit and activate cytotoxic T cells, and these cells attempt to destroy the antigen with a localized immune response that can be observed at the skin) and lymphocyte proliferation (a measure of clonal expansion of T cells after exposure to antigen).

The humoral immune response is dependent upon the production of antibodies by B cells. Naïve helper T cells differentiate into Th2 cells upon binding antigen presenting cells and in the presence of certain cytokines. These Th2 cells then bind B cells specific for certain antigens, thereby activating the B cells and increasing immunoglobulin production specific for that pathogen. Once the immunoglobulins are secreted, they are capable of binding directly to the pathogen or to complement, increasing phagocytosis and stimulating further inflammation.

4. The Immune System in Primary Malnutrition

The lymphatic tissues in animals and children suffering from primary malnutrition exhibit significant histologic changes. The thymus shows generalized atrophy and distorted architecture [14–16]. The peripheral lymph nodes and spleen also show generalized atrophy and distorted architecture [14–16], although to a lesser extent than that seen in the thymus [14,15]. The bone marrow frequently becomes hypo-cellular with decreased hematopoietic stem cells (HSC) (the precursor to the hematologic cells produced in the marrow) and increased adipocytes [17–19], contributing to lymphopenia, decreased myeloid cells (neutrophils and monocytes), and potentially other plasma hematologic changes (i.e., anemia) as found in murine models [17,20,21]. However, plasma leukocyte and lymphocyte levels in children with malnutrition are conflicting, likely related to recent or concomitant infection as well as the methodology employed [22,23]. Nonetheless, research suggests that leukopenia is present in human subjects when malnutrition is not associated with other processes such as infection [24,25].

Significant deficits in the functioning of the innate immune system are suggested in primary malnutrition. Neutrophil chemotaxis (cellular movement toward a stimulus) seems to be abnormal [15,23,26]. Neutrophil intracellular killing with various enzymatic activities is also likely to be impaired [15,23,27]. Results of phagocytosis are, however, contradictory [15,23] and may be related to whether activated neutrophils obtained from sites of inflammation versus neutrophils circulating in plasma are being studied [26,28]. Macrophage function including chemotaxis, phagocytosis, and intracellular killing all seem to be largely impaired in primary malnutrition [15,20,29]. Complement levels and function appear to be decreased [15,23,30,31], and DC function may be impaired [32]. In addition, NK cell cytotoxicity seems impaired in a minority of individuals with malnutrition, although collectively it is not statistically decreased [33,34]; it is likely that those select individuals with impairment are suffering from various micronutrient deficiencies [35–37].

Studies in primary malnutrition are also suggestive of abnormalities with cell-mediated immunity [38], resulting in a reduced cytotoxic T cell response [39] and reduced delayed cutaneous hypersensitivity [16]. The ratio of helper to cytotoxic T cells (CD4/CD8) seems abnormally low in this population [40,41]. CD4 counts seem to be more greatly decreased than CD8 counts in malnutrition when infection is not present [39,42]. Results examining lymphocyte proliferation depend on the antigen used, although this appears to be overall impaired in primary malnutrition [22,23].

Studies examining cytokine production in primary malnutrition can be contradictory based on the methodology used (in vitro or in vivo), but certain patterns are nonetheless suggested. Cytokine production in malnutrition favors the Th2 pathway with overall increased production of IL-4 and decreased production of IL-12 and IFN-gamma [23,43–46]. Stimulated and spontaneous production of IL-1 suggest either unchanged or decreased concentration [20,47–50]. Interpretation of IL-6 production in malnutrition is made difficult by the findings of decreased, unchanged, and elevated levels when compared to the controls; however, when controlling for infection, IL-6 seems to be overall decreased [20,45,47,48,51–53]. Studies also seem to suggest decreased stimulated production of tumor necrosis factor-alpha (TNF) when controlling for infection [20,49,51,53,54], without any suggestion of increased spontaneous release of TNF [49,55].

Abnormalities in humoral immunity are quite controversial in the setting of primary malnutrition due to limited research, but certain patterns are suggested. Diminished lymphopoiesis leads to decreased circulating B cells [15,23,56]. However, B cell function appears mostly intact when controlling for infection [15,22,23]. Studies are suggestive of decreased secretory IgA levels [15,23,57], which are important for mucosal immunity, but otherwise preserved immunoglobulin production and concentration (although it remains possible that these antibodies may have lower affinity to antigens) [58,59]. Research also suggests that abnormalities in the T cell-B cell interaction contribute to abnormalities with antibody production, although this appears to be secondary to helper T cell abnormalities with intact B cell function [41,60].

5. The Immune System in Anorexia Nervosa

The lymphoreticular system (spleen, lymph nodes, thymus, and bone marrow) is largely unstudied in anorexia nervosa except for findings regarding the bone marrow, wherein there is the frequently noted condition referred to as gelatinous marrow transformation (GMT) [61–63]. GMT is associated with an overall hypocellular marrow with decreased adiposity, and instead, the deposition of thick amorphous gelatinous substances in the extracellular spaces [62,64], contributing to the decreased red and white cell counts seen in these patients [61]. This differs from primary malnutrition, which is frequently associated with a hypocellular marrow, but increased marrow adiposity [17].

The innate immune system in anorexia nervosa has multiple abnormalities. A single study of ten individuals suffering from anorexia nervosa found deficits in neutrophil chemotaxis when compared to a control group of expanded size ($p < 0.05$, $n = 44$), with chemotaxis nearly absent in two patients with anorexia nervosa; neutrophil adherence was also decreased when compared to the controls ($p < 0.001$) [65]. Defects in granulocyte microbicidal activity were also suggested in one study, who found decreased alkaline phosphatase in five of six patients with anorexia nervosa [65]. Although limited in sample size ($n = 3$), another study found reduced ability of granulocytes to kill two bacterial species [66]. Similarly, neutrophil phagocytosis is poorly studied in anorexia nervosa, consisting of only a single small study ($n = 3$) that found intact opsonization with Staphylococcus aureus [66]; however, no studies have been completed on the phagocytic function of activated neutrophils obtained from sites of inflammation. Serum complement C3 levels were found to be decreased in anorexia nervosa compared to the controls ($p < 0.001$) in a small study ($n = 14$), but 50% hemolytic complement activity (CH50) was not statistically different [67]. Similarly, serum complement C3 ($p < 0.001$), along with C1q ($p < 0.05$) and C2 ($p < 0.001$), were all low in the anorexia nervosa group of another study ($n = 14$), but with normal serum levels of C4, C5, and C6 when compared to the controls [67]. Furthermore, C3 levels appear to correlate with nutritional status, improving with weight restoration [67,68]. NK cell quantity is reduced in anorexia nervosa when compared to the controls [69–71], but NK cell activity seems intact based on the few studies completed [72,73]. DC and macrophage function in anorexia nervosa are unstudied. These aforementioned findings of the innate immune system in patients with anorexia nervosa are thus similar to those noted in primary malnutrition.

Cell-mediated immunity in anorexia nervosa appears to be "dysregulated" when compared to the immunologic abnormalities observed in primary malnutrition. Nine patients with anorexia nervosa had insignificant skin reactions to various mitogens; however, four individuals were unresponsive (anergic) to the mitogen [74]. In addition, greater mitogen concentrations were required to elicit a similar reaction to the controls ($p < 0.005$), although still dependent on the mitogen used [74]. A study of 22 individuals with anorexia nervosa found anergy in six individuals, with five of these individuals weighing less than 60% of their ideal body weight [75]. Similarly, a study of 12 individuals with anorexia nervosa examining cell-mediated cytotoxicity found a significantly reduced response when compared to the controls ($p < 0.05$) [76]. T cell proliferation appears overall intact, if not increased, though still dependent upon the mitogen used [77–80]. Nagata et al. [77] and Silber et al. [78] reported similar responses to various mitogens when comparing individuals with anorexia nervosa to a control group. However, Golla et al. [79] and Bentdal et al. [80] both reported statistically significant increased T cell responsiveness, although dependent upon the mitogen used. Overall, these results suggest diminished delayed type hypersensitivity and cell-mediated cytotoxicity, similar to primary malnutrition. However, T cell proliferation seems intact, if not exaggerated, compared to the response observed in primary malnutrition.

T cell subtypes also appear to be "dysregulated" when comparing anorexia nervosa to primary malnutrition. The CD4/CD8 ratio in anorexia nervosa is seemingly increased, and this appears due to a greater reduction in CD8 counts compared to CD4 counts [70,77,81,82]. Elegido et al. [70] and Mustafa et al. [81] both attributed this abnormality in CD8 counts to a statistically significant decrease in memory CD8 cells as opposed to naïve CD8 cells ($p < 0.01$). Nagata et al. [77] also found greater elevation in the CD4/CD8 ratio with more significant weight loss ($p < 0.05$); indeed, these researchers suggest that with greater depletion in body weight, lymphocyte production is prioritized over other immune cells, especially naïve T helper cells, in the attempt to preserve the efficacy of the adaptive immune system [77]. Regulatory T cell function seems to be unaffected in anorexia nervosa based on a single study [83].

Fewer studies have been completed with regard to the humoral system in anorexia nervosa and are inconclusive. One study with 16 individuals suffering from anorexia nervosa found normal serum IgA, IgM, and IgG [84]. However, another small study ($n = 5$) found decreased IgG and IgM when comparing anorexia nervosa patients to healthy controls [67]. One study found only reduced IgG when comparing individuals with greater severity of anorexia nervosa (BMI less than 17.5) to the controls ($p < 0.05$) [69]. One study seems to suggest normal B cell counts [69], while another study found increased B cell counts in 46 anorexia nervosa patients when solely examining the restrictive subtype; indeed this population suffered greater weight loss than the individuals in the binge/purge subtype, and negative correlation between B cell counts and BMI was also found in this study [70]. T–B cell interaction has also been found to be abnormal in this population based on a single study [69].

Therefore, abnormalities in the innate immune system are largely similar between anorexia nervosa and primary malnutrition. Although a few differences seem to exist regarding cell-mediated immunity including potentially enhanced T cell proliferation in anorexia nervosa compared to primary malnutrition, and increased CD4/CD8 ratios in anorexia nervosa compared to primary malnutrition, the findings are largely similar between anorexia nervosa and primary malnutrition. Conclusions regarding the similarities and differences between the humoral immune system in anorexia nervosa and primary malnutrition are more difficult to determine with the current research.

These above aberrations in the immune system in anorexia nervosa and primary malnutrition are likely multifactorial, albeit expected, given the significant interaction between the state of nutrition and immune system function [85,86]. Leptin is an adipokine (secreted by adipocytes), similar in structure to multiple cytokines, that circulates at levels correlating with the density of adipose tissue and nutritional status. Adequate leptin levels are indeed needed for nearly all aspects of the immune system to function properly including cellular proliferation of the thymus and peripheral lymphoreticular system [14]; bone marrow cellular proliferation and hematopoiesis [87–89]; macrophage phagocytosis, chemotaxis, and microbicidal activity [86,90–92]; neutrophil chemotaxis and microbicidal activity [86,90]; complement function [93]; increasing CD4 T cell proliferation [94,95]; Th1 cytokine response (inadequate leptin favors Th2 response) [86,90,96,97]; cytotoxic T cell activity [90]; survival of B cells [56,86,90]; and NK cell proliferation [86]. The immune system changes in primary malnutrition can likely be explained by a leptin deficiency, which is low in primary malnutrition. Furthermore, serum leptin levels are known to be abnormally low in anorexia nervosa [98]. Moreover, with weight restoration in patients with anorexia nervosa, leptin levels rise back to a normal range. One must, therefore, question the etiology of the possibly increased CD4/CD8 ratios and intact lymphoproliferative response noted in anorexia nervosa when compared to primary malnutrition.

Furthermore, an examination of the cytokine profile in anorexia nervosa suggests a "dysregulated" immune system when compared to the cytokine profile present in primary malnutrition. Although the Th2 pathway seems to be favored in anorexia nervosa and primary malnutrition, with increased IL-4 as well as decreased IL-2 production [69,99,100], pro-inflammatory cytokines appear to be upregulated in anorexia nervosa. Studies examining IL-6 [82,100–103], IL-1 [100,101,104,105], and IFN-γ [101,102,106,107] have found decreased, unchanged, or increased levels, depending on the methodology employed. However, one meta-analysis was suggestive of overall increased IL-1 and IL-6 in anorexia nervosa when compared to healthy controls ($p = 0.003$ and $p = 0.009$, respectively) [106], while another meta-analysis reported increased IL-6 when compared to the controls ($p = 0.001$) [107], but elevated IL-1 only when comparing the restricting subtype of anorexia nervosa to the controls ($p = 0.018$); there was no statistical significance in this meta-analysis when comparing all subtypes of anorexia nervosa to healthy controls ($p = 0.110$).

Studies examining tumor necrosis factor (TNF) levels have also resulted in decreased, unchanged, or increased levels of this cytokine [55,69,76,100–104,108,109], but a majority of the studies suggest increased secretion of TNF by immune cells in anorexia nervosa [55,69,76,100,101,103,104,109]. Indeed, meta-analyses have found elevated levels of TNF in anorexia nervosa when compared to the controls ($p = 0.008$, $p = 0.015$) [106,107]. Furthermore, research is suggestive of increased spontaneous production of TNF from circulating monocytes and lymphocytes in individuals with anorexia nervosa when studied in vitro [55,69,76]. One study, directly comparing spontaneous TNF production in seven patients with anorexia nervosa and six patients with primary malnutrition (infection free), found significantly greater levels in anorexia nervosa when compared to primary malnutrition ($p < 0.0006$) [55]. In addition, the current research suggests that mRNA levels of TNF might remain elevated with refeeding and weight restoration, although other cytokines seem to normalize [104,106].

To summarize, there are similarities between anorexia nervosa and primary malnutrition, but there also exist the following immune system differences between anorexia nervosa and primary malnutrition: (1) anorexia nervosa is associated with the bone marrow changes of GMT and reduced marrow fat, which are not also seen in primary malnutrition; (2) T cell proliferation to various antigens appears decreased in primary malnutrition when compared to the response in anorexia nervosa; (3) CD8 cell counts seem to be more affected in anorexia nervosa without similar affects noted in primary malnutrition; (4) various pro-inflammatory cytokines (IL-1, IL-6, and TNF) seem to be elevated in anorexia nervosa when compared to levels in primary malnutrition (when adequately controlled for infection); and (5) there may be increased spontaneous production of TNF in anorexia nervosa that is not present in primary malnutrition (see Table 1).

Table 1. Immune system and cytokine concentration differences between anorexia nervosa and primary malnutrition.

	Bone Marrow	T Cell Proliferation	CD4/CD8 Ratio	IL-1	IL-6	TNF
Anorexia nervosa	Gelatinous Marrow Transformation (GMT) (low adiposity)	Unchanged to increased	High (greater effect on CD8 cells)	Normal to increased	Increased	High (including spontaneous production)
Primary malnutrition	Increased adiposity without GMT	Decreased	Low (greater effect on CD4 cells)	Low to normal	Decreased	Low (no spontaneous production)

Therefore, one is left to ponder the question as to the cause of these immunologic differences between anorexia nervosa and primary malnutrition if working under the assumption that the immune system changes are solely due to malnutrition. Furthermore, these changes may suggest a pro-inflammatory state in anorexia nervosa that does not appear to be present in primary malnutrition. The genetic studies discussed above suggest there may be some intrinsic abnormality within the immune system that contributes to this pro-inflammatory state; however, this remains speculative. Several potential contributors to this "dysregulated" immune system in anorexia nervosa are discussed below, although their contributions are highly speculative at this time. These include increased oxidative stress, a chronically activated sympathetic nervous system (SNS) and hypothalamic-pituitary-adrenal (HPA) axis, altered intestinal microbiota, and an abnormal bone marrow microenvironment.

6. Oxidative Stress

One potential contributor to an upregulated immune system in anorexia nervosa is increased free radical formation causing increased oxidative stress [110]. Briefly, free radicals are atoms with unpaired electrons, making them highly unstable and capable of causing damage to all tissues by disrupting cellular function. In the human body, reactive oxygen species (ROS) are constantly generated in mitochondria as electrons flow down the electron transport chain through the process of aerobic metabolism. Important sources of increased oxidation in anorexia nervosa include not only the aerobic metabolism of nutrients, but also the activation of the arachidonic acid cascade and activation of various enzymes used by phagocytes in pathogen killing [111]. Once generated, these ROS are capable of activating the inflammatory cascade and increasing production of pro-inflammatory cytokines [110]. This is largely accomplished through lipid peroxidation, which occurs when free radicals interact with cell membrane fatty acids, disrupting the lipid structure and thereby altering downstream intracellular signaling as well as propagating additional damage to proteins, DNA, and other cellular structures [112].

Individuals with anorexia nervosa have increased oxidative stress [113–116], partially attributed to decreased levels of anti-oxidants [113,117,118]. Studies in this population have also found abnormalities in the electron transport chain, likely further contributing to increased oxidative stress [119,120]. Changes in lipid peroxidation also contribute [121], as individuals with anorexia nervosa have various fatty acid deficiencies including the omega 3 fatty acids that have anti-inflammatory properties [122–124]. By increasing the ratio of omega 6 to omega 3 fatty acids within the cell membrane (the typical Western diet contains much greater amounts of omega 6 than omega 3 fatty acids), increased amounts of arachidonic acid are produced, thereby increasing the pro-inflammatory secondary signals [125].

Refeeding, critical to the sustained recovery of patients with anorexia nervosa, is another potential contributor to the upregulated immune system presumed in this condition. Although unstudied in eating disorders, oxidative stress is increased in animal models of starvation when undergoing refeeding and may potentially be related to increased adiposity (and associated adipokine secretion) with weight gain [126]. Increased central adiposity has indeed been found in anorexia nervosa with weight restoration [127], and this regional adiposity is very metabolically active [128]. Furthermore, "postprandial dysmetabolism", which is a function of increased oxidative stress following food consumption due to elevated plasma glucose and lipids, creates increased inflammation for several hours following oral consumption [129,130]. This dysmetabolism is believed to be secondary to the effects of glucagon [129]. Although postprandial dysmetabolism has not been directly studied in anorexia nervosa, individuals with anorexia nervosa behave similarly to diabetics before weight restoration in that they have higher plasma glucagon and greater plasma glucose levels during a glucose tolerance test [131], supporting a role for "postprandial dysmetabolism" in this population.

7. Chronic Stress

Stress, "a set of constructs representing stages in a process by which environmental demands that tax or exceed the adaptive capacity of an organism occasion psychological, behavioral, and biological responses that may place persons at risk for disease" [132], is another potential contributor to the upregulated immune system in anorexia nervosa. Both physiologic stressors and situations perceived as stressful are capable of activating the hypothalamic-pituitary-adrenal (HPA) system and sympathetic nervous system (SNS), ultimately resulting in increased cortisol and norepinephrine (NE)/epinephrine (EPI), respectively, and thereby affecting the immune system in anorexia nervosa. Cortisol affects the immune system through binding with glucocorticoid receptors, which downregulate gene transcription of inflammatory mediators. NE and EPI act through the mostly anti-inflammatory β2 receptors present on the innate and adaptive immune cells, although α1 receptors are also present and tend to upregulate the immune system. Under homeostatic conditions, the β2 receptor mediated signals predominate [133].

Research supports both pro- and anti-inflammatory effects with long-term stressors [134,135]. However, it is being increasingly suggested that the target tissue response is more important than circulating hormone levels [135]. Indeed, studies have found glucocorticoid receptor desensitization with long-term activation of the HPA system, mitigating the anti-inflammatory response to cortisol [134–136]. Although not as well studied and the implications of these findings are unclear, a similar mechanism is suggested for the long-term activation of the SNS. The β receptors become desensitized to NE and EPI, requiring higher levels of hormones to have the same effect [137,138]. Chronic binding of the hormone to the β receptors also causes them to become internalized [137], thereby increasing the concentration of the pro-inflammatory α1 receptors on the cell membrane. In addition, chronic activation of the β receptor alters intracellular signaling toward a pro-inflammatory state [137,139].

When examining target tissue response in those with anorexia nervosa, the findings are suggestive of increased activation of the stress response systems. Individuals with anorexia nervosa lose responsiveness to glucocorticoid stimulation [140–142], and decreased numbers of β adrenergic receptors have been found on immune cells [143], both of which would contribute to a pro-inflammatory state.

Furthermore, individuals with anorexia nervosa have high co-morbidity of obsessive compulsive disease, anxiety, depression, post-traumatic stress disorder, and other mental health disorders that are associated with a chronically upregulated HPA axis and SNS [144]. Depression has been found to be associated with abnormal β adrenergic responsiveness [145], anxiety is associated with downregulation of the β adrenergic receptors [146], and panic disorder is associated with decreased β adrenergic receptors on cell membranes as well as a reduced response to β agonists [147].

Although it would seem that chronic stress impacts immune function, the above discussion is overly simplified. Thus, the true effects of stress on immune function in anorexia nervosa and the comorbid illnesses are unknown. The other hormones/cytokines present in the local milieu of the immune cells, the timing of the stressor(s) on immune cell development, the type of immune cells studied, and whether the immune cells are obtained from lymph nodes or other sites all likely impact whether a pro- or anti-inflammatory effect is observed.

Stress has also been found to alter intestinal permeability through the actions of corticotropin releasing hormone and mast cell activation, causing increased gut permeability and translocation of commensal and pathogenic bacteria [148–150]. The implications of this are discussed below.

8. Intestinal Microbiota

The trillions of commensal bacteria normally inhabiting the human intestinal tract are very important for normal gut health and function and are referred to as the microbiota [151]. They play a role through the production of various metabolites such as the short chain fatty acid butyrate, which serve as nutrition for the epithelial cells of the gastrointestinal tract [152]. The commensal bacteria normally inhabiting the gastrointestinal tract are also very important for appropriate development of the immune system [153], and for maintenance of immune tolerance in this state of symbiosis [151]. However, non-commensal gut microbes have developed means to evade the mucosal barrier and interact with the intestinal epithelial cells [154]. These pathogenic bacteria are then capable of activating the immune system through multiple processes: direct activation of the immune system via the constant sampling of the luminal contents by the host's immune cells [153], activation of the various immune receptors located directly on the gut epithelial cells [153], loss of commensal bacterial metabolites that downregulate the immune response through cell signaling [155], and disruption of the intestinal barrier [156], leading to a proclivity toward sepsis and gastrointestinal infections. Increased production of pro-inflammatory cytokines by the epithelial and immune cells further disrupts the intestinal barrier [157], and a recurring pattern then develops [158].

The role of the microbiota is being increasingly studied in anorexia nervosa; however, it is beyond the scope of this article to adequately discuss the microbiota and how it relates to anorexia nervosa. For a good review on the topic of the microbiota and anorexia nervosa, see Roubalova et al. [159]. Briefly, microbiota changes do seem to occur in anorexia nervosa with weight loss and weight restoration [160–163] as well as decreases in short chain fatty acid production [161]. Weight loss alone is also capable of disrupting the intestinal epithelial barrier [158]. All of these changes would be expected to ultimately lead to upregulation of the immune system. However, one study examining intestinal permeability in anorexia nervosa actually found decreased intestinal permeability [164]. Ultimately, it is currently unknown how the microbiota changes impact the immune system in anorexia nervosa and is only speculative that these changes impact the functioning of the immune system.

9. Gelatinous Marrow Transformation and Mesenchymal Stem Cells

An appropriately functioning bone marrow is necessary not only for adequate hematopoiesis, but also for regulation of immune cell activity [165]. The mesenchymal stem cells (MSC), which are the precursors for the marrow stromal compartment, regulate growth and differentiation of hematopoietic stem cells, and have an immunomodulatory effect on the various immune cells [166,167]. Local cytokines [165,168,169], SNS input [170,171], and MSC interactions with other cells in the marrow [165,170] all impact factors produced by the MSCs. For example, IFN-γ appears to be the most important cytokine for "licensing" the largely immunosuppressive functions of the MSCs [166,167,172]. These MSCs are then capable of inhibiting nearly all cells of the immune system [173–179].

Although MSCs are largely immunosuppressive, they can also have immune stimulatory properties [166]. These cells are capable of phagocytosis and can have antigen presenting properties [180]. MSCs tend to lose their immunosuppressive properties with changes in the microenvironment including changes in MSC concentration [179,181], changes in various cytokine concentrations [180,182], and as a consequence of alterations in MSC interactions with other immune cells in the marrow [175].

The marrow microenvironment is also largely responsible for MSC differentiation into adipocytes and osteoblasts, amongst other cells [87,183]. MSC differentiation into osteoblasts is favored with exposure to various growth factors including leptin [87,184], while differentiation into adipocytes is favored with upregulation of the transcription factor peroxisome proliferator-activated receptor-γ (PPARγ) [183,184]. PPARγ appears to be upregulated in malnutrition and fasting, contributing to the increased marrow adiposity seen with malnutrition [17,185]. Similar to adipocytes throughout the rest of the body, these marrow adipocytes are capable of producing pro-inflammatory adipokines [186], which could alter the marrow microenvironment and immunomodulatory properties of the MSCs.

Although increased marrow adiposity can be seen in anorexia nervosa, frequently, the rule is that these patients develop GMT, associated with decreased adiposity. The pathogenesis of GMT is incompletely understood, but the microenvironment is highly altered, likely due to fat mobilization and secondary hyaluronic acid deposition [187]. Although in anorexia nervosa the development of this condition is dependent upon amount of weight loss [61], weight loss is not a pre-requisite as it has also been observed in individuals with other conditions without documented weight loss such as Hashimoto's thyroiditis, chronic heart failure, and acute severe infection [62]. Furthermore, GMT seems to be uncommon in individuals with kwashiorkor or marasmus [64], and seems to be very rare in children [159,187], even though there is a higher prevalence of primary malnutrition in this age group. Current evidence does seem to suggest that an upregulated immune response is a likely contributor toward the development of this condition [62,64,187]. Therefore, one is left to question how these bone marrow changes including a decreased amount of the bone marrow adipose tissue that is important for immune system regulation, impacts the immune system in anorexia nervosa, and, although speculative, whether this is a significant contributor to the immune system changes present in anorexia nervosa compared to primary malnutrition, given that GMT and low marrow adiposity is not noted in primary malnutrition.

10. Conclusions

The aforementioned increased secretion and concentration of the inflammatory cytokines as well as genetic studies strongly suggest a "dysregulated" immune system in anorexia nervosa. When comparing the immune system changes in protein malnutrition and anorexia nervosa, it is suggested that anorexia nervosa is associated with increased pro-inflammatory cytokines, an elevated CD4/CD8 ratio, and increased T cell proliferation. It is difficult to explain these immunologic changes as occurring solely secondary to malnutrition. Although the exact pathogenesis of these immunologic changes in anorexia nervosa is unclear, a potential primary immunologic defect contributing to the development of anorexia nervosa, which is possibly compounded by the conditions briefly discussed in this article, remains a strong possibility. However, this remains speculative at this time, and the contribution from oxidative stress, chronic psychological stress, an altered microbiota, and an abnormal bone marrow microenvironment, is currently unknown. Additional research must be completed to determine the etiology of the pro-inflammatory cytokine production as well as the effects of this pro-inflammatory state toward the development and maintenance of anorexia nervosa. Although heretofore anorexia nervosa was considered to have a bland state devoid of inflammation, as suggested by basic markers of inflammation such as sedimentation rates, it is becoming increasingly intriguing to consider that the immune system may actually be causal in the pathogenesis and maintenance of anorexia nervosa.

Author Contributions: G.D. drafted the manuscript, and critical revision of the manuscript was provided by M.P.S Both authors reviewed the final manuscript.

Conflicts of Interest: The authors declare no conflicts of interest.

References

1. Kerschensteiner, M.; Meinl, E.; Hohlfeld, R. Neuro-immune crosstalk in CNS diseases. *Neuroscience* **2009**, *158*, 1122–1132. [CrossRef] [PubMed]
2. Wang, Q.; Yang, C.; Gelernter, J.; Zhao, H. Pervasive pleiotropy between psychiatric disorders and immune disorders revealed by integrative analysis of multiple GWAS. *Hum. Genet.* **2015**, *134*, 1195–1209. [CrossRef] [PubMed]
3. Bowers, J.K.; Eckert, E. Leukopenia in anorexia nervosa: Lack of increased risk of infection. *Arch. Intern. Med.* **1978**, *138*, 1520–1523. [CrossRef] [PubMed]
4. Duncan, L.; Yilmaz, Z.; Gaspar, H.; Walters, R.; Goldstein, J.; Anttila, V.; Bulik-Sullivan, B.; Ripke, S.; Eating Disorders Working Group of the Psychiatric Genomics Consortium; Thornton, L.; et al. Significant locus and metabolic genetic correlations revealed in genome-wide association study of anorexia nervosa. *Am. J. Psychiatry* **2017**, *174*, 850–858. [CrossRef]
5. Wotton, C.J.; James, A.; Goldacre, M.J. Coexistence of eating disorders and autoimmune diseases: Record linkage cohort study, UK. *Int. J. Eat. Disord.* **2016**, *49*, 663–672. [CrossRef]
6. Zerwas, S.; Larsen, J.T.; Petersen, L.; Thornton, L.M.; Quaranta, M.; Koch, S.V.; Pisetsky, D.; Mortensen, P.B.; Bulik, C.M. Eating disorders, autoimmune, and autoinflammatory disease. *Pediatrics* **2017**, *140*, e20162089. [CrossRef]
7. Raevuori, A.; Haukka, J.; Vaarala, O.; Suvisaari, J.M.; Gissler, M.; Grainger, M.; Linna, M.S.; Suokas, J.T. The increased risk for autoimmune diseases in patients with eating disorders. *PLoS ONE* **2014**, *9*, e104845. [CrossRef]
8. Barber, J.; Sheeran, T.; Mulherin, D. Anti-tumor necrosis factor treatment in a patient with anorexia nervosa and juvenile idiopathic arthritis. *Ann. Rheum. Dis.* **2003**, *62*, 490–491. [CrossRef]
9. Solmi, M.; Santonastaso, P.; Caccaro, R.; Favaro, A. A case of anorexia nervosa with comorbid Crohn's disease: Beneficial effects of anti-TNF-alpha therapy? *Int. J. Eat. Disord.* **2013**, *46*, 639–641. [CrossRef]
10. Li, D.; Change, X.; Connolly, J.J.; Tian, L.; Liu, Y.; Bhoj, E.J.; Robinson, N.; Abrams, D.; Li, Y.R.; Bradfield, J.P.; et al. A genome-wide association study of anorexia nervosa suggests a risk locus implicated in dysregulated leptin signaling. *Sci. Rep.* **2017**, *7*, 3847. [CrossRef]
11. Wade, T.D.; Gordon, S.; Medland, S.; Bulik, C.; Heath, A.C.; Montgomery, G.W.; Martin, N.G. Genetic variants associated with disordered eating. *Int. J. Eat. Disord.* **2013**, *46*, 594–608. [CrossRef] [PubMed]
12. Turvey, S.E.; Broide, D.H. Innate immunity. *J. Allergy Clin. Immunol.* **2010**, *125*, S24–S32. [CrossRef] [PubMed]
13. Bonilla, F.A.; Oettgen, H.C. Adaptive immunity. *J. Allergy Clin. Immunol.* **2010**, *125*, S33–S40. [CrossRef] [PubMed]
14. Howard, J.K.; Lord, G.M.; Matarese, G.; Vendetti, S.; Ghatei, M.A.; Ritter, M.A.; Lechler, R.I.; Bloom, S.R. Leptin protects mice from starvation-induced lymphoid atrophy and increases thymic cellularity in ob/ob mice. *J. Clin. Investig.* **1999**, *104*, 1051–1059. [CrossRef] [PubMed]
15. Gross, R.L.; Newberne, P.M. Role of nutrition in immunologic function. *Physiol. Rev.* **1980**, *60*, 188–302. [CrossRef]
16. Smythe, P.M.; Brereton-Stiles, G.G.; Grace, H.J.; Mafoyane, A.; Schonland, M.; Coovadia, H.M.; Loening, W.E.K.; Parent, M.A.; Vos, G.H. Thymolymphatic deficiency and depression of cell-mediated immunity in protein-calorie malnutrition. *Lancet* **1971**, *298*, 939–944. [CrossRef]
17. Cunha, M.C.R.; Lima, F.D.S.; Vinolo, M.A.R.; Hastreiter, A.; Curi, R.; Borelli, P.; Fock, R.A. Protein malnutrition induces bone marrow mesenchymal stem cells commitment to adipogenic differentiation leading to hematopoietic failure. *PLoS ONE* **2013**, *8*, e58872. [CrossRef]
18. Naveiras, O.; Nardi, V.; Wenzel, P.L.; Hauschka, P.V.; Fahey, F.; Daley, G.Q. Bone-marrow adipocytes as negative regulators of the haematopoietic microenvironment. *Nature* **2009**, *460*, 259–263. [CrossRef]
19. Sandozai, M.K.; Rajeshvari, V.; Haquani, A.H.; Kaur, J. Kwashiorkor: A clinic-haematological study. *Br. Med. J.* **1963**, *2*, 93–96. [CrossRef]
20. Fock, R.A.; Vinolo, M.A.R.; Rocha, V.D.M.S.; Rocha, L.C.D.S.; Borelli, P. Protein-energy malnutrition decreases the expression of TLR-4/MD-2 and CD14 receptors in peritoneal macrophages and reduces the synthesis of TNF-alpha in response to lipopolysaccharide (LPS) in mice. *Cytokine* **2007**, *40*, 105–114. [CrossRef]

21. Vinolo, M.A.R.; Crisma, A.R.; Nakajima, K.; Rogero, M.M.; Fock, R.A.; Borelli, P. Malnourished mice display an impaired hematologic response to granulocyte colony-stimulating factor administration. *Nutr. Res.* **2008**, *28*, 791–797. [CrossRef] [PubMed]
22. Chandra, R.K.; Gupta, S.; Singh, B.Sc. Inducer and suppressor T cell subsets in protein-energy malnutrition: Analysis by monoclonal antibodies. *Nut. Res.* **1982**, *2*, 21–26. [CrossRef]
23. Rytter, M.J.H.; Kolte, L.; Briend, A.; Friis, H.; Christensen, V.B. The immune system in children with malnutrition—A systematic review. *PLoS ONE* **2014**, *9*, e105017. [CrossRef] [PubMed]
24. Borelli, P.; Mariano, M.; Borojevic, R. Protein malnutrition: Effect on myeloid cell production and mobilization into inflammatory reactions in mice. *Nutr. Res.* **1995**, *15*, 1477–1485. [CrossRef]
25. Catchatourian, R.; Eckerling, G.; Fried, W. Effect of short-term protein deprivation on hemopoietic functions of healthy volunteers. *Blood* **1980**, *55*, 625–628. [CrossRef] [PubMed]
26. Ikeda, S.; Saito, H.; Fukatsu, K.; Inoue, T.; Han, I.; Furukawa, S.; Matsuda, T.; Hidemura, A. Dietary restriction impairs neutrophil exudation by reducing CD11b/CD18 expression and chemokine production. *Arch. Surg.* **2001**, *136*, 297–304. [CrossRef]
27. Seth, V.; Chandra, R.K. Opsonic activity, phagocytosis, and bactericidal capacity of polymorphs in undernutrition. *Arch. Dis. Child.* **1972**, *47*, 282–284. [CrossRef]
28. Moore, S.I.; Huffnagle, G.B.; Chen, G.H.; White, E.S.; Mancuso, P. Leptin modulates neutrophil phagocytosis of Klebsiella pneumoniae. *Infect. Immun.* **2003**, *71*, 4182–4185. [CrossRef]
29. Santos, E.W.; de Oliveira, D.C.; Hastreiter, A.; Beltran, S.D.O.; Rogero, M.M.; Fock, F.A.; Borelli, P. High-fat diet or low-protein diet changes peritoneal macrophages function in mice. *Nutrire* **2016**, *41*, 6. [CrossRef]
30. Sakamoto, M.; Ishii, S.; Nishioka, K.; Shimada, K. Complement response after experimental bacterial infection in various nutritional states. *Immunology* **1979**, *38*, 421–427.
31. Sakamoto, M.; Fujisawa, Y.; Nishioka, K. Physiologic role of the complement system in host defense, disease, and malnutrition. *Nutrition* **1998**, *14*, 391–398. [CrossRef]
32. Niiya, T.; Akbar, F.; Yoshida, O.; Miyake, T.; Matsuura, B.; Murakami, H.; Abe, M.; Hiasa, Y.; Onji, M. Impaired dendritic cell function resulting from chronic undernutrition disrupts the antigen-specific immune response in mice. *J. Nutr.* **2007**, *137*, 671–675. [CrossRef] [PubMed]
33. Salimonu, L.S.; Ojo-Amaize, E.; Williams, A.I.O.; Johnson, A.O.K.; Cooke, A.R.; Adekunle, F.A.; Alm, G.V.; Wigzell, H. Depressed natural killer activity in children with protein-calorie malnutrition. *Clin. Immunol. Immunopathol.* **1982**, *24*, 1–7. [CrossRef]
34. Salimonu, L.S.; Ojo-Amaize, E.; Johnson, A.O.K.; Laditan, A.A.O.; Akinwolere, O.A.O.; Wigzell, H. Depressed natural killer cell activity in children with protein-calorie malnutrition: II. Correction of the impaired activity after nutritional recovery. *Cell. Immunol.* **1983**, *82*, 210–215. [CrossRef]
35. Bowman, T.A.; Goonewardene, I.M.; Pasatiempo, A.M.; Ross, A.C.; Taylor, C.E. Vitamin A deficiency decreases natural killer cell activity and interferon production in rats. *J. Nutr.* **1990**, *120*, 1264–1273. [CrossRef]
36. Kim, Y.I.; Hayek, M.; Mason, J.B.; Meydani, S.N. Severe folate deficiency impairs natural killer cell-mediated cytotoxicity in rats. *J. Nutr.* **2002**, *132*, 1361–1367. [CrossRef]
37. Dowd, P.S.; Kelleher, J.; Walker, B.E.; Guillou, P.J. Nutrition and cellular immunity in hospital patients. *Br. J. Nutr.* **1986**, *55*, 515–527. [CrossRef]
38. Edelman, R.; Suskind, R.; Olson, R.E.; Sirisinha, S. Mechanisms of defective delayed cutaneous hypersensitivity in children with protein-calorie malnutrition. *Lancet* **1973**, *301*, 506–509. [CrossRef]
39. Najera, O.; Gonzalez, C.; Cortes, E.; Toledo, G.; Ortiz, R. Effector T lymphocytes in well-nourished and malnourished infected children. *Clin. Exp. Immunol.* **2007**, *148*, 501–506. [CrossRef]
40. Najera, O.; Gonzalez, C.; Toledo, G.; Lopez, L.; Ortiz, R. Flow cytometry study of lymphocyte subsets in malnourished and well-nourished children with bacterial infections. *Clin. Diagn. Lab. Immunol.* **2004**, *11*, 577–580. [CrossRef]
41. Chandra, R.K. Numerical and functional deficiency in T helper cells in protein energy malnutrition. *Clin. Exp. Immunol.* **1983**, *51*, 126–132. [PubMed]
42. Iyer, S.S.; Chatraw, J.H.; Tan, W.G.; Wherry, E.J.; Becker, T.C.; Ahmed, R.; Kapasi, Z.F. Protein energy malnutrition impairs homeostatic proliferation of memory CD8 T cells. *J. Immunol.* **2012**, *188*, 77–84. [CrossRef] [PubMed]

43. Rodriguez, L.; Gonzalez, C.; Flores, L.; Jimenez-Zamudio, L.; Graniel, J.; Ortiz, R. Assessment by flow cytometry of cytokine production in malnourished children. *Clin. Diagn. Lab. Immunol.* **2005**, *12*, 502–507. [CrossRef] [PubMed]
44. Gonzalez-Torres, C.; Gonzalez-Martinez, H.; Miliar, A.; Najera, O.; Graniel, J.; Firo, V.; Alvarex, C.; Bonilla, E.; Rodriguez, L. Effect of malnutrition on the expression of cytokines involved in Th1 cell differentiation. *Nutrients* **2013**, *5*, 579–593. [CrossRef] [PubMed]
45. Gonzalez-Martinez, H.; Rodriguez, L.; Najera, O.; Cruz, D.; Miliar, A.; Dominguez, A.; Sanchez, F.; Graniel, J.; Gonzelez-Torres, M.C. Expression of cytokine mRNA in lymphocytes of malnourished children. *J. Clin. Immunol.* **2008**, *28*, 593–599. [CrossRef]
46. Bhaskaram, P.; Hemalatha, R.; Narayana Goud, B. Expression of messenger ribonucleic acid and production of cytokines in children with malnutrition. *Nutr. Res.* **2003**, *23*, 367–376. [CrossRef]
47. Sauerwein, R.W.; Mulder, J.A.; Mulder, L.; Lowe, B.; Peshu, N.; Demacker, P.N.M.; van der Meer, J.W.M.; Marsh, K. Inflammatory mediators in children with protein energy malnutrition. *Am. J. Clin. Nutr.* **1997**, *65*, 1534–1539. [CrossRef]
48. De Oliveira, D.C.; Hastreiter, A.A.; Mello, A.S.; Beltran, J.S.D.O.; Santos, E.W.C.O.; Borelli, P. The effects of protein malnutrition on the TNF-RI and NF-kB expression via the TNF-alpha signaling pathway. *Cytokine* **2014**, *6*, 218–225. [CrossRef]
49. Munoz, C.; Arevalo, M.; Lopez, M.; Schlesinger, L. Impaired interleukin-1 and tumor necrosis factor production in protein-calorie malnutrition. *Nutr. Res.* **1994**, *14*, 347–352. [CrossRef]
50. Bhaskaram, P.; Sivakumar, B. Interleukin-1 in malnutrition. *Arch. Dis. Child.* **1986**, *61*, 182–185. [CrossRef]
51. Anstead, G.M.; Chandrasekar, B.; Zhang, Q.; Melby, P.C. Multinutrient undernutrition dysregulates the resident macrophage proinflammatory cytokine network, nuclear factor-kB activation, and nitric oxide production. *J. Leukoc. Biol.* **2003**, *74*, 982–991. [CrossRef] [PubMed]
52. Dulger, H.; Arik, M.; Sekeroglu, M.R.; Tarakcioglu, M.; Noyan, T.; Cesur, Y.; Balahoroglu, B. Pro-inflammatory cytokines in Turkish children with protein-energy malnutrition. *Mediat. Inflamm.* **2002**, *11*, 363–365. [CrossRef] [PubMed]
53. McCarter, M.D.; Naama, H.A.; Shou, J.; Kwi, L.X.; Evoy, D.A.; Calvano, S.E.; Daly, J.M. Altered macrophage intracellular signaling induced by protein-calorie malnutrition. *Cell. Immunol.* **1998**, *183*, 131–136. [CrossRef] [PubMed]
54. Fock, R.A.; Rogero, M.M.; Vinolo, M.A.R.; Curi, R.; Borges, M.C.; Borelli, P. Effects of protein-energy malnutrition on NF-KappaB signaling in murine peritoneal macrophages. *Inflammation* **2010**, *33*, 101–109. [CrossRef]
55. Vaisman, N.; Hahn, T. Tumor necrosis factor-alpha and anorexia—Cause or effect. *Metabolism* **1991**, *40*, 720–723. [CrossRef]
56. Tanaka, M.; Suganami, T.; Kim-Saijo, M.; Toda, C.; Tsuiji, M.; Ochi, K.; Kamei, Y.; Minokoshi, Y.; Ogawa, Y. Role of central leptin signaling in the starvation-induced alteration of B-cell development. *J. Neurosci.* **2011**, *31*, 8370–8380. [CrossRef]
57. Douglas, S.D. Analytical review: Host defense mechanisms in protein-energy malnutrition. *Clin. Immunol. Immunopathol.* **1976**, *5*, 1–5. [CrossRef]
58. Passwell, J.H.; Steward, M.W.; Soothill, J.F. The effects of protein malnutrition on macrophage function and the amount and affinity of antibody response. *Clin. Exp. Immunol.* **1974**, *17*, 491–495.
59. Chandra, R.K. Protein-energy malnutrition and immunological responses. *J. Nutr.* **1992**, *122*, 597–600. [CrossRef]
60. Mathur, M.; Ramalingaswami, V.; Deo, M.G. Influence of protein deficiency on 19S antibody-forming cells in rats and mice. *J. Nutr.* **1972**, *102*, 841–846. [CrossRef]
61. Abella, E.; Feliu, E.; Granada, I.; Milla, F.; Oriol, A.; Ribera, J.M.; Sancehz-Planell, L.; Berga, L.; Reverter, J.C.; Rozman, C. Bone marrow changes in anorexia nervosa are correlated with the amount of weight loss and not with other clinical findings. *Am. J. Clin. Pathol.* **2002**, *118*, 582–588. [CrossRef] [PubMed]
62. Bohm, J. Gelatinous transformation of the bone marrow: The spectrum of underlying diseases. *Am. J. Surg. Pathol.* **2000**, *24*, 56–65. [CrossRef] [PubMed]
63. Mehler, P.S.; Howe, S.E. Serous fat atrophy with leukopenia in severe anorexia nervosa. *Am. J. Hematol.* **1995**, *49*, 171–172. [CrossRef] [PubMed]

64. Barbin, F.F.; Oliveira, C.C. Gelatinous transformation of bone marrow. *Autops. Case Rep.* **2017**, *7*, 5–8. [CrossRef]
65. Palmblad, J.; Fohlin, L.; Lundstrom, M. Anorexia nervosa and polymorphonuclear granulocyte reactions. *Scand. J. Haematol.* **1977**, *19*, 334–342. [CrossRef]
66. Gotch, F.M.; Spry, C.J.F.; Mowat, A.G.; Beeson, P.B.; Maclennan, I.C.M. Reversible granulocyte killing defect in anorexia nervosa. *Clin. Exp. Immunol.* **1975**, *21*, 244–249.
67. Wyatt, R.J.; Farrell, M.; Berry, P.; Forristal, J.; Maloney, M.J.; West, C.D. Reduced alternative complement pathway control protein levels in anorexia nervosa: Response to parenteral alimentation. *Am. J. Clin. Nutr.* **1982**, *35*, 973–980. [CrossRef]
68. Flierl, M.A.; Gaudiani, J.L.; Sabel, A.L.; Long, C.S.; Stahel, P.F.; Mehler, P.S. Complement C3 serum levels in anorexia nervosa: A potential biomarker for the severity of disease? *Ann. Gen. Psychiatry* **2011**, *10*, 16. [CrossRef]
69. Allende, L.M.; Corell, A.; Manzanares, J.; Madruga, D.; Marcos, A.; Madrono, A.; Lopez-Goyanes, A.; Garcia-Perez, A.; Moreno, J.M.; Rodrigo, M.; et al. Immunodeficiency associated with anorexia nervosa is secondary and improves after refeeding. *Immunology* **1998**, *94*, 543–551. [CrossRef]
70. Elegido, A.; Graell, M.; Andres, P.; Gheorghe, A.; Marcos, A.; Nova, E. Increased naïve CD4+ and B lymphocyte subsets are associated with body mass loss and drive relative lymphocytosis in anorexia nervosa patients. *Nutr. Res.* **2017**, *39*, 43–50. [CrossRef]
71. Omodei, D.; Pucino, V.; Labruna, G.; Procaccini, C.; Galgani, M.; Perna, F.; Pirozzi, D.; de Caprio, C.; Marone, G.; Fontana, L.; et al. Immune-metabolic profiling of anorexic patients reveals an anti-oxidant and anti-inflammatory phenotype. *Metabolism* **2015**, *64*, 396–405. [CrossRef] [PubMed]
72. Dowd, P.S.; Kelleher, J.; Walker, B.E.; Guillou, P.J. Nutritional and immunological assessment of patients with anorexia nervosa. *Proc. Nutr. Soc.* **1983**, *2*, 79–83. [CrossRef]
73. Staurenghi, A.H.; Masera, R.G.; Prolo, P.; Griot, G.; Sartori, M.L.; Ravizza, L.; Angeli, A. Hypothalamic-pituitary-adrenal axis function, psychopathological traits, and natural killer (NK) cell activity in anorexia nervosa. *Psychoneuroendocrinology* **1997**, *22*, 575–590. [CrossRef]
74. Cason, J.; Ainley, C.C.; Wolstencroft, R.A.; Norton, K.R.W.; Thompson, R.P.H. Cell-mediated immunity in anorexia nervosa. *Clin. Exp. Immunol.* **1986**, *64*, 370–375. [CrossRef]
75. Pertschuk, M.; Crosby, L.; Barot, L.; Mullen, J.L. Immunocompetency in anorexia nervosa. *Am. J. Clin. Nutr.* **1982**, *35*, 968–972. [CrossRef]
76. Schattner, A.; Steinbock, M.; Tepper, R.; Schonfeld, A.; Vaisman, N.; Hahn, T. Tumour necrosis factor production and cell-mediated immunity in anorexia nervosa. *Clin. Exp. Immunol.* **1999**, *79*, 62–66. [CrossRef]
77. Nagata, T.; Kiriike, N.; Tobitani, W.; Kawarada, Y.; Matsunaga, H.; Yamagami, S. Lymphocyte subset, lymphocyte proliferative response, and soluble interleukin-2 receptor in anorexic patients. *Biol. Psychiatry* **1999**, *45*, 471–474. [CrossRef]
78. Silber, T.J.; Chan, M. Immunologic cytofluorometric studies in adolescents with anorexia nervosa. *Int. J. Eat. Disord.* **1996**, *19*, 415–418. [CrossRef]
79. Golla, J.A.; Larson, L.A.; Anderson, C.F.; Lucas, A.R.; Wilson, W.R.; Tomasi, T.B. An immunological assessment of patients with anorexia nervosa. *Am. J. Clin. Nutr.* **1981**, *34*, 2756–2762. [CrossRef]
80. Bentdal, O.H.; Froland, S.S.; Larsen, S. Cell-mediated immunity in anorexia nervosa augmented lymphocyte transformation response to concanavalin A and lack of increased risk of infection. *Clin. Nutr.* **1989**, *8*, 253–258. [CrossRef]
81. Mustafa, A.; Ward, A.; Treasure, J.; Peakman, M. T lymphocyte subpopulations in anorexia nervosa and refeeding. *Clin. Immunol. Immunopathol.* **1997**, *82*, 282–289. [CrossRef] [PubMed]
82. Fink, S.; Eckert, E.; Mitchell, J.; Crosby, R.; Pomeroy, C. T-lymphocyte subsets in patients with abnormal body weight: Longitudinal studies in anorexia nervosa and obesity. *Int. J. Eat. Disord.* **1996**, *20*, 295–305. [CrossRef]
83. Paszthy, B.; Svec, P.; Vasarhelyi, B.; Tury, F.; Mazzag, J.; Tulassay, T.; Treszl, A. Investigation of regulatory T cells in anorexia nervosa. *Eur. J. Clin. Nutr.* **2007**, *61*, 1245–1249. [CrossRef] [PubMed]
84. Marcos, A.; Varela, P.; Santacruz, I.; Munoz-Velez, A.; Morande, G. Nutritional status and immunocompetence in eating disorders. A comparative study. *Eur. J. Clin. Nutr.* **1993**, *47*, 787–793. [PubMed]
85. Ponton, F.; Wilson, K.; Cotter, S.C.; Raubenheimer, D.; Simpson, S.J. Nutritional immunology: A multi-dimensional approach. *PLoS Pathog.* **2011**, *7*, e1002223. [CrossRef] [PubMed]

86. Perez-Perez, A.; Vilarino-Garcia, T.; Fernandez-Riejos, P.; Martin-Gonzalez, J.; Segura-Egea, J.J.; Sanchez-Margalet, V. Role of leptin as a link between metabolism and the immune system. *Cytokine Growth Factor Rev.* **2017**, *35*, 71–84. [CrossRef] [PubMed]
87. Noh, M. Interleukin-17A increases leptin production in human bone marrow mesenchymal stem cells. *Biochem. Pharmacol.* **2012**, *83*, 661–670. [CrossRef]
88. Devlin, M.J.; Brooks, D.J.; Conlon, C.; Vliet, M.V.; Louis, L.; Rosen, C.J.; Bouxsein, M.L. Daily leptin blunts marrow fat but does not impact bone mass in calorie restricted mice. *J. Endocrinol.* **2016**, *229*, 295–306. [CrossRef]
89. Bennett, B.D.; Solar, G.P.; Yuan, J.Q.; Mathias, J.; Thomas, G.R.; Matthews, W. A role for leptin and its cognate receptor in hematopoiesis. *Curr. Biol.* **1996**, *6*, 1170–1180. [CrossRef]
90. Procaccini, C.; La Rocca, C.; Carbone, F.; de Rosa, V.; Galgani, M.; Matarese, G. Leptin as immune mediator: Interaction between neuroendocrine and immune system. *Dev. Comp. Immunol.* **2017**, *66*, 120–129. [CrossRef]
91. Dayakar, A.; Chandrasekaran, S.; Veronica, J.; Maurya, R. Leptin induces the phagocytosis and protective immune response in Leishmania donovani infected THP-cell line and human PBMCs. *Exp. Parasitol.* **2016**, *160*, 54–59. [CrossRef] [PubMed]
92. Mancuso, P.; Myers Jr, M.G.; Goel, D.; Serezani, C.H.; O'Brien, E.; Goldberg, J.; Aronoff, D.M.; Peters-Golden, M. Ablation of leptin receptor-mediated ERK activation impairs host defense against gram-negative pneumonia. *J. Immunol.* **2012**, *189*, 867–875. [CrossRef] [PubMed]
93. Chang, M.L.; Kuo, C.J.; Huang, H.C.; Chu, Y.Y.; Chiu, C.T. Association between leptin and complement in hepatitis C patients with viral clearance: Homeostasis of metabolism and immunity. *PLoS ONE* **2016**, *11*, e0166712. [CrossRef] [PubMed]
94. Matarese, G.; La Rocca, C.; Moon, H.S.; Huh, J.Y.; Brinkoetter, M.T.; Chou, S.; Perna, F.; Greco, D.; Kilim, H.P.; Gao, C.; et al. Selective capacity of metreleptin administration to reconstitute CD4+ T-cell number in females with acquired hypoleptinemia. *Proc. Natl. Acad. Sci. USA* **2013**, *110*, E818–E827. [CrossRef]
95. Saucillo, D.C.; Gerriets, V.A.; Sheng, J.; Rathmell, J.C.; MacIver, N.J. Leptin metabolically licenses T cells for activation to link nutrition and immunity. *J. Immunol.* **2014**, *192*, 136–144. [CrossRef]
96. Naylor, C.; Petri, W.A., Jr. Leptin regulation of immune responses. *Trends Mol. Med.* **2016**, *22*, 88–98. [CrossRef]
97. Rodriguez, L.; Graniel, J.; Ortiz, R. Effect of leptin on activation and cytokine synthesis in peripheral blood lymphocytes of malnourished infected children. *Clin. Exp. Immunol.* **2007**, *148*, 478–485. [CrossRef]
98. Mehler, P.S.; Eckel, R.H.; Donahoo, W.T. Leptin levels in restricting and purging anorectics. *Int. J. Eat. Disord.* **1999**, *26*, 189–194. [CrossRef]
99. Komorowska-Pietrzykowska, R.; Rajewski, A.; Sobieska, M.; Wiktorowicz, K.P. Serum concentrations of interleukin 4 and interleukin 10 in patients suffering from anorexia nervosa. *Eur. Neuropsychopharmacol.* **2006**, *16*, S534. [CrossRef]
100. Corcos, M.; Guilbaud, O.; Chaouat, G.; Cayol, V.; Speranza, M.; Chambry, J.; Paterniti, S.; Moussa, M.; Flament, M.; Jeammet, P. Cytokines and anorexia nervosa. *Psychosom. Med.* **2001**, *63*, 502–504. [CrossRef]
101. Nova, E.; Gomez-Martinez, S.; Morande, G.; Marcos, A. Cytokine production by blood mononuclear cells from in-patients with anorexia nervosa. *Br. J. Nutr.* **2002**, *88*, 183–188. [CrossRef] [PubMed]
102. Pisetsky, D.S.; Trace, S.E.; Brownley, K.A.; Hamer, R.M.; Zucker, N.L.; Roux-Lombard, P.; Dayer, J.M.; Bulik, C.M. The expression of cytokines and chemokines in the blood of patients with severe weight loss from anorexia nervosa: An exploratory study. *Cytokine* **2014**, *69*, 110–115. [CrossRef] [PubMed]
103. Brambilla, F.; Bellodi, L.; Brunetta, M.; Perna, G. Plasma concentrations of interleukin-1b, interleukin-6 and tumor necrosis factor-alpha in anorexia nervosa and bulimia nervosa. *Psychoneuroendocrinology* **1998**, *23*, 439–447. [CrossRef]
104. Kahl, K.G.; Kruse, N.; Rieckmann, P.; Schmidt, M.H. Cytokine mRNA expression patterns in the disease course of female adolescents with anorexia nervosa. *Psychoneuroendocrinology* **2004**, *29*, 13–20. [CrossRef]
105. Raymond, N.C.; Dysken, M.; Bettin, K.; Eckert, E.D.; Crow, S.J.; Markus, K.; Pomeroy, C. Cytokine production in patients with anorexia nervosa, bulimia nervosa, and obesity. *Int. J. Eat. Disord.* **2000**, *28*, 293–302. [CrossRef]
106. Solmi, M.; Veronese, N.; Favaro, A.; Santonastaso, P.; Manzato, E.; Sergi, G.; Correll, C.U. Inflammatory cytokines and anorexia nervosa: A meta-analysis of cross-sectional and longitudinal studies. *Psychoneuroendocrinology* **2015**, *51*, 237–252. [CrossRef]

107. Dalton, B.; Bartholdy, S.; Robinson, L.; Solmi, M.; Ibrahim, M.A.A.; Breen, G.; Schmidt, U.; Himmerich, H. A meta-analysis of cytokine concentrations in eating disorders. *J. Psychiatry Res.* **2018**, *103*, 252–264. [CrossRef]
108. Nakai, Y.; Hamagaki, S.; Takagi, R.; Taniguchi, A.; Kurimoto, F. Plasma concentrations of tumor necrosis factor-alpha (TNF-alpha) and soluble TNF receptors in patients with anorexia nervosa. *J. Clin. Endocrinol. Metab.* **1999**, *84*, 1226–1228. [CrossRef]
109. Vaisman, N.; Schattner, A.; Hahn, T. Tumor necrosis factor production during starvation. *Am. J. Med.* **1989**, *87*, 115. [CrossRef]
110. Chapple, I.L.C. Reactive oxygen species and antioxidants in inflammatory diseases. *J. Clin. Periodontol.* **1997**, *24*, 287–296. [CrossRef]
111. Rosen, G.M.; Pou, S.; Ramos, C.L.; Cohen, M.S.; Britigan, B.E. Free radicals and phagocytic cells. *FASEB J.* **1995**, *9*, 200–209. [CrossRef] [PubMed]
112. Higdon, A.; Diers, A.R.; Oh, J.Y.; Landar, A.; Darley-Usmar, V.M. Cell signaling by reactive lipid species: New concepts and molecular mechanisms. *Biochem. J.* **2012**, *442*, 453–464. [CrossRef] [PubMed]
113. Solmi, M.; Veronese, N.; Manzato, E.; Sergi, G.; Favaro, A.; Santonastaso, P.; Correll, C.U. Oxidative stress and antioxidant levels in patients with anorexia nervosa: A systematic review and exploratory meta-analysis. *Int. J. Eat. Disord.* **2015**, *48*, 826–841. [CrossRef] [PubMed]
114. Vignini, A.; Canibus, P.; Nanetti, L.; Montecchiani, G.; Faloia, E.; Cester, A.M.; Boscaro, M.; Mazzanti, L. Lipoproteins obtained from anorexia nervosa patients induce higher oxidative stress in U373MG astrocytes through nitric oxide production. *Neuromol. Med.* **2008**, *10*, 17–23. [CrossRef]
115. Vannacci, A.; Ravaldi, C.; Giannini, L.; Rotella, C.M.; Masini, E.; Faravelli, C.; Ricca, V. Increased nitric oxide production in eating disorders. *Neurosci. Lett.* **2006**, *399*, 230–233. [CrossRef]
116. Vignini, A.; D'Angelo, M.; Nanetti, L.; Camilloni, M.A.; Cester, A.M.; Faloia, E.; Salvolini, E.; Mazzanti, L. Anorexia nervosa: A role for L-arginine supplementation in cardiovascular risk factors? *Int. J. Eat. Disord.* **2010**, *43*, 464–471. [CrossRef]
117. Paszynska, E.; Tyszkiewicz-Nwafor, M.; Slopien, A.; Dmitrzak-Weglarz, M.; Dutkiewicz, A.; Grzelak, T. Study of salivary and serum vaspin and total antioxidants in anorexia nervosa. *Clin. Oral Investig.* **2018**, *22*, 2837–2845. [CrossRef]
118. Moyano, D.; Sierra, C.; Brandi, N.; Artuch, R.; Mira, A.; Garcia-Tornel, S.; Vilaseca, M.A. Antioxidant status in anorexia nervosa. *Int. J. Eat. Disord.* **1999**, *25*, 99–103. [CrossRef]
119. Bohm, M.; Papezova, H.; Hansikova, H.; Wenchich, L.; Zeman, J. Activities of respiratory chain complexes in isolated platelets in females with anorexia nervosa. *Int. J. Eat. Disord.* **2007**, *40*, 659–663. [CrossRef]
120. Victor, V.M.; Rovira-Llopis, S.; Saiz-Alarcon, V.; Sanguesa, MC.; Rojo-Bofill, L.; Banuls, C.; Falcon, R.; Castello, R.; Rojo, L.; Rocha, M.; et al. Altered mitochondrial function and oxidative stress in leukocytes of anorexia nervosa patients. *PLoS ONE* **2014**, *9*, e106463. [CrossRef]
121. Tajiri, K.; Shimizu, Y.; Tsuneyama, K.; Sugiyama, T. A case report of oxidative stress in a patient with anorexia nervosa. *Int. J. Eat. Disord.* **2006**, *39*, 616–618. [CrossRef] [PubMed]
122. Caspar-Bauguil, S.C.; Montastier, E.; Galinon, F.; Frisch-Benarous, D.; Salvayre, R.; Ritz, P. Anorexia nervosa patients display a deficit in membrane long chain poly-unsaturated fatty acids. *Clin. Nutr.* **2012**, *31*, 386–390. [CrossRef] [PubMed]
123. Holman, R.T.; Adams, C.E.; Nelson, R.A.; Grater, S.J.E.; Jaskiewicz, J.A.; Johnson, S.B.; Erdman, J.W. Patients with anorexia nervosa demonstrate deficiencies of selected essential fatty acids, compensatory changes in nonessential fatty acids and decreased fluidity of plasma lipids. *J. Nutr.* **1995**, *125*, 901–907. [PubMed]
124. Langan, S.M.; Farrell, P.M. Vitamin E, vitamin A and essential fatty acid status of patients hospitalized for anorexia nervosa. *Am. J. Clin. Nutr.* **1985**, *41*, 1054–1060. [CrossRef]
125. Davis, T.A.; Gao, L.; Yin, H.; Morrow, J.; Porter, N.A. In vivo and in vitro lipid peroxidation of arachidonate esters: The effect of fish oil omega-3 lipids on product distribution. *J. Am. Chem. Soc.* **2006**, *128*, 14897–14904. [CrossRef]
126. Omidi, A.; Namazi, F.; Jabire, S.; Afsar, M.; Honarmand, M.; Nazifi, S. The effects of starvation and refeeding on oxidative stress parameters (MDA, SOD, GPx), lipid profile, thyroid hormones and thyroid histopathology in male Wistar rats. *Int. Arch. Med.* **2016**, *9*. [CrossRef]
127. Mayer, L.; Walsh, B.T.; Pierson, R.N., Jr.; Heymsfield, S.B.; Gallagher, D.; Wang, J.; Parides, M.K.; Leibel, R.L.; Warren, M.P.; Killory, E.; et al. Body fat redistribution after weight gain in women with anorexia nervosa. *Am. J. Clin. Nutr.* **2005**, *81*, 1286–1291. [CrossRef]

128. Anoop, M.; Vikram, N.K. Clinical and pathophysiological consequences of abdominal adiposity and abdominal adipose tissue depots. *Nutrition* **2003**, *19*, 457–466.
129. Pappas, C.; Kandaraki, E.A.; Tsirona, S.; Kountouras, D.; Kassi, G.; Diamanti-Kandarakis, E. Postprandial dysmetabolism: Too early or too late? *Hormones* **2016**, *15*, 321–344. [CrossRef]
130. Sies, H.; Stahl, W.; Sevanian, A. Nutritional, dietary and postprandial oxidative stress. *J. Nutr.* **2005**, *1135*, 969–972. [CrossRef]
131. Kumai, M.; Tamai, H.; Fujii, S.; Nakagawa, J.; Aoki, T.T. Glucagon secretion in anorexia nervosa. *Am. J. Clin. Nutr.* **1988**, *47*, 239–242. [CrossRef] [PubMed]
132. Cohen, S.; Gianaros, P.J.; Manuck, S.B. A stage model of stress and disease. *Perspect. Psychol. Sci.* **2016**, *11*, 456–463. [CrossRef] [PubMed]
133. Bellinger, D.L.; Lorton, D. Autonomic regulation of cellular immune function. *Auton. Neurosci.* **2014**, *182*, 15–41. [CrossRef] [PubMed]
134. Rohleder, N. Acute and chronic stress induced changes in sensitivity of peripheral inflammatory pathways to the signals of multiple stress systems—2011 Curt Richter Award Winner. *Psychoneuroendocrinology* **2012**, *37*, 307–316. [CrossRef]
135. Cohen, S.; Janicki-Deverts, D.; Doyle, W.J.; Miller, G.E.; Frank, E.; Rabin, B.S.; Turner, R.B. Chronic stress, glucocorticoid receptor resistance, inflammation, and disease risk. *Proc. Natl. Acad. Sci. USA* **2012**, *109*, 5995–5999. [CrossRef]
136. Miller, G.E.; Chen, E.; Sze, J.; Marin, T.; Arevalo, J.M.G.; Doll, R.; Ma, R.; Cole, S.W. A functional genomic fingerprint of chronic stress in humans: Blunted glucocorticoid and increased NF-kB signaling. *Biol. Psychiatry* **2008**, *64*, 266–272. [CrossRef]
137. Lorton, D.; Bellinger, D.L. Molecular mechanisms underlying B-adrenergic receptor-mediated cross-talk between sympathetic neurons and immune cells. *Int. J. Mol. Sci.* **2015**, *16*, 5635–5665. [CrossRef]
138. Lefkowitz, R.J. G protein coupled receptors. III. New roles for receptor kinases and beta-arrestins in receptor signaling and desensitization. *J. Biol. Chem.* **1998**, *273*, 18677–18680. [CrossRef]
139. Daaka, Y.; Luttrell, L.M.; Lefkowitz, R.J. Switching of the coupling of the Beta2-adrenergic receptor to different G proteins by protein kinase A. *Nature* **1997**, *390*, 88–91. [CrossRef]
140. Het, S.; Vocks, S.; Wolf, J.M.; Hammelstein, P.; Herpertz, S.; Wolf, O.T. Blunted neuroendocrine stress reactivity in young women with eating disorders. *J. Psychosom. Res.* **2015**, *78*, 260–267. [CrossRef]
141. Walsh, B.T.; Roose, S.P.; Katz, J.L.; Dyrenfurth, I.; Wright, L.; Wiele, R.V.; Glassman, A.H. Hypothalamic-pituitary-adrenal-cortical activity in anorexia nervosa and bulimia. *Psychoneuroendocrinology* **1987**, *12*, 131–140. [CrossRef]
142. Kontula, K.; Andersson, L.C.; Huttunen, M.; Pelkonen, R. Reduced level of cellular glucocorticoid receptors in patients with anorexia nervosa. *Horm. Metab. Res.* **1982**, *14*, 619–620. [CrossRef] [PubMed]
143. Lonati-Galligani, M.; Pirke, K.M. Beta2-adrenergic receptor regulation in circulating mononuclear leukocytes in anorexia nervosa and bulimia. *Psychiatry Res.* **1986**, *19*, 189–198. [CrossRef]
144. Furtado, M.; Katzman, M.A. Neuroinflammatory pathways in anxiety, posttraumatic stress, and obsessive compulsive disorders. *Psychiatry Res.* **2015**, *229*, 37–48. [CrossRef] [PubMed]
145. Magliozzi, J.R.; Gietzen, D.; Maddock, R.J.; Haack, D.; Doran, A.R.; Goodman, T.; Weiler, P.G. Lymphocyte beta-adrenoceptor density in patients with unipolar depression and normal controls. *Biol. Psychiatry* **1989**, *26*, 15–25. [CrossRef]
146. Yu, B.H.; Dimsdale, J.E.; Mills, P.J. Psychological states and lymphocyte beta-adrenergic receptor responsiveness. *Neuropsychopharmacology* **1999**, *21*, 147–152. [CrossRef]
147. Maddock, R.J.; Carter, C.S.; Magliozzi, J.R.; Gietzen, D.W. Evidence that decreased function of lymphocyte beta-adrenoceptors reflects regulatory and adaptive processes in panic disorder with agoraphobia. *Am. J. Psychiatry* **1993**, *150*, 1219–1225.
148. Wallon, C.; Yang, P.C.; Keita, A.V.; Ericson, A.C.; McKay, D.M.; Sherman, P.M.; Perdue, M.H.; Soderholm, J.D. Corticotropin-releasing hormone (CRH) regulates macromolecular permeability via mast cells in normal human colonic biopsies in vitro. *Gut* **2008**, *57*, 50–58. [CrossRef]
149. Vanuytsel, T.; van Wanrooy, S.; Vanheel, H.; Vanormelingen, C.; Verschueren, S.; Houben, E.; Rasoel, S.S.; Toth, J.; Holvoet, L.; Farre, R.; et al. Psychological stress and corticotropin-releasing hormone increase intestinal permeability in humans by a mast cell-dependent mechanism. *Gut* **2014**, *63*, 1293–1299. [CrossRef]

150. Soderholm, J.D.; Perdue, M.H. Stress and the gastrointestinal tract. II. Stress and intestinal barrier function. *Am. J. Physiol. Gastrointest. Liver Physiol.* **2001**, *280*, 7–13. [CrossRef]
151. Maynard, C.L.; Elson, C.O.; Hatton, R.D.; Weaver, C.T. Reciprocal interactions of the intestinal microbiota and immune system. *Nature* **2012**, *489*, 231–241. [CrossRef] [PubMed]
152. Pryde, S.E.; Duncan, S.H.; Hold, G.L.; Steward, C.S.; Flint, H.J. The microbiology of butyrate formation in the human colon. *FEMS Microbiol. Lett.* **2002**, *217*, 133–139. [CrossRef] [PubMed]
153. Spasova, D.S.; Surh, C.D. Blowing on embers: Commensal microbiota and our immune system. *Front. Immunol.* **2014**, *5*, 318. [CrossRef] [PubMed]
154. McGuckin, M.A.; Linden, S.K.; Sutton, P.; Florin, T.H. Mucin dynamics and enteric pathogens. *Nat. Rev. Microbiol.* **2011**, *9*, 265–278. [CrossRef]
155. Maslowski, K.M.; Vieira, A.T.; Ng, A.; Kranich, J.; Sierro, F.; Yu, D.; Schilter, H.C.; Rolph, M.S.; Mackay, F.; Artis, D.; et al. Regulation of inflammatory responses by gut microbiota and chemoattractant receptor GPR43. *Nature* **2009**, *461*, 1282–1287. [CrossRef]
156. Kimura, H.; Sawada, N.; Tobioka, H.; Isomura, H.; Kokai, Y.; Hirata, K.; Mori, M. Bacterial lipopolysaccharide reduced intestinal barrier function and altered localization of 7H6 antigen in IEC-6 rat intestinal crypt cells. *J. Cell. Physiol.* **1997**, *171*, 284–290. [CrossRef]
157. Bruewer, M.; Luegering, A.; Kucharzik, T.; Parkos, C.A.; Madara, J.L.; Hopkins, A.M.; Nusrat, A. Proinflammatory cytokines disrupt epithelial barrier function by apoptosis-independent mechanisms. *J. Immunol.* **2003**, *171*, 6164–6172. [CrossRef]
158. Genton, L.; Cani, P.D.; Schrenzel, J. Alterations of gut barrier and gut microbiota in food restriction, food deprivation and protein-energy wasting. *Clin. Nutr.* **2015**, *34*, 341–349. [CrossRef]
159. Roubalova, R.; Prochazkova, P.; Papezova, H.; Smitka, K.; Bilej, M.; Tlaskalova-Hogenova, H. Anorexia nervosa: Gut-microbiota-immune-brain interactions. *Clin. Nutr.* **2019**. [CrossRef]
160. Kleiman, S.C.; Watson, H.J.; Bulik-Sullivan, E.C.; Huh, E.Y.; Tarantino, L.M.; Bulik, C.M.; Carroll, I.M. The intestinal microbiota in acute anorexia nervosa and during renourishment: Relationship to depression, anxiety, and eating disorder psychopathology. *Psychosom. Med.* **2015**, *77*, 969–981. [CrossRef]
161. Borgo, F.; Riva, A.; Benetti, A.; Casiraghi, M.C.; Bertelli, S.; Garbossa, S.; Anselmetti, S.; Scarone, S.; Pontiroli, A.E.; Morace, G.; et al. Microbiota in anorexia nervosa: The triangle between bacterial species, metabolites, and psychological tests. *PLoS ONE* **2017**, *12*, e0179739. [CrossRef] [PubMed]
162. Morita, C.; Tsuji, H.; Hata, T.; Gondo, M.; Takakura, S.; Kawai, K.; Yoshihara, K.; Ogata, K.; Nomoto, K.; Miyazaki, K.; et al. Gut dysbiosis in patients with anorexia nervosa. *PLoS ONE* **2015**, *19*, e0145274. [CrossRef] [PubMed]
163. Morkl, S.; Lackner, S.; Muller, W.; Gorkiewicz, G.; Kashofer, K.; Oberascher, A.; Painold, A.; Holl, A.; Holzer, P.; Meinitzer, A.; et al. Gut microbiota and body composition in anorexia nervosa inpatients in comparison to athletes, overweight, obese, and normal weight controls. *Int. J. Eat. Disord.* **2017**, *50*, 1421–1431. [CrossRef] [PubMed]
164. Monteleone, P.; Carratu, R.; Carteni, M.; Generoso, M.; Lamberti, M.; De Magistris, L.; Brambilla, F.; Colurcio, B.; Secondulfo, M.; Maj, M. Intestinal permeability is decreased in anorexia nervosa. *Mol. Psychiatry* **2004**, *9*, 76–80. [CrossRef]
165. Li, T.; Wu, Y. Paracrine molecules of mesenchymal stem cells for hematopoietic stem cell niche. *Bone Marrow Res.* **2011**, *2011*, 353878. [CrossRef]
166. Marigo, I.; Dazzi, F. The immunomodulatory properties of mesenchymal stem cells. *Semin. Immunopathol.* **2011**, *33*, 593–602. [CrossRef]
167. Shi, Y.; Su, J.; Roberts, A.I.; Shou, P.; Rabson, A.B.; Ren, G. How mesenchymal stem cells interact with tissue immune responses. *Trends Immunol.* **2012**, *33*, 136–143. [CrossRef]
168. Sugiyama, T.; Kohara, H.; Noda, M.; Nagasawa, T. Maintenance of the hematopoietic stem cell pool by CXCL12-CXCR4 chemokine signaling in bone marrow stromal cell niches. *Immunity* **2006**, *25*, 977–988. [CrossRef]
169. Haynesworth, S.E.; Baber, M.A.; Caplan, A.I. Cytokine expression by human marrow-derived mesenchymal progenitor cells in vitro: Effects of dexamethasone and IL-1alpha. *J. Cell. Physiol.* **1996**, *166*, 585–592. [CrossRef]

170. Mendez-Ferrer, S.; Michurina, T.V.; Ferraro, F.; Mazloom, A.R.; MacArthur, B.D.; Lira, S.A.; Scadden, D.T.; Ma'ayan, A.; Enikolopov, G.N.; Frenette, P.S. Mesenchymal and haematopoietic stem cells form a unique bone marrow niche. *Nature* **2010**, *12*, 829–836. [CrossRef]
171. Katayama, Y.; Battista, M.; Kao, W.M.; Hidalgo, A.; Peired, A.J.; Thomas, S.A.; Frenette, P.S. Signals from the sympathetic nervous system regulate hematopoietic stem cell egress from bone marrow. *Cell* **2006**, *124*, 407–421. [CrossRef] [PubMed]
172. Ren, G.; Su, J.; Zhang, L.; Zhao, X.; Ling, W.; L'Huillie, A.; Zhang, J.; Lu, Y.; Roberts, A.I.; Ji, W.; et al. Species variation in the mechanisms of mesenchymal stem cell-mediated immunosuppression. *Stem Cells* **2009**, *27*, 1954–1962. [CrossRef] [PubMed]
173. Corcione, A.; Benvenuto, F.; Ferretti, E.; Giunti, D.; Cappiello, V.; Cazzanti, F.; Risso, M.; Gualandi, F.; Mancardi, G.L.; Pistoia, V.; et al. Human mesenchymal stem cells modulate B-cell functions. *Blood* **2006**, *107*, 367–372. [CrossRef] [PubMed]
174. Dos Santos, G.G.; Batool, S.; Hastreiter, A.; Sartori, T.; Nogueira-Pedro, A.; Borelli, P.; Fock, R.A. The influence of protein malnutrition on biological and immunomodulatory aspects of bone marrow mesenchymal stem cells. *Clin. Nutr.* **2017**, *36*, 1149–1157. [CrossRef]
175. Laranjeira, P.; Pedrosa, M.; Pedreiro, S.; Gomes, J.; Martinho, A.; Antunes, B.; Ribeiro, T.; Santos, F.; Trindade, H.; Paiva, A. Effect of human bone marrow mesenchymal stromal cells on cytokine production by peripheral blood naïve, memory, and effector T cells. *Stem Cell Res. Ther.* **2015**, *6*, 3. [CrossRef]
176. Spaggiari, G.M.; Capobianco, A.; Abdelrazik, H.; Becchetti, F.; Mingari, M.C.; Moretta, L. Mesenchymal stem cells inhibit natural killer-cell proliferation, cytotoxicity, and cytokine production: Role of indoleamine 2,3-dioxygenase and prostaglandin E2. *Blood* **2008**, *111*, 1327–1333. [CrossRef]
177. Krampera, M.; Glennie, S.; Dyson, J.; Scott, D.; Laylor, R.; Simpson, E.; Dazzi, F. Bone marrow mesenchymal stem cells inhibit the response of naïve and memory antigen-specific T cells to their cognate peptide. *Blood* **2003**, *101*, 3722–3729. [CrossRef]
178. Jiang, X.X.; Zhang, Y.; Liu, B.; Zhang, S.X.; Wu, Y.; Yu, X.D.; Mao, N. Human mesenchymal stem cells inhibit differentiation and function of monocyte-derived dendritic cells. *Blood* **2005**, *105*, 4120–4126. [CrossRef]
179. Chiesa, S.; Mobelli, S.; Morando, S.; Massollo, M.; Marini, C.; Bertoni, A.; Frassoni, F.; Bartolome, S.T.; Sambuceti, G.; Traggiai, E.; et al. Mesenchymal stem cells impair in vivo T-cell priming by dendritic cells. *Proc. Natl. Acad. Sci. USA* **2011**, *108*, 17384–17389. [CrossRef]
180. Chan, J.L.; Tang, K.C.; Patel, A.P.; Bonilla, L.M.; Pierobon, N.; Ponzio, N.M.; Rameshwar, P. Antigen-presenting property of mesenchymal stem cells occurs during a narrow window at low levels of interferon-gamma. *Blood* **2006**, *107*, 4817–4824. [CrossRef]
181. Le Blanc, K.; Tammik, L.; Sundberg, B.; Haynesworth, S.E.; Ringden, O. Mesenchymal stem cells inhibit and stimulate mixed lymphocyte cultures and mitogenic responses independently of the major histocompatibility complex. *Scand. J. Immunol.* **2003**, *57*, 11–20. [CrossRef] [PubMed]
182. Romieu-Mourez, R.; Francois, M.; Boivin, M.N.; Stagg, J.; Galipeau, J. Regulation of MHC class II expression and antigen processing in murine and human mesenchymal stromal cells by IFN-gamma, TGF-beta, and cell density. *J. Immunol.* **2007**, *179*, 1549–1558. [CrossRef]
183. Pittenger, M.F.; Mackay, A.M.; Beck, S.C.; Jaiswal, R.K.; Douglas, R.; Mosca, J.D.; Moorman, M.A.; Simonetti, D.W.; Craig, S.; Marshak, D.R. Multilineage potential of adult human mesenchymal stem cells. *Science* **1999**, *284*, 143–147. [CrossRef] [PubMed]
184. Hardouin, P.; Pansini, V.; Cortet, B. Bone marrow fat. *Jt. Bone Spine* **2014**, *81*, 313–319. [CrossRef] [PubMed]
185. Vidal-Puig, A.; Jimenez-Linan, M.; Lowell, B.B.; Hamann, A.; Hu, E.; Spiegelman, B.; Flier, J.J.; Moller, D.E. Regulation of PPAR gamma gene expression by nutrition and obesity in rodents. *J. Clin. Investig.* **1996**, *97*, 2553–2561. [CrossRef]
186. Liu, L.; Shen, W.J.; Ueno, M.; Patel, S.; Kraemer, F.B. Characterization of age-related gene expression profiling in bone marrow and epididymal adipocytes. *BMC Genom.* **2011**, *12*, 212. [CrossRef]
187. Shergill, K.K.; Shergill, G.S.; Pillai, H.J. Gelatinous transformation of bone marrow: Rare or underdiagnosed? *Autops. Case Rep.* **2017**, *7*, 8–17. [CrossRef]

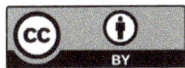

© 2019 by the authors. Licensee MDPI, Basel, Switzerland. This article is an open access article distributed under the terms and conditions of the Creative Commons Attribution (CC BY) license (http://creativecommons.org/licenses/by/4.0/).

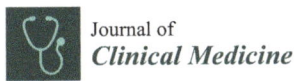
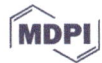

Review

Neural Processing of Disorder-Related Stimuli in Patients with Anorexia Nervosa: A Narrative Review of Brain Imaging Studies

Joe J. Simon *, Marion A. Stopyra and Hans-Christoph Friederich

Department of General Internal Medicine and Psychosomatics, Centre for Psychosocial Medicine, University Hospital Heidelberg, 69120 Heidelberg, Germany
* Correspondence: Joe.simon@med.uni-heidelberg.de; Tel.: +49-(0)6221-56-38667; Fax: +49-(0)6221-56-5988

Received: 22 May 2019; Accepted: 10 July 2019; Published: 18 July 2019

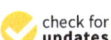

Abstract: Abnormalities and alterations in brain function are commonly associated with the etiology and maintenance of anorexia nervosa (AN). Different symptom categories of AN have been correlated with distinct neurobiological patterns in previous studies. The aim of this literature review is to provide a narrative overview of the investigations into neural correlates of disorder-specific stimuli in patients with AN. Although findings vary across studies, a summary of neuroimaging results according to stimulus category allows us to account for methodological differences in experimental paradigms. Based on the available evidence, the following conclusions can be made: (a) the neural processing of visual food cues is characterized by increased top-down control, which enables restrictive eating, (b) increased emotional and reward processing during gustatory stimulation triggers disorder-specific thought patterns, (c) hunger ceases to motivate food foraging but instead reinforces disorder-related behaviors, (d) body image processing is related to increased emotional and hedonic reactions, (e) emotional stimuli provoke increased saliency associated with decreased top-down control and (f) neural hypersensitivity during interoceptive processing reinforces avoidance behavior. Taken together, studies that investigated symptom-specific neural processing have contributed to a better understanding of the underlying mechanisms of AN.

Keywords: anorexia nervosa; functional magnetic resonance imaging; disorder-specific stimuli; narrative review

1. Introduction

Anorexia nervosa (AN) is a serious mental disorder characterized by self-induced starvation and excessive weight loss, fear of weight gain, body image concerns and food aversion [1]. Psychiatric comorbidities are common in patients with AN, as well as an increased mortality rate due to medical complications and suicide [2,3]. Previous research has identified numerous factors involved in the etiology of AN, where psychological, sociocultural and biological factors contribute to both the onset and maintenance of this disorder [4,5]. Recently, neurobiological alterations have been proposed as major factors contributing to AN [6]. Specifically, various studies have begun to employ neuroimaging techniques to elucidate the underlying pathophysiology and neurobiological substrate of AN [7–10]. Altered neural activity is observed throughout the brain in patients with AN, including cortical- and subcortical regions [7,11,12]. Based on neuroimaging investigations, theories have been proposed to explain the contribution of aberrant brain function to the development and maintenance of AN. For example, hyperactivity in cognitive control networks and a cooccurring reduction in motivational responses to food has been proposed as a core neural mechanism underlying the development of AN [5,12–14]. In contrast, reduced somatosensory and insula processing of taste stimuli may relate to a failure to accurately recognize hunger signals [15,16]. However, due to methodological differences between neuroimaging studies, as well as a paucity of studies employing a longitudinal design to differentiate between the state and trait, the exact neurobiological mechanisms of AN remain unclear. The aim of this review is to provide a narrative overview of recent studies investigating alterations in brain function related to disorder-specific stimuli in patients with AN and to provide a better characterization of the pathophysiological mechanisms underlying AN. Specifically, we focused on neuroimaging studies employing experimental designs drawing on symptom provocation to assess neural aberrations associated with AN. Symptom provocation has been extensively analyzed in patients with AN since the advent of fMRI-techniques [17] and has played an important role in the elaboration of neurobiological theories of AN. The following section will outline results from previous neuroimaging investigations grouped by stimulus type and relate these findings to current approaches examining neuroanatomical biomarkers of AN. Specifically, we describe studies investigating the following: (1) the responsivity to food-related stimuli, (2) hunger, (3) body image, (4) emotional processing and (5) interoceptive processing.

2. Neural Processing of Food-Related Stimuli

Food restriction and avoidance are cornerstones of AN, since patients are able to limit food intake even in the presence of prolonged food deprivation. Although the causative mechanisms are not completely understood, a relation to increased inhibition, alterations in the rewarding effect of food and a conditioned relationship between food and aversive emotional states have all been proposed as possible explanations [13,18]. Numerous studies have investigated brain alterations related to the exposure to different types of food stimuli in patients with AN. The experimental paradigms employed in these studies have been broadly classified as using either visual depictions of food or gustatory stimulation.

2.1. Visual Food Stimuli

The majority of studies investigating the neural processing of food have employed visual depictions of food [19,20]. Visual stimuli are used in a wide array of different experimental tasks, and they allow researchers to probe psychopathology-related neural processing in an efficient and economical manner.

Previous studies employing *passive viewing of visual food stimuli* have yielded conflicting results, since a number different processes may be captured when passively viewing food stimuli [21]. However, altered activation of the amygdala and insula has been consistently observed in patients with AN during passive viewing of visual food stimuli [17,22,23]. Holsen and colleagues [24] investigated neural processing when patients viewed high- and low calorie food images and the relation to hormone mediated hunger signaling (i.e., by assessing the level of the hunger-inducing peptide hormone Ghrelin). They aimed to investigate potential neurobiological mechanisms underlying appetite dysregulation in AN. The authors observed a strong connection between hormone-mediated hunger signaling and the neural processing of food pictures in the amygdala and insula in healthy controls but were unable to detect the same relation in patients with acute AN and weight-recovered AN. These results suggest a link between the often observed resistance to hunger-inducing hormones in patients with AN and reduced motivational processing of food as a mechanism of restrictive eating.

When instructing participants to *imagine eating the depicted food stimuli* or to *rate stimuli* according to their pleasantness, patients with AN commonly display aberrant activation in different regions of the prefrontal cortex [25–29]. Specifically, as outlined in two recent reviews [20,21], hypoactivity during food picture processing in regions such as the inferior parietal lobule and lateral prefrontal cortex may indicate weight and body shape concerns induced by the exposure to visual food stimuli [27,30,31]. The cooccurring increased activation of medial prefrontal regions during picture processing may be related to increased top-down control and efforts to restrain eating and food avoidance [27,30,32,33]. For example, Scaife and colleagues [28] instructed patients with AN to look at images of food with a high caloric content and to focus on how much they want to eat the depicted items. As predicted, patients displayed increased activation in inhibitory brain regions (i.e., the lateral prefrontal cortex), consistent with the persistent avoidance of high-calorie food observed in patients with AN. These results are in line with eye-tracking data showing avoidance of food pictures by patients with AN [34]. Finally, decreased activation in the medial orbitofrontal cortex and insula during food picture processing has been interpreted as reduced hedonic reactivity to food stimuli in in patients with AN [20,31].

Foerde and colleagues [35] asked patients with AN to *choose between different visually depicted food items to assess the neural correlates of disorder-specific food choices in these patients*. When choosing low-fat foods, patients with AN displayed an increased connectivity between the dorsal striatum and dorsolateral prefrontal cortex [35]. Furthermore, this association was related to subsequent food intake, where a stronger connectivity was coupled with lower caloric intake on the following day [35]. The authors concluded that frontal-striatal networks are crucial in the development of habitual behaviors [36] and may subserve maladaptive eating behavior in patients with AN [35]. However, the authors did not clearly determine whether this observation was a risk factor for the development of AN or is simply caused by prolonged periods of self-starvation, particularly since adolescent patients with AN display hyperactivation in both reward-related and inhibitory control regions when viewing pictures of high calorie food [37].

Taken together, the results from studies investigating visual food stimuli note a pronounced top-down control mediated by medial prefrontal regions, which may override both somatosensory and hedonic-related brain signals.

2.2. Gustatory Stimulation

Studies employing real taste stimuli are able to probe disorder-specific neural reactions to food in a more natural setting. Behavioral investigations using gustatory stimulation have reported lower taste sensitivity in patients with AN [38], although patients report an increased subjective perception of taste stimuli [39]. Similarly, reduced taste classification accuracy in the insula during the tasting of sucrose has been observed in patients with AN [40], although conflicting results exist [32].

The majority of studies using gustatory stimulation to investigate the neural processing of taste found altered activation profiles in patients with AN compared to healthy controls. Interestingly, with a few exceptions, (e.g., [41]), most studies consistently detected increased activation in reward-related regions in patients with AN [15,42]. For example, Cowdrey and colleagues [32] compared the neural responses to rewarding and aversive tastes in participants who had recovered from AN and healthy controls. They did not observe differences between groups in subjective ratings of pleasantness and taste processing in the primary gustatory cortex, which indicates similar sensory experiences in both groups. However, the authors observed increased activation of brain regions processing reward and aversion (i.e., the ventral striatum and posterior insula, respectively) in response to both pleasant and aversive tastes.

Increased activation of reward-related brain regions during taste processing has been discussed as an increased salience attribution to taste stimuli and is considered a potential neural biomarker for AN [32]. Similarly, Frank and colleagues observed increased reward-related activity during the processing of taste in both adolescent and adult patients with AN [43,44]. They propose a conflict between an innate starvation-induced approach mechanism to food and a strong drive for thinness. Specifically, the authors suggest that a starvation-induced sensitization of the dopamine system stimulates food intake, which is in direct conflict with a high drive for thinness and body dissatisfaction. Thus, neural reward processing may then become associated with a fear-driven mechanism that overrides homeostatic signals that would normally initiate feeding behavior [43]. These results are in part corroborated by a study by Vocks and colleagues [15], where patients with AN displayed higher activation in the amygdala and medial temporal gyrus when drinking chocolate milk than healthy controls during hunger. Since the amygdala is related to the processing of aversive stimuli and in the acquisition of conditioned emotional responses [45], the authors postulated that this finding indicated an increased fear of weight gain.

Horndasch et al. [46] used an incentive delay task, allowing the measurement of both anticipation and receipt of pleasant and aversive tastes. In a group of first-degree relatives of patients with AN, the authors observed increased neural reward processing during the anticipation of both pleasant and unpleasant tastes, but they observed a decreased reward processing during the receipt of aversive taste. They interpret this finding as increased emotional arousal in response to food anticipation and a bias towards reduced liking of food, with both observations representing a potential biomarker for AN.

Taken together, the results from studies investigating taste processing indicate an increased salience of taste stimuli in patients with AN, which appears to be strongly correlated with disorder-specific reactions to food stimuli, such as fear of weight gain and a drive for thinness.

3. Hunger

As stated above, since self-starvation allows the maintenance of the desired low body weight, this behavior develops rewarding qualities in patients with AN and reinforces the illness [13]. Hunger promotes foraging by inducing increased mesolimbic dopaminergic signaling, which increases the motivational value of foraging behaviors [47]. This mechanism is thought to facilitate the progression to anorexia nervosa, where the constant fasting-induced dopamine stimulation reinforces disorder-related behaviors that are otherwise perceived as aversive [48–50]. However, few neuroimaging studies have directly compared the effects of both hunger and satiety on the processing of disorder-related stimuli in patients with AN.

Using *visual depictions of food*, Santel and colleagues [51] observed decreased somatosensory processing during satiation in the parietal cortex and decreased processing in the visual cortex during hunger when subjected rated food pictures. Similarly, when passively viewing food pictures, Gizewski and colleagues [52] observed satiety state-dependent differences in brain activation in the cingulate cortex, insula and prefrontal cortex in patients with AN compared to healthy controls. Furthermore, both patients with AN and weight-restored patients show a general hypo-activation pattern in regions associated with motivational processing when viewing pictures of food while they are hungry [53]. The authors conclude that hunger loses its ability to induce an increased motivational drive for food consumption, thereby facilitating food restriction.

By presenting *taste stimuli* during both hunger and satiety, Vocks and colleagues [15] found that patients with AN display increased activation in the amygdala and medial temporal gyrus while tasting chocolate milk during hunger. Within the patient group, satiety led to an increased activation of the right inferior temporal gyrus, a region that is typically activated during the processing of body images, compared to the hungry state [54]. Together with the observed activation of the amygdala and its relevance to the processing of aversive and fear-inducing stimuli [45,55], the authors propose that the observed results possibly reflect a fear of weight gain in patients with AN.

Taken together, studies investigating the effect of hunger on brain activation in patients with AN observe decreased activation in areas related to motivational processing and an interaction with emotional processing related to a fear of weight gain. However, these results relate exclusively to visual and gustatory food cues, since the influence of the satiety state on the processing of additional disorder-related stimuli remains to be investigated.

4. Body Image

Body image distortion is a hallmark feature of AN. The subjective perception of body weight or shape is disturbed, together with increased attention to particular details or parts of the body [1]. Body image disturbances are persistent symptoms of AN and are negatively correlated with patients' long-term outcomes [56]. In healthy participants, a network of brain regions is associated with body image processing. Studies investigating brain activation when participants compare their own body with slim-idealized bodies or when they are presented with distorted images of their own body typically observe increased activation in regions such as the extrastriate body area (a subportion of the extrastriate visual cortex), the fusiform body area located in the fusiform gyrus [54,57], the dorsolateral prefrontal cortex and parietal lobe [58]. Previous studies have observed alterations in this network in patients with AN, although the direction of differences has been inconsistent [59–62]. For example, when viewing body images of other women, patients with AN display both similar and differing brain activation patterns compared with healthy controls [59,63]. Furthermore, studies have observed both activation in fear-related networks [64,65], and reward-related networks during body image processing [66].

During the *passive viewing of body images*, patients with AN display reduced connectivity between the extrastriate and fusiform body areas and a negative correlation between the magnitude of connectivity and body size misjudgment [67]. Vocks and colleagues observed reduced activation in the inferior parietal lobule when patients viewed their own body, but increased activation of the amygdala when viewing pictures of another woman's thin body [63]. The authors hypothesize correlations between decreased attentional processing towards the patient's own body and an increased emotional response when viewing other bodies with an inherent bias towards social comparison.

When asked to *compare their own body to slim, idealized female bodies*, patients with AN display reduced activation in the rostral anterior cingulate cortex, but increased activation in the insula and premotor cortex [64]. Thus, body image perception in patients with AN may be related to alterations in regions associated with interoceptive awareness. Furthermore, participants who have recovered from AN show increased activation in the rostral anterior cingulate cortex during a comparison of their own body with an underweight body [68]. This change may be viewed as a recovery of top-down control of the emotional impact of body comparisons with others. Fladung and colleagues [66] employed pictures of a female body corresponding to different weight categories; when patients with AN were asked to imagine having the same weight as featured in the picture, they showed increased activation in the bilateral ventral striatum when imagining having an underweight body shape compared to healthy controls.

When shown pictures of their *own body digitally modified to be oversized*, patients with AN show increased activation in the dorsolateral prefrontal cortex compared to healthy controls [69]. Furthermore, this activation was related to eating disorder psychopathology (i.e., shape concerns). These results suggest an increase in top-down control when patients are facing emotionally aversive stimuli, such as distorted images of their own body. When asked to rate modified pictures of their own body, patients with AN display increased activation in the insula and lateral prefrontal cortex during the evaluation of thin self-images, which may indicate a stronger emotional involvement, although this claim remains inconclusive since both regions are associated with a number of differing functions [70–72].

Taken together, studies examining the passive viewing of body shapes, body comparison and modified images of one's own body detected dysfunctional activation in neural body image networks and regions associated with interoception, and top-down control, as well as increased activation in regions associated with emotional processing and reward. Furthermore, the existing studies indicate a correlation between reduced top-down control and body-comparison in patients with AN, whereas the viewing of modified images of their own body is characterized by increased top-down control. These results highlight the importance of disturbed body image processing in patients with AN, indicating that underweight body images possess a rewarding effect and an increased emotional relevance for patients with AN.

5. Emotional Processing

Dysfunctional emotional processing is prevalent in patients with AN and is related to both the onset and prevalence of the disorder [73,74]. Dietary restrictions and binging/purging may facilitate the avoidance or reduction of negative emotions [75–77]. Accordingly, a broad range of emotion regulation deficits have been observed in patients with AN [78,79] and have been shown to correlate with AN psychopathology [80,81]. For example, behavioral investigations suggest an increase in disorder-related thoughts during an induced negative mood [82]. However, vast differences in emotion regulation exist across different types of eating disorders. Patients with binge eating/purging compared to restrictive eating behaviour experience greater difficulties in emotion regulation in the domains of goal-directed behaviour, impulse control and have limited access to regulatory strategies. In fact, the emotion regulation profile of patients with AN-binge eating/purging type (AN-BP) is similar to patients diagnosed with bulimia nervosa [83]. In contrast, patients with restrictive AN (AN-R) experience greater difficulties in recognizing and expressing of emotions than patients with AN-BP [84].

When assessing neural emotional processing in response to *affective facial expressions*, Fonville and colleagues [85] observed increased activation of the fusiform gyrus in patients with AN during exposure to happy facial expressions. This observation may indicate the increased saliency of facial expressions in patients with AN. However, Cowdrey and colleagues [86] failed to identify differences during the neural processing of happy and fearful faces in participants who had recovered from AN, leading the authors to conclude that deficits in the processing of emotional faces in patients with AN might be state-dependent and improve with recovery. In contrast, Rangaprakash and colleagues [87] reported reduced connectivity between the amygdala and prefrontal cortex when patients who had recovered from AN viewed fearful facial expressions. These findings suggest that a decrease in top-down control during the processing of emotional facial expressions represents a trait marker of AN, indicating that aberrations in emotion regulation persist at neurobiological and behavioural levels [88] in weight-recovered patients with AN. Leppanen and colleagues [89] investigated neural responses to faces of infants displaying positive and negative emotions, and found that patients with AN exhibit increased prefrontal downregulation of limbic regions when viewing of positive emotions, but increased activation of the posterior insula when viewing of negative emotions. The latter finding suggests an increased saliency of negative emotions in patients AN, due to the frequently observed association of insula activation and emotion processing [90]. Taken together, studies employing facial stimuli commonly observe increased neural saliency processing and suggest the presence of different activation profiles, depending on the emotional valence of facial stimuli, where negative emotional stimuli tend to be associated with decreased top-down control.

Neural processing during *social interactions* also appears to be impaired in patients with AN. During positive social interactions in an economic exchange game, patients with AN and participants who had recovered from AN displayed diminished neural responses in the precuneus and right angular gyrus. However, only patients with current AN showed reduced activation in the fusiform gyrus during negative interactions [91]. The authors discuss a potential role of aberrant neural responses during positive social interactions as a predisposing trait for the development of AN, whereas changes in the neural processing of negative interactions may be important for weight recovery following AN. Via and colleagues used a social judgement task where participants received feedback on whether other participants would like to meet them [92]. Patients exhibited reduced activation of the dorsal prefrontal cortex when receiving positive feedback, but hyperactivation of visual regions and, surprisingly, a positive correlation between reward-related brain regions and clinical severity scores when receiving negative feedback. These results suggest the presence of dysfunctional self-evaluative processes and reduced perceptions of social rewards, and finally, they highlight the importance of brain reward networks for pathological behaviors in patients with AN. Consistent with the frequently observed disturbances in interpersonal relationships in patients with AN [93], Maier and colleagues [94] found that both patients with AN and participants who had recovered from AN display decreased activation in the superior parietal cortex and a reduced responsivity in the dorsolateral prefrontal cortex when viewing pictures displaying intimate situations. Similarly, Miyake and colleagues [95] observed a negative relationship between alexithymia, or the inability to articulate and interpret emotional experiences, and activation of the amygdala and posterior and anterior cingulate cortices during the processing of negative interpersonal words. Furthermore, reduced processing in the medial prefrontal cortex during a theory of mind task negatively correlates with treatment outcome [96]. This finding further corroborates the observed relation between social functioning and therapy outcomes in patients with AN [97] and confirms the importance and potential effectiveness of social skills training and family-based interventions for patients with AN [98,99].

Altered neural processing during the *active regulation of emotions* has also been observed in patients with AN. According to Seidel and colleagues, when patients with AN are asked to "distance" themselves from aversive pictures, they display the same neural activation pattern as healthy controls, but increased activation of the amygdala and dorsolateral prefrontal cortex is detected when they passively view aversive pictures [100]. However, in a subsequent study, Seidel and colleagues [101] reported a positive correlation between activation of the ventral striatum during distancing from positive pictures and body-related rumination, but this activation pattern negatively correlates with negative affect and treatment outcomes in patients with AN. Although the neural regulation of emotions is partially preserved in patients with AN, the authors emphasized the need to focus on adaptive emotion regulation strategies during the treatment of AN.

Taken together, studies investigating neural activation related to the processing of emotions in patients with AN reported contradictory results, but suggest increased salience processing and a concurrent dysfunctional top-down control during emotional processing. However, heterogeneity in studies investigating emotion regulation in patients with AN might explain the fact that more than 55% of patients with AN exhibit at least one comorbid disorder [102], with approximately a 73% lifetime prevalence of depressive disorders among patients with AN [103]. Comorbid depression is associated with increased emotion regulation difficulties [104] and researchers have not clearly determined how these comorbidities, particularly mood disorders, interact with the neural processing of emotional stimuli in patients with AN. In previous functional imaging studies, little emphasis was placed on the contributions of comorbid disorders, which might play an essential role when examining disorder-specific stimuli, as these disorders might moderate the patient's emotion regulation capacities.

6. Interoceptive Processing

Interoception refers to the perception and integration of visceral and homeostatic signals representing internal physiological body states [105]. Altered interoceptive awareness is viewed as a vulnerability factor for the development of AN, where overactive cognitive control enables the development of maladaptive food habits that do not subserve the homeostatic weight balance [13]. Decreased interoceptive awareness is associated with alexithymia, which is the to describe and identify one's own feelings [106]. Alexithymia is related to impaired emotional regulation and is as risk factor for the development and maintenance of AN [107]. Several neuropsychological models of alexithymia have been proposed. According to an early hypothesis proposed by MacLean [108], an altered communication between limbic and neocortical brain areas exists, leading to impairments in identifying and describing one's own emotions and feelings. As shown in recent studies, individuals with alexithymia display decreased activation of limbic and paralimbic brain areas in response to affective stimuli or increased activity in somatosensory/sensorimotor areas. The former indicates a low emotional arousal to external emotional stimuli, while the latter suggests a hypersensitivity and overreliance on physical stimulation [109].

Employing an interoceptive attention task where participants must focus on *internal bodily sensations* such as heartbeat or stomach distension, Kerr and colleagues [110] observed altered activity in the insula in weight-restored patients with AN. Furthermore, insula activity during stomach interoception negatively correlates with eating disorder psychopathology and anxiety. The authors postulate a visceral hypersensitivity entailing increased perception of gastrointestinal discomfort during food consumption, particularly during the weight restoration process. In a subsequent study, Kerr and colleagues [23] investigated the effect of interoceptive sensation on the neural processing of food pictures in weight-restored patients with AN. During the neural processing of food pictures, stomach sensation ratings recorded before scanning positively correlated with activity in the insula, anterior cingulate cortex and amygdala, but negatively correlated with activity in the ventral pallidum and ventral tegmental area. The authors concluded that gastric sensations may interfere with food reward processing and may be related to an aversive response to food pictures in patients with AN.

Two studies have investigated neural processing during unpleasant bodily sensations in patients with AN. Strigo and colleagues [111] investigated the neural processing of *pain* in patients recovered from AN and observed increased activity in the insula and dorsolateral prefrontal cortex (DLPFC) during the anticipation of pain, whereas the experience of pain was associated with decreased insula but increased DLPFC activity. Increased insular activity during the anticipation of pain was also related to high levels of alexithymia. The authors concluded that the results suggest an abnormal integration of interoceptive signals, and the increase in DLPFC activity is an attempt to control the increased distress caused by the subsequent pain stimulation.

Similarly, Berner and colleagues assessed neural processing in women who had remitted from AN during an *inspiratory breathing load paradigm*, where participants' breathing was intermittently restricted, causing mild discomfort [112]. When anticipating breathing restriction, patients displayed reduced insular activation, whereas they showed stronger activation of the striatum, cingulate cortex and prefrontal cortex during the actual breathing restriction. These results may reflect difficulties in predicting and adapting to changes in interoceptive states in patients with AN, and highlight eating restriction as a method for preventing unpredictable and/or unpleasant internal changes.

Bischoff-Grethe and colleagues investigated neural processing during a *pleasant affective touch* task (i.e., gentle strokes with a soft brush administered to the forearm or palm), where participants who had recovered from AN displayed an increased response in the right ventral mid-insula, but a decreased response in the same region during the anticipation of a pleasant touch [113]. These results indicate an impaired ability of patients with AN to predict and interpret physiological stimuli. Furthermore, since reduced activity in the insula during anticipation is related to increased harm avoidance and higher body dissatisfaction, aberrant interoceptive processing might contribute to an altered subjective body experience and avoidance behavior [113].

In summary, the results from studies investigating neural interoceptive processing have identified a pronounced relation between neural hypersensitivity to bodily sensations and concurrent avoidance behavior, which is partially mediated by dysfunctional prefrontal processing. Importantly, since all of the aforementioned studies recruited women who had recovered from AN, dysfunctional interoceptive processing might be a potential trait of AN.

7. Summary and Conclusions

This narrative review aimed to provide a general overview of the neuroimaging literature investigating symptom-specific neural processing in patients with AN. In recent years, a number of studies have investigated the neural profiles of different symptom-categories in patients with AN using fMRI. While the obtained results sometimes differ and certain disorder-related stimuli have not yet been investigated, the findings provide a better understanding of the underlying neurobiological correlates of AN. Based on the reviewed literature, we provide the following summary of the different symptom categories.

Neural processing of visual *food* cues in patients with AN is characterized by increased top-down control, enabling restrictive eating habits and a concurrent reduction in hedonic and somatosensory reactivity. On the other hand, studies using real tastants typically observe increased activation of brain areas related to saliency and reward processing, as well as emotional arousal, namely, a fear of weight gain and drive for thinness. Thus, although an increase in neural cognitive control in response to food cues allows patients to avoid food and consistently reduce their cravings for food, the actual consumption of food is associated with a number of disorder-specific neural reactions that collectively increase the saliency of food.

In patients with AN, *hunger* is associated with a decrease in neural motivational processing in response to food cues, and the observed activation patterns suggest an increase in emotional sensitivity related to a fear of weight gain. This finding is also consistent with the results from animal models suggesting that conditioned fear cues inhibit food consumption by food-deprived rats; therefore, signals from the amygdala may potentially override the homeostatic signaling of hunger in the hypothalamus and inhibit eating [114]. Therefore, the frequently observed strong effect of top-down control regions on food reward processing [115] has also been observed on homeostatic signals driving food consumption.

When using stimuli related to *body image*, studies identified a number of aberrations in brain regions related to emotion and reward processing, as well as interoceptive processing and top-down control. Body images gain increased emotional relevance, and exposure to thin body figures can become rewarding. These results are consistent with the "reward contamination theory" proposed by Keating [49], which hypothesizes that the observed reduction in neural food reward processing is caused by a pronounced fear of weight gain, but illness-related stimuli and behaviors, such as emaciated body shapes or food restriction, become rewarding and activate reward-related brain regions in patients with AN [50]. Furthermore, the observed activation of brain regions related to interoception in patients with AN who are confronted with body images supports the hypothesis that dysfunctional interoceptive awareness is linked and contributes to body image concerns [116].

The processing of *emotions* in patients with AN is characterized by increased saliency processing and dysfunctional top-down control. These observations extend to visual depictions of emotional facial expressions, social interactions and emotion regulation but are more pronounced for negative emotional stimuli. Neural activation in corticolimbic regions during the processing of social stimuli and emotion regulation are related to treatment outcomes. However, a number of open questions related to emotional processing in patients with AN remain, such as the effect of the satiety state, since no neuroimaging study has yet investigated the specific interaction between the hunger state and neural emotional processing in patients with AN. An investigation of this interaction would be very interesting because dietary restriction represents an important method avoiding or reducing negative emotions in patients with AN [77].

The neural processing of *interoception* is related to a dysfunctional integration of interoceptive signals in the insula and an increased general neural sensitivity to interoceptive and somatosensory stimuli, which facilitates restrictive and avoidant behaviors in patients with AN. These results are consistent with previous studies showing that anxiety associated with food intake in patients with AN is related to intensified interoceptive sensations [117].

Taken together, studies using symptom provocation paradigms to assess disorder-specific neurobiological alterations in patients with AN observed a number of alterations in different brain networks. Some of these activation patterns are related to the acute phase of AN and some have been identified as state-independent risk factors. Specifically, an increase in top-down control observed in response to *visual food cues* appears to enable restrictive eating; a concurrent increase in the activation of reward- and emotion related areas during *gustatory stimulation* triggers disorder-specific thought patterns, such as a fear of weight gain. *Hunger* loses its ability to motivate food foraging but instead reinforces disorder-related behaviors. Dysfunctional neural processing of *body images* is a central feature of AN, where increased emotional and hedonic processing are prevalent, and neural activation during *emotional stimuli* indicates decreased top-down control but increased salience, particularly for negative stimuli. Finally, dysfunctional *interoceptive processing* is a trait of AN, where neural hypersensitivity to bodily sensations promotes avoidance behavior.

Studies investigating the neurobiological correlates of disorder-specific stimuli in patients with other psychiatric disorders might provide information about the pathophysiological mechanisms underlying shared symptomatology of psychiatric disorders. Given the high prevalence of comorbidities in patients with AN, studies investigating patients with anxiety disorders (e.g. obsessive-compulsive disorder or social phobia), affective disorders or substance abuse disorder can contribute to a better understanding of the psychopathology of AN. For example, patients with OCD show increased activation of fronto-striato-limbic regions and the amygdala upon exposure to symptom-provoking stimuli [118]. The authors concluded that amygdala hyperactivation in response to disorder-related stimuli reflects an exaggerated fear response. This finding is similar to the observed amygdala hyperactivation in patients with AN upon exposure to taste stimuli [15], food [22], and their own body image [65]. Similar findings of exaggerated limbic activation in response to disorder-specific stimuli have been observed in individuals with substance use disorder [119], panic disorder with agoraphobia [120] and social anxiety disorder [121]. These results suggest a potential shared functional neural basis of symptom-provoking stimuli across patients with different psychiatric disorders. However, researchers have not clearly determined whether these commonalities are a causal factor for the response to disorder-specific stimuli or reflect an overlap of symptomatology underlying the high prevalence of comorbidities.

Conclusions drawn from neuroimaging data often remain ambiguous since using observed brain activation to infer conclusions about cognitive processes can be problematic. Specifically, reverse inference, or "reasoning backwards from brain activation to the engagement of a particular cognitive function" [122] is only valid when the selectivity of activation in the observed brain regions is high. Furthermore, a number of limitations are present in fMRI-studies and should be taken into account when drawing general conclusions. General limitations relate to small sample sizes and an almost exclusive focus on female patients with AN. Contradictory results across studies could in part be caused by differences in experimental paradigms and sample heterogeneity such as illness state (acute vs. recovered AN) and duration, pharmacological treatment and psychiatric comorbidities. A number of studies have included patients recovered from AN to avoid the confounding effects of starvation. However, this approach can produce misleading findings, since patients often continue to display core symptoms even after recovery [123,124] and the definition of recovery varies substantially in the literature [125]. Furthermore, AN is characterized by alexithymia and high prevalence rates of affective disorders which likely moderate neural response to disorder-related stimuli and tasks [126]. Finally, emotion regulation difficulties differ across subtypes of AN [84] and future neuroimaging studies should address the influence of both comorbid disorders as well as differences in emotion regulation strategies across the eating disorder spectrum. A combination of neurophysiological techniques could contribute to the understanding of the interactive effect of neurobiology and disorder eating behavior underlying the psychopathology of AN.

Our conclusions are preliminary, since no systematic literature search or formal assessment of methodological quality was performed. However, the aim of this review was to reconcile findings derived from differing neural stimuli and to provide a parsimonious account of the underlying neurobiological alterations associated with AN. Alterations in brain networks subserving various functions jointly contribute to AN-specific symptoms and behaviors. Studies investigating symptom-specific neural processing will provide a better understanding of the mechanisms underlying AN and important suggestions for targets for neurobiologically informed treatments. In fact, treatment options integrating neurobiological contributions have already been described [127,128].

Author Contributions: Conceptualization, J.J.S.; writing-original draft preparation, J.J.S., M.A.S. and H.-C.F.; writing-review and editing, M.A.S. and H.-C.F.

Funding: German Research Foundation (Deutsche Forschungsgemeinschaft), Grant/Award Number: SI 2087/3-1.

Conflicts of Interest: The authors report no potential conflicts of interest or any types of commercial or financial involvement.

References

1. American Psychiatric Association. *Diagnostic and Statistical Manual of Mental Disorders (DSM-5®)*; American Psychiatric Association: Washington, DC, USA, 2013.
2. Mehler, P.S.; Brown, C. Anorexia nervosa—Medical complications. *J. Eat. Disord.* **2015**, *3*, 11. [CrossRef] [PubMed]
3. Kask, J.; Ekselius, L.; Brandt, L.; Kollia, N.; Ekbom, A.; Papadopoulos, F.C. Mortality in Women with Anorexia Nervosa: The Role of Comorbid Psychiatric Disorders. *Psychosom. Med.* **2016**, *78*, 910–919. [CrossRef] [PubMed]
4. Zipfel, S.; Giel, K.E.; Bulik, C.M.; Hay, P.; Schmidt, U. Anorexia nervosa: Aetiology, assessment, and treatment. *Lancet Psychiat.* **2015**, *2*, 1099–1111. [CrossRef]

5. Kaye, W.H.; Wierenga, C.E.; Bailer, U.F.; Simmons, A.N.; Bischoff-Grethe, A. Nothing tastes as good as skinny feels: The neurobiology of anorexia nervosa. *Trends Neurosci.* **2013**, *36*, 110–120. [CrossRef] [PubMed]
6. Frank, G.K.W. Altered brain reward circuits in eating disorders: Chicken or egg? *Curr. Psychiat. Rep.* **2013**, *15*, 396. [CrossRef] [PubMed]
7. Fuglset, T.S.; Landrø, N.I.; Reas, D.L.; Rø, Ø. Functional brain alterations in anorexia nervosa: A scoping review. *J. Eat. Disord.* **2016**, *4*, 32. [CrossRef]
8. King, J.A.; Frank, G.K.W.; Thompson, P.M.; Ehrlich, S. Structural Neuroimaging of Anorexia Nervosa: Future Directions in the Quest for Mechanisms Underlying Dynamic Alterations. *Biol. Psychiat.* **2018**, *83*, 224–234. [CrossRef]
9. Gaudio, S.; Wiemerslage, L.; Brooks, S.J.; Schioth, H.B. A systematic review of resting-state functional-MRI studies in anorexia nervosa: Evidence for functional connectivity impairment in cognitive control and visuospatial and body-signal integration. *Neurosci. Biobehav. Rev.* **2016**, *71*, 578–589. [CrossRef]
10. Kullmann, S.; Giel, K.E.; Hu, X.; Bischoff, S.C.; Teufel, M.; Thiel, A.; Zipfel, S.; Preissl, H. Impaired inhibitory control in anorexia nervosa elicited by physical activity stimuli. *Soc. Cogn. Affect. Neurosci.* **2014**, *9*, 917–923. [CrossRef]
11. Lipsman, N.; Woodside, D.B.; Lozano, A.M. Neurocircuitry of limbic dysfunction in anorexia nervosa. *Cortex* **2015**, *62*, 109–118. [CrossRef]
12. Friederich, H.-C.; Wu, M.; Simon, J.J.; Herzog, W. Neurocircuit function in eating disorders. *Int. J. Eat. Disord.* **2013**, *46*, 425–432. [CrossRef] [PubMed]
13. Kaye, W.H.; Fudge, J.L.; Paulus, M. New insights into symptoms and neurocircuit function of anorexia nervosa. *Nat. Rev. Neurosci.* **2009**, *10*, 573–584. [CrossRef] [PubMed]
14. Klein, D.A.; Schebendach, J.E.; Gershkovich, M.; Smith, G.P.; Walsh, B.T. Modified sham feeding of sweet solutions in women with anorexia nervosa. *Physiol. Behav.* **2010**, *101*, 132–140. [CrossRef]
15. Vocks, S.; Herpertz, S.; Rosenberger, C.; Senf, W.; Gizewski, E.R. Effects of gustatory stimulation on brain activity during hunger and satiety in females with restricting-type anorexia nervosa: An fMRI study. *J. Psychiatr. Res.* **2011**, *45*, 395–403. [CrossRef] [PubMed]
16. Oberndorfer, T.A.; Frank, G.K.W.; Simmons, A.N.; Wagner, A.; McCurdy, D.; Fudge, J.L.; Yang, T.T.; Paulus, M.P.; Kaye, W.H. Altered Insula Response to Sweet Taste Processing After Recovery From Anorexia and Bulimia Nervosa. *Am. J. Psychiat.* **2013**, *170*, 1143–1151. [CrossRef] [PubMed]
17. Ellison, Z.; Foong, J.; Howard, R.; Bullmore, E.; Williams, S.; Treasure, J. Functional anatomy of calorie fear in anorexia nervosa. *Lancet* **1998**, *352*, 1192. [CrossRef]
18. Hildebrandt, T.; Grotzinger, A.; Reddan, M.; Greif, R.; Levy, I.; Goodman, W.; Schiller, D. Testing the disgust conditioning theory of food-avoidance in adolescents with recent onset anorexia nervosa. *Behav. Res. Ther.* **2015**, *71*, 131–138. [CrossRef]
19. Frank, G.K.W. Recent Advances in Neuroimaging to Model Eating Disorder Neurobiology. *Curr. Psychiat. Rep.* **2015**, *17*, 22. [CrossRef] [PubMed]
20. García-García, I.; Narberhaus, A.; Marqués-Iturria, I.; Garolera, M.; Rădoi, A.; Segura, B.; Pueyo, R.; Ariza, M.; Jurado, M.A. Neural Responses to Visual Food Cues: Insights from Functional Magnetic Resonance Imaging. *Europ. Eat. Disord. Rev.* **2013**, *21*, 89–98. [CrossRef] [PubMed]
21. Lloyd, E.C.; Steinglass, J.E. What can food-image tasks teach us about anorexia nervosa? A systematic review. *J. Eat. Disord.* **2018**, *6*, 31. [CrossRef]
22. Joos, A.A.; Saum, B.; van Elst, L.T.; Perlov, E.; Glauche, V.; Hartmann, A.; Freyer, T.; Tuscher, O.; Zeeck, A. Amygdala hyperreactivity in restrictive anorexia nervosa. *Psychiat. Res.* **2011**, *191*, 189–195. [CrossRef] [PubMed]
23. Kerr, K.L.; Moseman, S.E.; Avery, J.A.; Bodurka, J.; Simmons, W.K. Influence of Visceral Interoceptive Experience on the Brain's Response to Food Images in Anorexia Nervosa. *Psychosom. Med.* **2017**, *79*, 777–784. [CrossRef] [PubMed]
24. Holsen, L.M.; Lawson, E.A.; Christensen, K.; Klibanski, A.; Goldstein, J.M. Abnormal relationships between the neural response to high- and low-calorie foods and endogenous acylated ghrelin in women with active and weight-recovered anorexia nervosa. *Psychiat. Res.* **2014**, *223*, 94–103. [CrossRef] [PubMed]
25. Sanders, N.; Smeets, P.A.; van Elburg, A.A.; Danner, U.N.; van Meer, F.; Hoek, H.W.; Adan, R.A. Altered food-cue processing in chronically ill and recovered women with anorexia nervosa. *Front. Behav. Neurosci.* **2015**, *9*, 46. [CrossRef] [PubMed]

26. Brooks, S.J.; O'Daly, O.G.; Uher, R.; Friederich, H.C.; Giampietro, V.; Brammer, M.; Williams, S.C.; Schioth, H.B.; Treasure, J.; Campbell, I.C. Differential neural responses to food images in women with bulimia versus anorexia nervosa. *PLoS ONE* **2011**, *6*, e22259. [CrossRef] [PubMed]
27. Uher, R.; Murphy, T.; Brammer, M.J.; Dalgleish, T.; Phillips, M.L.; Ng, V.W.; Andrew, C.M.; Williams, S.C.; Campbell, I.C.; Treasure, J. Medial prefrontal cortex activity associated with symptom provocation in eating disorders. *Am. J. Psychiat.* **2004**, *161*, 1238–1246. [CrossRef] [PubMed]
28. Scaife, J.C.; Godier, L.R.; Reinecke, A.; Harmer, C.J.; Park, R.J. Differential activation of the frontal pole to high vs low calorie foods: The neural basis of food preference in Anorexia Nervosa? *Psychiat. Res. Neuroimag.* **2016**, *258*, 44–53. [CrossRef] [PubMed]
29. Brooks, S.J.; O'Daly, O.; Uher, R.; Friederich, H.C.; Giampietro, V.; Brammer, M.; Williams, S.C.; Schioth, H.B.; Treasure, J.; Campbell, I.C. Thinking about eating food activates visual cortex with reduced bilateral cerebellar activation in females with anorexia nervosa: An fMRI study. *PLoS ONE* **2012**, *7*, e34000. [CrossRef]
30. Kim, K.R.; Ku, J.; Lee, J.-H.; Lee, H.; Jung, Y.-C. Functional and effective connectivity of anterior insula in anorexia nervosa and bulimia nervosa. *Neurosci. Lett.* **2012**, *521*, 152–157. [CrossRef]
31. Uher, R.; Brammer, M.J.; Murphy, T.; Campbell, I.C.; Ng, V.W.; Williams, S.C.R.; Treasure, J. Recovery and chronicity in anorexia nervosa: Brain activity associated with differential outcomes. *Biol. Psychiat.* **2003**, *54*, 934–942. [CrossRef]
32. Cowdrey, F.A.; Park, R.J.; Harmer, C.J.; McCabe, C. Increased neural processing of rewarding and aversive food stimuli in recovered anorexia nervosa. *Biol. Psychiatry* **2011**, *70*, 736–743. [CrossRef] [PubMed]
33. Rothemund, Y.; Buchwald, C.; Georgiewa, P.; Bohner, G.; Bauknecht, H.C.; Ballmaier, M.; Klapp, B.F.; Klingebiel, R. Compulsivity predicts fronto striatal activation in severely anorectic individuals. *Neuroscience* **2011**, *197*, 242–250. [CrossRef] [PubMed]
34. Giel, K.E.; Friederich, H.C.; Teufel, M.; Hautzinger, M.; Enck, P.; Zipfel, S. Attentional processing of food pictures in individuals with anorexia nervosa—An eye-tracking study. *Biol. Psychiat.* **2011**, *69*, 661–667. [CrossRef]
35. Foerde, K.; Steinglass, J.E.; Shohamy, D.; Walsh, B.T. Neural mechanisms supporting maladaptive food choices in anorexia nervosa. *Nat. Neurosci.* **2015**, *18*, 1571–1573. [CrossRef] [PubMed]
36. Tricomi, E.; Balleine, B.W.; O'Doherty, J.P. A specific role for posterior dorsolateral striatum in human habit learning. *Eur. J. Neurosci.* **2009**, *29*, 2225–2232. [CrossRef] [PubMed]
37. Horndasch, S.; Roesch, J.; Forster, C.; Dorfler, A.; Lindsiepe, S.; Heinrich, H.; Graap, H.; Moll, G.H.; Kratz, O. Neural processing of food and emotional stimuli in adolescent and adult anorexia nervosa patients. *PLoS ONE* **2018**, *13*, e0191059. [CrossRef] [PubMed]
38. Kinnaird, E.; Stewart, C.; Tchanturia, K. Taste sensitivity in anorexia nervosa: A systematic review. *Int. J. Eat. Disord.* **2018**, *51*, 771–784. [CrossRef] [PubMed]
39. Brand-Gothelf, A.; Parush, S.; Eitan, Y.; Admoni, S.; Gur, E.; Stein, D. Sensory modulation disorder symptoms in anorexia nervosa and bulimia nervosa: A pilot study. *Int. J. Eat. Disord.* **2016**, *49*, 59–68. [CrossRef]
40. Frank, G.K.W.; Shott, M.E.; Keffler, C.; Cornier, M.A. Extremes of eating are associated with reduced neural taste discrimination. *Int. J. Eat. Disord.* **2016**, *49*, 603–612. [CrossRef]
41. Wagner, A.; Aizenstein, H.; Mazurkewicz, L.; Fudge, J.; Frank, G.K.; Putnam, K.; Bailer, U.F.; Fischer, L.; Kaye, W.H. Altered Insula Response to Taste Stimuli in Individuals Recovered from Restricting-Type Anorexia Nervosa. *Neuropsychopharmacology* **2008**, *33*, 513–523. [CrossRef]
42. Monteleone, A.M.; Monteleone, P.; Esposito, F.; Prinster, A.; Volpe, U.; Cantone, E.; Pellegrino, F.; Canna, A.; Milano, W.; Aiello, M.; et al. Altered processing of rewarding and aversive basic taste stimuli in symptomatic women with anorexia nervosa and bulimia nervosa: An fMRI study. *J. Psychiatr. Res.* **2017**, *90*, 94–101. [CrossRef] [PubMed]
43. Frank, G.K.W.; DeGuzman, M.C.; Shott, M.E.; Laudenslager, M.L.; Rossi, B.; Pryor, T. Association of Brain Reward Learning Response with Harm Avoidance, Weight Gain, and Hypothalamic Effective Connectivity in Adolescent Anorexia Nervosa. *JAMA Psychiat.* **2018**, *75*, 1071–1080. [CrossRef] [PubMed]
44. Frank, G.K.W.; Reynolds, J.R.; Shott, M.E.; Jappe, L.; Yang, T.T.; Tregellas, J.R.; O'Reilly, R.C. Anorexia Nervosa and Obesity are Associated with Opposite Brain Reward Response. *Neuropsychopharmacology* **2012**, *37*, 2031–2046. [CrossRef]
45. Zald, D.H.; Lee, J.T.; Fluegel, K.W.; Pardo, J.V. Aversive gustatory stimulation activates limbic circuits in humans. *Brain* **1998**, *121*, 1143–1154. [CrossRef] [PubMed]

46. Horndasch, S.; O'Keefe, S.; Lamond, A.; Brown, K.; McCabe, C. Increased anticipatory but decreased consummatory brain responses to food in sisters of anorexia nervosa patients. *BJPsych Open* **2016**, *2*, 255–261. [CrossRef]
47. Berridge, K.C.; Kringelbach, M.L. Pleasure Systems in the Brain. *Neuron* **2015**, *86*, 646–664. [CrossRef] [PubMed]
48. Sodersten, P.; Bergh, C.; Leon, M.; Zandian, M. Dopamine and anorexia nervosa. *Neurosci. Biobehav. Rev.* **2016**, *60*, 26–30. [CrossRef]
49. Keating, C. Theoretical perspective on anorexia nervosa: The conflict of reward. *Neurosci. Biobehav. Rev.* **2010**, *34*, 73–79. [CrossRef]
50. Keating, C.; Tilbrook, A.J.; Rossell, S.L.; Enticott, P.G.; Fitzgerald, P.B. Reward processing in anorexia nervosa. *Neuropsychologia* **2012**, *50*, 567–575. [CrossRef]
51. Santel, S.; Baving, L.; Krauel, K.; Munte, T.F.; Rotte, M. Hunger and satiety in anorexia nervosa: fMRI during cognitive processing of food pictures. *Brain Res.* **2006**, *1114*, 138–148. [CrossRef]
52. Gizewski, E.R.; Rosenberger, C.; de Greiff, A.; Moll, A.; Senf, W.; Wanke, I.; Forsting, M.; Herpertz, S. Influence of satiety and subjective valence rating on cerebral activation patterns in response to visual stimulation with high-calorie stimuli among restrictive anorectic and control women. *Neuropsychobiology* **2010**, *62*, 182–192. [CrossRef] [PubMed]
53. Holsen, L.M.; Lawson, E.A.; Blum, J.; Ko, E.; Makris, N.; Fazeli, P.K.; Klibanski, A.; Goldstein, J.M. Food motivation circuitry hypoactivation related to hedonic and nonhedonic aspects of hunger and satiety in women with active anorexia nervosa and weight-restored women with anorexia nervosa. *J. Psychiat. Neurosci.* **2012**, *37*, 322–332. [CrossRef] [PubMed]
54. Hummel, D.; Rudolf, A.K.; Brandi, M.L.; Untch, K.H.; Grabhorn, R.; Hampel, H.; Mohr, H.M. Neural adaptation to thin and fat bodies in the fusiform body area and middle occipital gyrus: An fMRI adaptation study. *Hum. Brain Mapp.* **2013**, *34*, 3233–3246. [CrossRef] [PubMed]
55. Schienle, A.; Schafer, A.; Hermann, A.; Rohrmann, S.; Vaitl, D. Symptom provocation and reduction in patients suffering from spider phobia: An fMRI study on exposure therapy. *Eur. Arch. Psychiat. Clin. Neurosci.* **2007**, *257*, 486–493. [CrossRef] [PubMed]
56. Boehm, I.; Finke, B.; Tam, F.I.; Fittig, E.; Scholz, M.; Gantchev, K.; Roessner, V.; Ehrlich, S. Effects of perceptual body image distortion and early weight gain on long-term outcome of adolescent anorexia nervosa. *Eur. Child Adolesc. Psychiat.* **2016**, *25*, 1319–1326. [CrossRef] [PubMed]
57. van Koningsbruggen, M.G.; Peelen, M.V.; Downing, P.E. A causal role for the extrastriate body area in detecting people in real-world scenes. *J. Neurosci.* **2013**, *33*, 7003–7010. [CrossRef] [PubMed]
58. Friederich, H.-C.; Uher, R.; Brooks, S.; Giampietro, V.; Brammer, M.; Williams, S.C.R.; Herzog, W.; Treasure, J.; Campbell, I.C. I'm not as slim as that girl: Neural bases of body shape self-comparison to media images. *Neuroimage* **2007**, *37*, 674–681. [CrossRef]
59. Sachdev, P.; Mondraty, N.; Wen, W.; Gulliford, K. Brains of anorexia nervosa patients process self-images differently from non-self-images: An fMRI study. *Neuropsychologia* **2008**, *46*, 2161–2168. [CrossRef]
60. Uher, R.; Murphy, T.; Friederich, H.C.; Dalgleish, T.; Brammer, M.J.; Giampietro, V.; Phillips, M.L.; Andrew, C.M.; Ng, V.W.; Williams, S.C.; et al. Functional neuroanatomy of body shape perception in healthy and eating-disordered women. *Biol. Psychiat.* **2005**, *58*, 990–997. [CrossRef]
61. Wagner, A.; Ruf, M.; Braus, D.F.; Schmidt, M.H. Neuronal activity changes and body image distortion in anorexia nervosa. *Neuroreport* **2003**, *14*, 2193–2197. [CrossRef]
62. Gaudio, S.; Quattrocchi, C.C. Neural basis of a multidimensional model of body image distortion in anorexia nervosa. *Neurosci. Biobehav. Rev.* **2012**, *36*, 1839–1847. [CrossRef] [PubMed]
63. Vocks, S.; Busch, M.; Gronemeyer, D.; Schulte, D.; Herpertz, S.; Suchan, B. Neural correlates of viewing photographs of one's own body and another woman's body in anorexia and bulimia nervosa: An fMRI study. *J. Psychiat. Neurosci.* **2010**, *35*, 163–176. [CrossRef]
64. Friederich, H.-C.; Brooks, S.; Uher, R.; Campbell, I.C.; Giampietro, V.; Brammer, M.; Williams, S.C.R.; Herzog, W.; Treasure, J. Neural correlates of body dissatisfaction in anorexia nervosa. *Neuropsychologia* **2010**, *48*, 2878–2885. [CrossRef] [PubMed]
65. Seeger, G.; Braus, D.F.; Ruf, M.; Goldberger, U.; Schmidt, M.H. Body image distortion reveals amygdala activation in patients with anorexia nervosa—A functional magnetic resonance imaging study. *Neurosci. Lett.* **2002**, *326*, 25–28. [CrossRef]

66. Fladung, A.K.; Gron, G.; Grammer, K.; Herrnberger, B.; Schilly, E.; Grasteit, S.; Wolf, R.C.; Walter, H.; von Wietersheim, J. A neural signature of anorexia nervosa in the ventral striatal reward system. *Am. J. Psychiat.* **2010**, *167*, 206–212. [CrossRef] [PubMed]
67. Suchan, B.; Bauser, D.S.; Busch, M.; Schulte, D.; Gronemeyer, D.; Herpertz, S.; Vocks, S. Reduced connectivity between the left fusiform body area and the extrastriate body area in anorexia nervosa is associated with body image distortion. *Behav. Brain Res.* **2013**, *241*, 80–85. [CrossRef] [PubMed]
68. Kodama, N.; Moriguchi, Y.; Takeda, A.; Maeda, M.; Ando, T.; Kikuchi, H.; Gondo, M.; Adachi, H.; Komaki, G. Neural correlates of body comparison and weight estimation in weight-recovered anorexia nervosa: A functional magnetic resonance imaging study. *Biopsychosoc. Med.* **2018**, *12*, 15. [CrossRef]
69. Castellini, G.; Polito, C.; Bolognesi, E.; D'Argenio, A.; Ginestroni, A.; Mascalchi, M.; Pellicano, G.; Mazzoni, L.N.; Rotella, F.; Faravelli, C.; et al. Looking at my body. Similarities and differences between anorexia nervosa patients and controls in body image visual processing. *Eur. Psychiat.* **2013**, *28*, 427–435. [CrossRef]
70. Mohr, H.M.; Zimmermann, J.; Roder, C.; Lenz, C.; Overbeck, G.; Grabhorn, R. Separating two components of body image in anorexia nervosa using fMRI. *Psychol. Med.* **2010**, *40*, 1519–1529. [CrossRef]
71. Reynolds, J.R.; O'Reilly, R.C.; Cohen, J.D.; Braver, T.S. The function and organization of lateral prefrontal cortex: A test of competing hypotheses. *PLoS ONE* **2012**, *7*, e30284. [CrossRef]
72. Nieuwenhuys, R. The insular cortex: A review. *Prog. Brain Res.* **2012**, *195*, 123–163. [CrossRef] [PubMed]
73. Treasure, J.; Schmidt, U. The cognitive-interpersonal maintenance model of anorexia nervosa revisited: A summary of the evidence for cognitive, socio-emotional and interpersonal predisposing and perpetuating factors. *J. Eat. Disord.* **2013**, *1*, 13. [CrossRef] [PubMed]
74. Haynos, A.F.; Fruzzetti, A.E. Anorexia nervosa as a disorder of emotion dysregulation: Evidence and treatment implications. *Clin.l Psychol.* **2011**, *18*, 183–202. [CrossRef]
75. Racine, S.E.; Wildes, J.E. Emotion dysregulation and symptoms of anorexia nervosa: The unique roles of lack of emotional awareness and impulse control difficulties when upset. *Int. J. Eat. Disord.* **2013**, *46*, 713–720. [CrossRef] [PubMed]
76. Brockmeyer, T.; Holtforth, M.G.; Bents, H.; Kammerer, A.; Herzog, W.; Friederich, H.C. Starvation and emotion regulation in anorexia nervosa. *Compr. Psychiat.* **2012**, *53*, 496–501. [CrossRef]
77. Schmidt, U.; Treasure, J. Anorexia nervosa: Valued and visible. A cognitive-interpersonal maintenance model and its implications for research and practice. *Br. J. Clin. Psychol.* **2006**, *45*, 343–366. [CrossRef] [PubMed]
78. Lavender, J.M.; Wonderlich, S.A.; Engel, S.G.; Gordon, K.H.; Kaye, W.H.; Mitchell, J.E. Dimensions of emotion dysregulation in anorexia nervosa and bulimia nervosa: A conceptual review of the empirical literature. *Clin. Psychol. Rev.* **2015**, *40*, 111–122. [CrossRef]
79. Oldershaw, A.; Hambrook, D.; Stahl, D.; Tchanturia, K.; Treasure, J.; Schmidt, U. The socio-emotional processing stream in Anorexia Nervosa. *Neurosci. Biobehav. Rev.* **2011**, *35*, 970–988. [CrossRef]
80. Stroe-Kunold, E.; Friederich, H.C.; Stadnitski, T.; Wesche, D.; Herzog, W.; Schwab, M.; Wild, B. Emotional Intolerance and Core Features of Anorexia Nervosa: A Dynamic Interaction during Inpatient Treatment? Results from a Longitudinal Diary Study. *PLoS ONE* **2016**, *11*, e0154701. [CrossRef]
81. Engel, S.G.; Wonderlich, S.A.; Crosby, R.D.; Mitchell, J.E.; Crow, S.; Peterson, C.B.; Le Grange, D.; Simonich, H.K.; Cao, L.; Lavender, J.M.; et al. The role of affect in the maintenance of anorexia nervosa: Evidence from a naturalistic assessment of momentary behaviors and emotion. *J. Abnorm. Psychol.* **2013**, *122*, 709–719. [CrossRef]
82. Wildes, J.E.; Marcus, M.D.; Bright, A.C.; Dapelo, M.M.; Psychol, M.C. Emotion and eating disorder symptoms in patients with anorexia nervosa: An experimental study. *Int. J. Eat. Disord.* **2012**, *45*, 876–882. [CrossRef] [PubMed]
83. Weinbach, N.; Sher, H.; Bohon, C. Differences in Emotion Regulation Difficulties Across Types of Eating Disorders During Adolescence. *J. Abnorm. Child Psychol.* **2018**, *46*, 1351–1358. [CrossRef] [PubMed]
84. Harrison, A.; Sullivan, S.; Tchanturia, K.; Treasure, J. Emotional functioning in eating disorders: Attentional bias, emotion recognition and emotion regulation. *Psychol. Med.* **2010**, *40*, 1887–1897. [CrossRef] [PubMed]
85. Fonville, L.; Giampietro, V.; Surguladze, S.; Williams, S.; Tchanturia, K. Increased BOLD signal in the fusiform gyrus during implicit emotion processing in anorexia nervosa. *Neuroimage Clin.* **2014**, *4*, 266–273. [CrossRef]

86. Cowdrey, F.A.; Harmer, C.J.; Park, R.J.; McCabe, C. Neural responses to emotional faces in women recovered from anorexia nervosa. *Psychiat. Res.* **2012**, *201*, 190–195. [CrossRef]
87. Rangaprakash, D.; Bohon, C.; Lawrence, K.E.; Moody, T.; Morfini, F.; Khalsa, S.S.; Strober, M.; Feusner, J.D. Aberrant Dynamic Connectivity for Fear Processing in Anorexia Nervosa and Body Dysmorphic Disorder. *Front. Psychiat.* **2018**, *9*, 273. [CrossRef]
88. Rowsell, M.; MacDonald, D.E.; Carter, J.C. Emotion regulation difficulties in anorexia nervosa: Associations with improvements in eating psychopathology. *J. Eat. Disord.* **2016**, *4*, 17. [CrossRef]
89. Leppanen, J.; Cardi, V.; Paloyelis, Y.; Simmons, A.; Tchanturia, K.; Treasure, J. FMRI Study of Neural Responses to Implicit Infant Emotion in Anorexia Nervosa. *Front. Psychol.* **2017**, *8*, 780. [CrossRef]
90. Menon, V.; Uddin, L.Q. Saliency, switching, attention and control: A network model of insula function. *Brain Struct. Funct.* **2010**, *214*, 655–667. [CrossRef]
91. McAdams, C.J.; Lohrenz, T.; Montague, P.R. Neural responses to kindness and malevolence differ in illness and recovery in women with anorexia nervosa. *Hum. Brain Mapp.* **2015**, *36*, 5207–5219. [CrossRef]
92. Via, E.; Soriano-Mas, C.; Sanchez, I.; Forcano, L.; Harrison, B.J.; Davey, C.G.; Pujol, J.; Martinez-Zalacain, I.; Menchon, J.M.; Fernandez-Aranda, F.; et al. Abnormal Social Reward Responses in Anorexia Nervosa: An fMRI Study. *PLoS ONE* **2015**, *10*, e0133539. [CrossRef] [PubMed]
93. Treasure, J.; Cardi, V. Anorexia Nervosa, Theory and Treatment: Where Are We 35 Years on from Hilde Bruch's Foundation Lecture? *Europ. Eat. Disord. Rev.* **2017**, *25*, 139–147. [CrossRef] [PubMed]
94. Maier, S.; Spiegelberg, J.; van Zutphen, L.; Zeeck, A.; Tebartz van Elst, L.; Hartmann, A.; Holovics, L.; Reinert, E.; Sandholz, A.; Lahmann, C.; et al. Neurobiological signature of intimacy in anorexia nervosa. *Europ. Eat. Disord. Rev.* **2019**, *27*, 315–322. [CrossRef] [PubMed]
95. Miyake, Y.; Okamoto, Y.; Onoda, K.; Shirao, N.; Okamoto, Y.; Yamawaki, S. Brain activation during the perception of stressful word stimuli concerning interpersonal relationships in anorexia nervosa patients with high degrees of alexithymia in an fMRI paradigm. *Psychiat. Res.* **2012**, *201*, 113–119. [CrossRef] [PubMed]
96. Schulte-Ruther, M.; Mainz, V.; Fink, G.R.; Herpertz-Dahlmann, B.; Konrad, K. Theory of mind and the brain in anorexia nervosa: Relation to treatment outcome. *J. Am. Acad. Child Adolesc. Psychiat.* **2012**, *51*, 832–841.e11. [CrossRef] [PubMed]
97. Strober, M.; Freeman, R.; Morrell, W. The long-term course of severe anorexia nervosa in adolescents: Survival analysis of recovery, relapse, and outcome predictors over 10–15 years in a prospective study. *Int. J. Eat. Disord.* **1997**, *22*, 339–360. [CrossRef]
98. Lock, J. Evaluation of family treatment models for eating disorders. *Curr. Opin. Psychiat.* **2011**, *24*, 274–279. [CrossRef]
99. Davies, H.; Fox, J.; Naumann, U.; Treasure, J.; Schmidt, U.; Tchanturia, K. Cognitive remediation and emotion skills training for anorexia nervosa: An observational study using neuropsychological outcomes. *Europ. Eat. Disord. Rev.* **2012**, *20*, 211–217. [CrossRef]
100. Seidel, M.; King, J.A.; Ritschel, F.; Boehm, I.; Geisler, D.; Bernardoni, F.; Beck, M.; Pauligk, S.; Biemann, R.; Strobel, A.; et al. Processing and regulation of negative emotions in anorexia nervosa: An fMRI study. *Neuroimage Clin.* **2018**, *18*, 1–8. [CrossRef]
101. Seidel, M.; King, J.A.; Ritschel, F.; Boehm, I.; Geisler, D.; Bernardoni, F.; Holzapfel, L.; Diestel, S.; Diers, K.; Strobel, A.; et al. The real-life costs of emotion regulation in anorexia nervosa: A combined ecological momentary assessment and fMRI study. *Transl. Psychiat.* **2018**, *8*, 28. [CrossRef]
102. Swanson, S.A.; Crow, S.J.; Le Grange, D.; Swendsen, J.; Merikangas, K.R. Prevalence and correlates of eating disorders in adolescents. Results from the national comorbidity survey replication adolescent supplement. *Arch. Gen. Psychiat.* **2011**, *68*, 714–723. [CrossRef]
103. Godart, N.; Radon, L.; Curt, F.; Duclos, J.; Perdereau, F.; Lang, F.; Venisse, J.L.; Halfon, O.; Bizouard, P.; Loas, G.; et al. Mood disorders in eating disorder patients: Prevalence and chronology of ONSET. *J. Affect. Disord.* **2015**, *185*, 115–122. [CrossRef] [PubMed]
104. Visted, E.; Vollestad, J.; Nielsen, M.B.; Schanche, E. Emotion Regulation in Current and Remitted Depression: A Systematic Review and Meta-Analysis. *Front. Psychol.* **2018**, *9*, 756. [CrossRef] [PubMed]
105. Barrett, L.F.; Simmons, W.K. Interoceptive predictions in the brain. *Nat. Rev. Neurosci.* **2015**, *16*, 419–429. [CrossRef] [PubMed]

106. Herbert, B.M.; Herbert, C.; Pollatos, O. On the Relationship Between Interoceptive Awareness and Alexithymia: Is Interoceptive Awareness Related to Emotional Awareness? *J. Personal.* **2011**, *79*, 1149–1175. [CrossRef] [PubMed]
107. Westwood, H.; Kerr-Gaffney, J.; Stahl, D.; Tchanturia, K. Alexithymia in eating disorders: Systematic review and meta-analyses of studies using the Toronto Alexithymia Scale. *J. Psychosom. Res.* **2017**, *99*, 66–81. [CrossRef]
108. MacLean, P.D. Psychosomatic disease and the "visceral brain"; recent developments bearing on the Papez theory of emotion. *Psychosom. Med.* **1949**, *11*, 338–353. [CrossRef]
109. Moriguchi, Y.; Komaki, G. Neuroimaging studies of alexithymia: Physical, affective, and social perspectives. *Biopsychosoc. Med.* **2013**, *7*, 8. [CrossRef]
110. Kerr, K.L.; Moseman, S.E.; Avery, J.A.; Bodurka, J.; Zucker, N.L.; Simmons, W.K. Altered Insula Activity during Visceral Interoception in Weight-Restored Patients with Anorexia Nervosa. *Neuropsychopharmacology* **2016**, *41*, 521–528. [CrossRef]
111. Strigo, I.A.; Matthews, S.C.; Simmons, A.N.; Oberndorfer, T.; Klabunde, M.; Reinhardt, L.E.; Kaye, W.H. Altered insula activation during pain anticipation in individuals recovered from anorexia nervosa: Evidence of interoceptive dysregulation. *Int. J. Eat. Disord.* **2013**, *46*, 23–33. [CrossRef]
112. Berner, L.A.; Simmons, A.N.; Wierenga, C.E.; Bischoff-Grethe, A.; Paulus, M.P.; Bailer, U.F.; Ely, A.V.; Kaye, W.H. Altered interoceptive activation before, during, and after aversive breathing load in women remitted from anorexia nervosa. *Psychol. Med.* **2018**, *48*, 142–154. [CrossRef] [PubMed]
113. Bischoff-Grethe, A.; Wierenga, C.E.; Berner, L.A.; Simmons, A.N.; Bailer, U.; Paulus, M.P.; Kaye, W.H. Neural hypersensitivity to pleasant touch in women remitted from anorexia nervosa. *Transl. Psychiat.* **2018**, *8*, 161. [CrossRef]
114. Petrovich, G.D. Learning and the motivation to eat: Forebrain circuitry. *Physiol. Behav.* **2011**, *104*, 582–589. [CrossRef] [PubMed]
115. Steward, T.; Menchon, J.M.; Jimenez-Murcia, S.; Soriano-Mas, C.; Fernandez-Aranda, F. Neural Network Alterations Across Eating Disorders: A Narrative Review of fMRI Studies. *Curr. Neuropharmacol.* **2018**, *16*, 1150–1163. [CrossRef]
116. Badoud, D.; Tsakiris, M. From the body's viscera to the body's image: Is there a link between interoception and body image concerns? *Neurosci. Biobehav. Rev.* **2017**, *77*, 237–246. [CrossRef]
117. Khalsa, S.S.; Craske, M.G.; Li, W.; Vangala, S.; Strober, M.; Feusner, J.D. Altered interoceptive awareness in anorexia nervosa: Effects of meal anticipation, consumption and bodily arousal. *Int. J. Eat. Disord.* **2015**, *48*, 889–897. [CrossRef]
118. Simon, D.; Adler, N.; Kaufmann, C.; Kathmann, N. Amygdala hyperactivation during symptom provocation in obsessive-compulsive disorder and its modulation by distraction. *Neuroimage Clin.* **2014**, *4*, 549–557. [CrossRef]
119. Jasinska, A.J.; Stein, E.A.; Kaiser, J.; Naumer, M.J.; Yalachkov, Y. Factors modulating neural reactivity to drug cues in addiction: A survey of human neuroimaging studies. *Neurosci. Biobehav. Rev.* **2014**, *38*, 1–16. [CrossRef] [PubMed]
120. Wittmann, A.; Schlagenhauf, F.; Guhn, A.; Lueken, U.; Elle, M.; Stoy, M.; Liebscher, C.; Bermpohl, F.; Fydrich, T.; Pfleiderer, B.; et al. Effects of Cognitive Behavioral Therapy on Neural Processing of Agoraphobia-Specific Stimuli in Panic Disorder and Agoraphobia. *Psychother. Psychosom.* **2018**, *87*, 350–365. [CrossRef]
121. Schulz, C.; Mothes-Lasch, M.; Straube, T. Automatic neural processing of disorder-related stimuli in social anxiety disorder: Faces and more. *Front. Psychol.* **2013**, *4*, 282. [CrossRef] [PubMed]
122. Poldrack, R.A. Can cognitive processes be inferred from neuroimaging data? *Trends Cogn. Sci.* **2006**, *10*, 59–63. [CrossRef] [PubMed]
123. Bulik, C.M.; Sullivan, P.F.; Fear, J.L.; Pickering, A. Outcome of anorexia nervosa: Eating attitudes, personality, and parental bonding. *Int. J. Eat. Disord.* **2000**, *28*, 139–147. [CrossRef]
124. Wagner, A.; Barbarich-Marsteller, N.C.; Frank, G.K.; Bailer, U.F.; Wonderlich, S.A.; Crosby, R.D.; Henry, S.E.; Vogel, V.; Plotnicov, K.; McConaha, C.; et al. Personality traits after recovery from eating disorders: Do subtypes differ? *Int. J. Eat. Disord.* **2006**, *39*, 276–284. [CrossRef] [PubMed]
125. Khalsa, S.S.; Portnoff, L.C.; McCurdy-McKinnon, D.; Feusner, J.D. What happens after treatment? A systematic review of relapse, remission, and recovery in anorexia nervosa. *J. Eat. Disord.* **2017**, *5*, 20. [CrossRef]

126. Hudson, J.I.; Hiripi, E.; Pope, H.G., Jr.; Kessler, R.C. The prevalence and correlates of eating disorders in the National Comorbidity Survey Replication. *Biol. Psychiat.* **2007**, *61*, 348–358. [CrossRef] [PubMed]
127. Hill, L.; Peck, S.K.; Wierenga, C.E.; Kaye, W.H. Applying neurobiology to the treatment of adults with anorexia nervosa. *J. Eat. Disord.* **2016**, *4*, 31. [CrossRef]
128. Wierenga, C.E.; Hill, L.; Knatz Peck, S.; McCray, J.; Greathouse, L.; Peterson, D.; Scott, A.; Eisler, I.; Kaye, W.H. The acceptability, feasibility, and possible benefits of a neurobiologically-informed 5-day multifamily treatment for adults with anorexia nervosa. *Int. J. Eat. Disord.* **2018**, *51*, 863–869. [CrossRef] [PubMed]

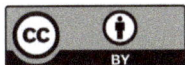

© 2019 by the authors. Licensee MDPI, Basel, Switzerland. This article is an open access article distributed under the terms and conditions of the Creative Commons Attribution (CC BY) license (http://creativecommons.org/licenses/by/4.0/).

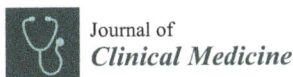 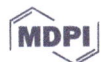

Review

Medication in AN: A Multidisciplinary Overview of Meta-Analyses and Systematic Reviews

Corinne Blanchet [1,2,3], Sébastien Guillaume [3,4,5], Flora Bat-Pitault [3,6,7], Marie-Emilie Carles [1], Julia Clarke [3,8,9], Vincent Dodin [3,10,11], Philibert Duriez [3,9,12], Priscille Gerardin [3,13,14], Mouna Hanachi-Guidoum [3,15,16], Sylvain Iceta [3,17,18], Juliane Leger [19,20,21], Bérénice Segrestin [3,17,22], Chantal Stheneur [3,23,24] and Nathalie Godart [3,16,25,26,*]

1. Maison de Solenn-Maison des Adolescents, Cochin Hospital, Assistance Publique-Hôpitaux de Paris, 75014 Paris, France; corinne.blanchet@aphp.fr (C.B.); marie-emilie.carles@aphp.fr (M.-E.C.)
2. CESP, INSERM 1178, Paris-Descartes University, USPC, 75014 Paris, France
3. French Federation Anorexia Bulimia (FFAB), 75014 Paris, France; s-guillaume@chu-montpellier.fr (S.G.); flora.bat@ap-hm.fr (F.B.-P.); julia.clarke@aphp.fr (J.C.); dodin.vincent@ghicl.net (V.D.); phduriez@gmail.com (P.D.); priscille.gerardin@chu-rouen.fr (P.G.); mouna.hanachi@aphp.fr (M.H.-G.); sylvain.iceta@chu-lyon.fr (S.I.); berenice.segrestin@chu-lyon.fr (B.S.); chantal.stheneur@fsef.net (C.S.)
4. Department of Psychiatric Emergency & Acute Care, Lapeyronie Hospital, CHRU Montpellier, 34090 Montpellier, France
5. INSERM U1061, University of Montpellier, 34090 Montpellier, France
6. Child and Adolescent Psychopathology Unit, Salvator Hospital, Public Assistance-Marseille Hospitals, 13009 Marseille, France
7. Institut de la Timone, CNRS, Aix-Marseille University, 13005 Marseille, France
8. Child and Adolescent Psychiatry Department, Robert Debré Hospital, Assistance Publique-Hôpitaux de Paris, 75019 Paris, France
9. INSERM U894, Institute of Psychiatry and Neuroscience of Paris (IPNP), 75013 Paris, France
10. Clinique Médico-Psychologique, Neurosciences Hôpital Saint Vincent de Paul, 59000 Lille, France
11. Faculté de Médecine et de Maïeutique de Lille, 59800 Lille, France
12. Sainte-Anne Hospital (CMME), Paris Descartes University, 75014 Paris, France
13. Pôle universitaire de psychiatrie de l'enfant et de l'adolescent CH du Rouvray-CHU de Rouen, 76300 Rouen, France
14. CRFDP, UFR des Sciences de l'Homme et de la Société, Rouen University, 76130 Mont-Saint-Aignan, France
15. Clinical Nutrition Unit, Raymond Poincaré University Hospital, Assistance Publique-Hôpitaux de Paris, 92380 Garches, France
16. CESP, INSERM, UMR 1018, University Paris-Sud, UVSQ, University Paris-Saclay, 94800 Villejuif, France
17. Referral Center for Eating Disorder, Hospices Civils de Lyon, 69677 Bron, France
18. Equipe PSYR2, INSERM U1028, CNRS UMR5292, Université Lyon 1, 69002 Lyon, France
19. Pediatric Endocrinology Diabetology Department, Reference Centre for Endocrine Growth and Development Diseases, Robert Debré University Hospital, Assistance Publique-Hôpitaux de Paris, 75019 Paris, France; juliane.leger@aphp.fr
20. Paris Diderot University, Sorbonne Paris Cité, F-75019 Paris, France
21. Institut National de la Santé et de la Recherche Médicale (INSERM), UMR 1141, DHU Protect, F-75019 Paris, France
22. INSERM 1060, Laboratoire CARMEN, Centre de Recherche en Nutrition Humaine Rhône-Alpes, Claude Bernard University, Lyon 1, Pierre Bénite, 69310 Lyon, France
23. Centre Médical et Pédagogique, Fondation Santé des Etudiants de France, 91480 Varennes Jarcy, France
24. Faculté de Médecine, Université de Montréal, Quebec, QC H3C 3J7, Canada
25. Adolescent and Young Adult mental health department, Fondation Santé des Etudiants de France, 75014 Paris, France
26. UFR Simone Veil-Santé, 78690 Saint-Quentin en Yvelines, France
* Correspondence: nathalie.godart@fsef.net; Tel.: +33-6-2186-6601

Received: 15 January 2019; Accepted: 20 February 2019; Published: 25 February 2019

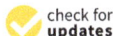

Abstract: Drugs are widely prescribed for anorexia nervosa in the nutritional, somatic, and psychiatric fields. There is no systematic overview in the literature, which simultaneously covers all these types of medication. The main aims of this paper are (1) to offer clinicians an overview of the evidence-based data in the literature concerning the medication (psychotropic drugs and medication for somatic and nutritional complications) in the field of anorexia nervosa since the 1960s, (2) to draw practical conclusions for everyday practise and future research. Searches were performed on three online databases, namely MEDLINE, Epistemonikos and Web of Science. Papers published between September 2011 and January 2019 were considered. Evidence-based data were identified from meta-analyses, if there were none, from systematic reviews, and otherwise from trials (randomized or if not open-label studies). Evidence-based results are scarce. No psychotropic medication has proved efficacious in terms of weight gain, and there is only weak data suggesting it can alleviate certain psychiatric symptoms. Concerning nutritional and somatic conditions, while there is no specific, approved medication, it seems essential not to neglect the interest of innovative therapeutic strategies to treat multi-organic comorbidities. In the final section we discuss how to use these medications in the overall approach to the treatment of anorexia nervosa.

Keywords: anorexia nervosa; drug-treatment; pharmacotherapy; medication; nutrition; comorbidity; complication

1. Introduction

Anorexia nervosa (AN) is a severe condition with high morbidity and mortality rates resulting from both somatic and psychiatric aspects of the disorder [1]. International guidelines recommend treatment based on a multidisciplinary approach, including nutritional, somatic, psychiatric, and social aspects [2–5]. This global treatment is mainly based on nutritional and psychotherapeutic approaches associated with the treatment of medical and socio-familial complications. In the National Institute for Health and Care Excellence (NICE) guidelines [4] it is clearly mentioned that medications cannot be seen as the sole treatment for anorexia nervosa (Number 1.3.24 see Table 1).

As stated by Aigner et al. [6] the treatment objectives in AN include weight gain, prevention of weight loss, a change in eating behaviours, reduction of associated psychopathologies (e.g., preoccupations with body image, depression, anxiety, obsessive compulsive symptoms) and the treatment of associated medical conditions (e.g., disturbances of the gonadal axis, infertility, osteoporosis). Medication for its part is used to treat AN symptoms including eating disorder symptoms (eating attitudes, refusal to gain weight, preoccupation about shape and weight, obsessions about food ...) and psychiatric symptoms (depression, anxiety, obsessions, and compulsions.). In addition, AN patients frequently have severe malnutrition and medical complications that can be treated by medication. Indeed, while the return to a normal weight by re-feeding associated with multidisciplinary care is crucial and enables the correction of many somatic functional disorders, it seems essential not to neglect the usefulness of somatic medication in limiting the short and long-term physical complications, optimizing quality of life and promoting a favourable outcome in all fields affected by AN (somatic, psychiatric and social).

In 2011 the World Federation of Societies of Biological Psychiatry (WFSBP) guidelines for the pharmacological treatment of eating disorders [6] concluded that the majority of the drugs to treat AN are used off-label [6]. These drugs are widely prescribed, but not in compliance with international guidelines [7,8], and can therefore be potentially unsafe for patients with AN.

For everyday practice, clinicians need improved recommendations about what medications can be used, for what purpose and in which conditions. Current guidelines give some indications for the use of different medications, but they lack precision and do not define who can be treated, when, and with which medication (as seen in Table 1, NICE recommendations for medication in AN). When clinicians try to find information in the literature, it is not easy, as there are numerous publications on the subject. For example, since the WFSBP guidelines were established for the pharmacological treatment of eating disorders, there have been around 300 reports on the topic of medication and AN, and no review covering all drugs used in the nutritional, somatic, and psychiatric fields.

The main aim of this work is to offer clinicians a multidisciplinary overview of the evidence-based published literature concerning drug treatments in the field of AN. This overview is based on the conclusions of meta-analyses, failing that on systematic reviews, and otherwise on trials (randomized or if not open-label studies). Unlike other reviews, this one is not restricted to drugs used to treat AN symptoms or psychiatric symptoms, but also includes the treatment of the medical conditions and the nutritional aspects associated with AN.

Table 1. Extract from the National Institute for Health and Care Excellence (NICE) recommendations [4] for medication in anorexia nervosa (chapter 1.3) and eating disorders in general including anorexia nervosa (chapter 1.8).

Recommendations
Medication for anorexia nervosa
1.3.24 Do not offer medication as the sole treatment for anorexia nervosa.
Dietary advice for people with anorexia nervosa [...]
1.3.21 Encourage people with anorexia nervosa to take an age-appropriate oral multi-vitamin and multi-mineral supplement until their diet includes enough to meet their dietary reference values.
Comorbid mental health problems
1.8.12 When deciding in which order to treat an eating disorder and a comorbid mental health condition (in parallel, as part of the same treatment plan or one after the other), take the following into account:
- The severity and complexity of the eating disorder and comorbidity.
- The person's level of functioning.
- The preferences of the person with the eating disorder and (if appropriate) those of their family members or carers.
1.8.13 Refer to the NICE guidelines on specific mental health problems for further guidance on treatment.
Medication risk management
1.8.14 When prescribing medication for people with an eating disorder, and comorbid mental or physical health conditions, take into account the impact that malnutrition and compensatory behaviours can have on medication effectiveness and the risk of side effects.
1.8.15 When prescribing for people with an eating disorder and comorbidity assess how the eating disorder will affect medication adherence (for example, for medication that can affect body weight).
1.8.16 When prescribing for people with an eating disorder, take into account the risks of medication that can compromise physical health due to pre-existing medical complications.
1.8.17 Offer electrocardiogram (ECG) monitoring for people with an eating disorder who are taking medication that could compromise cardiac functioning (including medication that could cause electrolyte imbalance, bradycardia below 40 beats per minute, hypokalaemia, or a prolonged QT interval).
Substance or medication misuse
1.8.18 For people with an eating disorder, who are misusing substances, or over-the-counter or prescribed medication, provide treatment for the eating disorder unless the substance misuse is interfering with this treatment.
1.8.19 If substance misuse or medication is interfering with treatment, consider a multidisciplinary approach with substance misuse services.
Growth and development
1.8.20 Seek specialist paediatric or endocrinology advice for delayed physical development or faltering growth in children and young people with an eating disorder.

2. Methods

A systematic literature search was performed on the topic of medication in AN in order to perform a systematic overview, according to the following method.

2.1. Data Sources and Search Strategies

Searches were performed on online databases, namely MEDLINE, Epistemonikos and Web of Science. Inclusion and exclusion criteria are described in Table 2.

Table 2. Inclusion and exclusion criteria for the systematic overview of systematic reviews, meta-analyses and selected trials (Population Intervention Control Outcome and Study design (PICOS) criteria and other elements).

Parameters	Inclusion Criteria	Exclusion Criteria
Patients	- AN [1] (with or without the mention of the restrictive or binging/purging types) - Human studies - All ages	- BN [2], BED [3], other ED [4] - Mixed eating disorder samples (AN and any other ED)
Interventions	- Medication for AN (psychotropic or somatic or nutritional)	- Medication for refeeding complications
Comparators	- All comparison groups (placebo or active drug or treatment as usual)	
Outcomes	- All criteria linked to ED symptoms, psychiatric -and somatic symptoms, and nutritional aspects, as appropriate	
Study design	- Meta-analyses and systematic reviews with a detailed methodology, including RCTs [5] and/or open trials	- Narrative or qualitative reviews - Overviews - Reviews of unpublished data
Period considered	- Papers published between September 2011 (since the publication of The World Federation of Societies of Biological Psychiatry Guidelines for the Pharmacological Treatment of Eating Disorders) [6] and 30th January 2019	
Language	- English and French	

[1] AN: Anorexia Nervosa; [2] BN: Bulimia Nervosa; [3] BED: Binge Eating Disorders; [4] ED: Eating Disorder; [5] RCT: Randomized Controlled Trial.

Only meta-analyses and systematic reviews with a detailed methodology were retained; narrative or qualitative reviews were excluded, as they provide elements only on some studies, and can be biased by a lack of information. We excluded studies that investigated mixed eating disorder groups, as their conclusions cannot be extended to AN.

The searches were complemented by a manual search: reference lists of articles were manually investigated to identify reviews or meta-analyses potentially relevant for inclusion that were not detected by electronic search.

The search strategies were conducted in two phases by two of the investigators (C.B., N.G.).

First, we defined a search in order to identify all reviews and meta-analyses published on the topic of drug treatments in AN with the following terms and algorithm, which, among the algorithms tested with different key words and combinations, proved to be the one that retrieved the largest corpus of papers: "anorexia nervosa and pharmacotherapy or drug treatment or medication or nutrition or enteral nutrition or weight restoration".

The search on the three databases previously mentioned selected 289 papers, 45 of which were reviews or meta-analyses on the topic (see Preferred Reporting Items for Systematic Reviews and Meta-Analyses (PRISMA) flow-chart Figure 1). Two further papers were identified by manual research.

Among the 45 reviews or meta-analyses, 26 were excluded for the following reasons: 16 were overviews and/or not systematic reviews with no explicit methodology for the selection of the papers mentioned [9–24], one review [25] predated the World Federation of Societies of Biological Psychiatry review, one [26] reviewed the same eight studies as a meta-analysis included [27], five focused on unpublished data, or studies that were reviewed in later papers included here [28–32], one mainly focused on emerging treatment research or perspectives [33], two concerned oxytocin but with no specific results in AN [34,35].

The 19 selected papers (15 systematic reviews and four meta-analyses) are presented in Table 3.

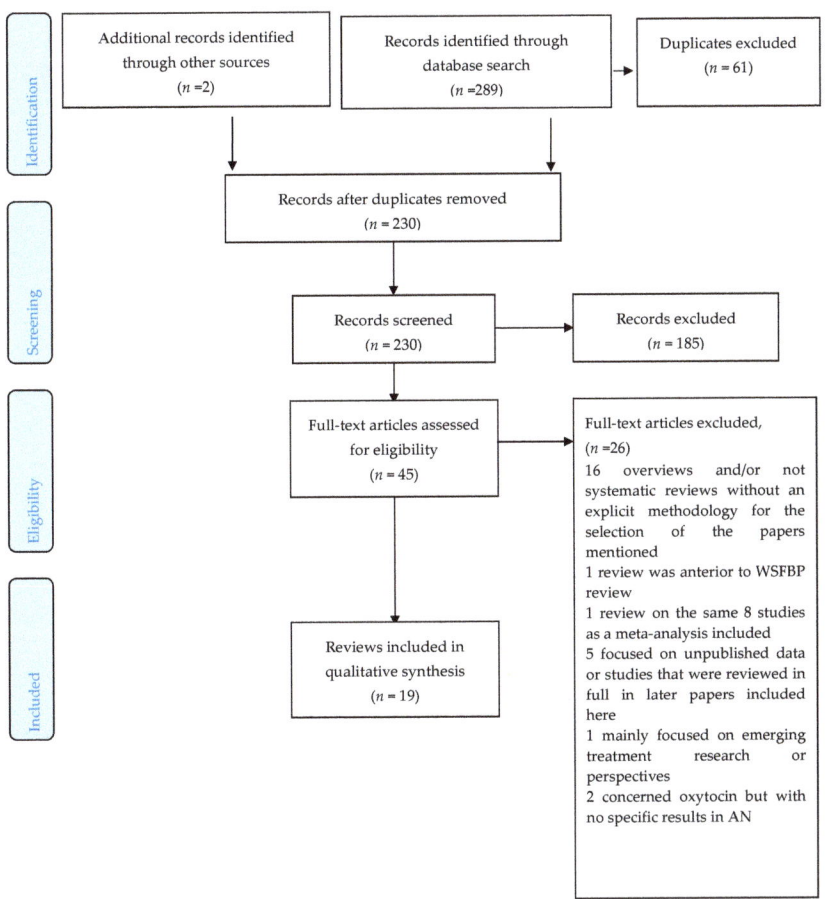

Figure 1. Preferred Reporting Items for Systematic Reviews and Meta-Analyses (PRISMA) Flow Diagram [36].

Table 3. Meta-analyses and systematic reviews selected.

Author	Year	Method	Database	Type of Study	Participant Age	Review Period from	Review Period to	Medication
Aigner, M. et al. [6]	2011	Systematic review	MEDLINE	45 studies = 19 open or case studies 26 RCTs	All	1977	2011	Antidepressants; Antipsychotics (typical and atypical); Prokinetic agents; Cannabinoids; Antihistaminics; Naltrexone; Clonidine; Tube feeding; Lithium; Growth Hormone; Zinc
Flament, M. et al. [37]	2012	Systematic review	MEDLINE; PsycINFO	11 RCTs; if none were available (e.g. for paediatric EDs) open trials or case reports suggesting benefits; systemic reviews; meta-analyses; and guidelines	All	1960	May 2010	Antidepressants; Antipsychotics (typical and atypical); Mood stabilizers and anticonvulsivants; Prokinetic agents; Opiate agonists; Appetite enhancers
Kishi, T. et al. [27]	2012	Meta-analysis	PubMed; PsycINFO; Cochrane	8 RCTs	All	No limitation	March 2012	Antipsychotics (typical and atypical)
Lebow et al. [38]	2013	Meta-analysis	Cochrane; MEDLINE; Embase; Scopus; Web of Science; PsychINFO	8 RCTs on atypical antipsychotics (in any form, used for at least 4 weeks) compared to any control intervention on BMI, eating disorder, and psychiatric symptoms in adolescents and adults with AN Eligible studies assessed BMI before, during, and/or after treatment. We excluded studies that enrolled patients who had a primary psychotic disorder.	All	1998	November 2011	Atypical antipsychotics
Lebow, J. et al. [39]	2013	Systematic review	Not reported	10 studies = 8 RCTs, 2 prospective cohort studies	11–42.5 years	Not reported	Not reported	Estrogen therapies
Watson, T. et al. [40]	2013	Systematic review	MEDLINE; PsycINFO; The Cumulative Index to Nursing and Applied Health; Educational Resources Information Center; National Agricultural OnLine; Embase Scopus Access; Cochrane Collaboration libraries	32 RCTs	All	1960	October 2011	Antidepressants; Antipsychotics; Cyproheptadine; Recombinant human growth hormone (rhGH); Risedronate; Testosterone; Nasogastric tube
De Vos et al. [41]	2014	Meta-analysis	PubMed; PsycINFO; Embase; Cochrane Library	18 studies = (a) RCTs and (b) comparing pharmacotherapy with a placebo controlled condition and reported on (c) patients with Anorexia Nervosa and an age minimum of 12 years. Outcome was measured in (d) terms of weight gain	All	No limitation	October 2012	Antidepressants; Antipsychotics; Hormonal therapy
Rocks, T. et al. [42]	2014	Systematic review	PubMed; Scopus; Web of Science ClinicalTrials.gov; Clinicaltrialsregister.eu;	7 observational studies	≤19 years	No limitation	May 2012	Nutrition therapy
Dold et al. [43]	2015	Meta-analysis	Cochrane Central Register of Controlled Trials (CENTRAL); Embase; PubMed/MEDLINE; PsycINFO	7 RCTs second generation antipsychotics efficacy, acceptability, and tolerability in comparison to placebo/no treatment, even unpublished studies	All	No limitation	August 2014	Atypical antipsychotics

Table 3. Cont.

Author	Year	Method	Database	Type of Study	Participant Age	Review Period from	Review Period to	Medication
El Ghoch, M. et al. [44]	2016	Systematic review	PubMed	19 studies = 11 prospective non-controlled, 4 prospective controlled, 4 retrospective non-controlled	11–19 years	No limitation	No limitation	Weight gain and restoration
Frank, G.K. et al. [45]	2016	Systematic review	National Center for Biotechnology Information database	66 studies = 25 double-blind, placebo-controlled studies; 7 double-blind, placebo-controlled crossover studies; 5 single-blind, placebo-controlled studies; 23 open-label studies; and 6 retrospective systematic chart reviews	All	No limitation	2014	Antidepressants; Antipsychotics (typical and atypical); Mood Stabilizers; Zinc; Opiates and Cannabinoids; Benzodiazepines and Alpha 2 Adrenergics; D-Cycloserine; Amantadine; DHEA; Ghrelin; Growth Hormone; Testosterone; Estrogen
Garber, A.K. et al. [46]	2016	Systematic review	PubMed; Scopus; PsycINFO; Clinical trials database	27 studies = 1 RCT, 6 prospective, 14 retrospective, 6 observational	13–38 years	1960	15 March 2015	Refeeding approaches
Kells, M. et al. [47]	2016	Systematic review (integrative)	PubMed; Embase; Cochrane CINAHL	18 studies = 2 RCTs, 6 retrospective, 5 cohort, 1 observational, 4 case reports	11–57 years	No limitation	May 2016	Tube feeding
Miniati, M. et al. [48]	2016	Systematic review	MEDLINE; PsycINFO	41 studies = 17 RCTs, 9 open trials, 12 case series and case reports, 2 retrospective observations, 1 single-blind RCT	Adults	January 1966	January 2014	Antidepressants; Antipsychotics (typical and atypical); Lithium; Clonidine; Cyproheptadine
Misra, M. et al. [49]	2016	Systematic review	PubMed	20 studies = 10 RCTs, 8 prospective observational studies, 1 retrospective cohort study, 1 prospective study	11–45 years	1995	2015	Weight gain and restoration, Estrogen replacement therapy, recombinant h-GH, recombinant h-IgF1, DHEA, Biphosphonates, Teriparatide
Robinson, L. et al. [50]	2017	Systematic review	MEDLINE; PsycINFO; Embase; Cochrane Database	19 studies =10 double-blind RCTs, 2 prospective observational studies, 1 retrospective cohort study, 1 case-control study and 5 non-randomised control trials	All	No limitation	3 March 2017	DHEA, various OC (EE or EE/levonorgestrel or EE/ progestin or EE/Norgestimate), various oestrogen replacement treatments (transdermal 17βPE/progesterone or oral EE/progesterone), Teriparatide (TPt), Alendronate, rhIgF1, Menateterenone (MED) (vitamin K2), risedronate, transdermal testosterone
Brockmeyer, T. et al. [51]	2018	Systematic review	PubMed; Scopus; Web of Science	6 RCTs on medication (including one unpublished study)	All	October 2011 (post Watson 2012)	31 December 2016	Antipsychotics; Dronabinol; Tube feeding
Hale, M.D. et al. [52]	2018	Systematic review	PubMed; PsycINFO; CINAHL; Web of Science; Cochrane Library; Dissertations and Theses (ProQuest); Google Scholar	19 open, prospective RCTs, non-randomized controlled trials, prospective cohort studies, retrospective chart reviews	All	No limitation	September 2017	Tube feeding
Rizzo, S.M. et al. [53]	2018	Systematic review	PubMed; Scopus;Web of Science; PsycINFO	10 studies = 1 RCT, 1 prospective cohort study, 8 retrospective cohort studies	10–57 years	No limitation	May 2018	Enteral Nutrition via Nasogastric Tube

ED: Eating Disorder; BMI: Body Mass Index; EE: Ethinyl Estradiol; GH: Growth Hormone; OC: Oral Contraceptive; DHEA: Dehydroepiandrosterone; RCT(s): randomized controlled trial(s).

Secondly, the overview was completed by original research (RCTs, open studies as mentioned previously) published after the last review or meta-analysis reviewed. In addition, for nutritional and somatic aspects, as there was no meta-analysis nor systematic review on some of the subjects (vitamin D and calcium, micronutrients supplementation and functional digestive disorders), we reviewed published papers (RCTs, and if not open studies as mentioned previously), and retrospective or case studies if no other information existed on the topic of AN. For functional digestive disorders, as there were no papers about their treatment in the AN literature, reviews including this topic (in general and not in AN) were selected.

2.2. Study selection and Quality Assessment

From the French Anorexia and Bulimia Federation (http://www.anorexieboulimie-afdas.fr/), we recruited a group of eating disorder specialists participating on a voluntary basis, including nutritionists, an endocrinologist, an adolescent paediatrician, psychiatrists, and child and adolescent psychiatrists (see authors of the paper).

Eligible papers were screened in the literature search by their title and abstract by two reviewers working together (C.B. and N.G.). The papers were selected by agreement on the basis of the inclusion exclusion criteria (Table 2). Then, the screened papers (meta-analyses or systematic reviews) were read in full and again selected or not, according to inclusion and exclusion criteria. If there was any uncertainty regarding the eligibility of a paper, it was referred to the rest of team for further discussion.

Disagreements between reviewers were resolved by consensus; they mainly concerned the suitability of studies for the purpose of the review.

3. Results

3.1. Papers Selected

The 19 selected systematic reviews are presented in Table 3.

We gave priority here to meta-analyses and systematic reviews rather than to study reports, according to the following rules. For each topic, meta-analysis results are presented first when available. Then, if the meta-analyses only focused on a particular period or a specific question, or if there was no meta-analysis on the topic, the results of the more recent systematic reviews on the topic based on RCTs were described, and completed by previous ones if they provided more information. If reviews on the topic were not available, existing trials on the topic are reported, RCTs are reported in priority if available, if not open trials are reported. Study reports are only cited if they were not referenced in the cited meta-analyses or reviews and were published after the reviews (we did not take into account papers excluded from the reviews for methodological reasons).

We do not report on case reports, or retrospective chart studies, as they are based on the local practice of the teams involved, and are more a reflection of their practice than an evaluation of treatments. In case of numerous reviews or meta-analyses on a topic, results are completed by earlier reviews if they provide complementary information. When samples only involved adolescents, this is mentioned, and any specifics concerning the adolescents are also mentioned.

3.2. Results: Psychotropic Medications

3.2.1. Methodological Issues

The reviews and meta-analyses selected in this overview reviewed from six [51] to 66 studies [45] (see Table 3). This wide range results from numerous factors (aim of the review; types of study considered: ranging from only RCTs to all types of study; period; methodology for selection of studies: ranging from all published studies to a selection based on quality guidelines; type and number of databases used). For example, Brockmeyer et al. used the Cochrane Handbook and the National Institute of Heath Criteria for a quality assessment of controlled intervention studies [51] between October 2011 and the end of 2016 and selected only three good quality RCTs on psychotropic medication. Conversely, Franck et al. [45] were exhaustive and included all studies (except case reports) published in the past 50 years. Miniati et al. [48] underlined the impossibility of applying quality criteria to select studies in their review. In addition, samples were very different in terms of age (see Table 3), some focused on adolescents, others on adults, and some on both.

Psychotropic medications have been used since the 1960s to treat AN. For the studies included in the reviews, Miniati et al [48] underlined the paucity of reports, including the small number of RCTs, the small numbers of subjects included in the studies (one to maximum 93 in this review), the heterogeneity of sample composition, treatments, and treatment settings, and the small number of males to enable comparisons based on gender, which are all aspects that impact the conclusions.

The variable settings (inpatient/outpatient) had an impact on patient characteristics; for example in the studies, these authors observed that the age of inpatients was significantly younger than that of outpatients [48]. In addition, in cases of positive results in favour of a medication, the results had never been replicated. The conclusions of these studies were based on small samples and the fact that they derived no significant results could be partly explained by a lack of power; the results were often extrapolated across patient groups of different ages, illness durations, and severity. Another important limitation of these studies is their duration [48]. Most of the studies were based on short term follow-up in an illness requiring long-term management [48]. The majority of the studies were conducted on inpatient samples, whereas the majority of patients are treated on an ambulatory basis [48]. Not all symptom dimensions of AN, nor all the comorbidities, nor the impact of the medication on these elements were systematically reported.

A small number of studies specially focused on children and adolescents. The majority of the studies were conducted in the acute phase of AN and a minority in the maintenance phase [40]. Below we provide information in terms of dose, duration of treatment, and sample size, for comparative studies only.

3.2.2. Antidepressants (AD)

The rationale for treating AN with antidepressants was initially that AN and depression had clinical and biological similarities, including comorbidity and symptom overlap with anxiety disorders, obsessive compulsive disorders and depression, and a hypothetical dysfunction in the serotonergic and noradrenergic systems in the pathophysiology of AN. The earliest studies mostly concerned tricyclics and monoamine oxydase inhibitors and the more recent mostly concerned selective serotonin reuptake inhibitors (SSRI) [6,37,45,48]. We found one small meta-analysis [41] pooling two studies on tricyclics [54,55], two on selective serotonin reuptake inhibitors [56,57], and five reviews concerning each different class of antidepressant separately [6,37,40,45,48]. No other recent study was found.

Meta-analyses

The meta-analyses (see Table 3 for details) concerned all antidepressant RCTs versus placebo evaluating the impact on either weight restoration or maintenance, with various doses, durations and evaluation criteria. It pooled four RCTs. One was on clomipramine (50 mg, duration not mentioned, there were eight placebo subjects and there were eight AD subjects, evaluation criterion: weight gain in kg) [54], one was on amitriptyline (160 mg max, for 32–45 days, there were 25 placebo subjects, and 24 AD subjects, evaluation criterion: weight gain per day) [55]. Two were on fluoxetine [56,57] (respectively 60 mg and 20 to 60mg, for 7 weeks and 1 year, 16 placebo and 44 subjects, 15 AD and 49 subjects, evaluation criteria, respectively: ideal body weight and body mass index) involving 96 patients in the antidepressant groups and 94 patients in the placebo groups. No impact of antidepressants on weight gain or maintenance in AN was found [41]; because of the small sample sizes no meta regression or subgroup analyses were conducted.

Tricyclics

On the basis of an analysis of three RCTs versus placebo [45,48], there is no clear evidence for the general use of tricyclics among patients with AN in terms of weight gain and depressive symptoms, according to two studies on amitryptiline (160 mg max and 2.8 ± 0.3mg/kg, respectively for 32–45 days and five weeks, placebo 25 subjects and 11, AD 24 and 11 subjects, evaluation criteria: weight gain per day and weight plus psychological outcome) [58] and one with clomipramine (50 mg, 76 days clomipramine and 72 days placebo, placebo eight and AD eight subjects, evaluation criterion: weight gain in kg) [54,59]. These drugs only showed some impact on hunger, appetite, and energy intake at the beginning of treatment, but with no effect on weight, as mentioned previously. Although clomipramine tended in one study [54] to be associated with lower weight gain compared to the placebo, this was hypothesised to be linked to more physical activity. An open trial comparing paroxetine to clomipramine (respectively 18.4 ± 4.7 mg and 75.3 ± 7.6 mg, duration 39 ± 26 and 58 ± 30, 39 and AD 57 subjects, evaluation criteria: BMI, duration to weight gain) found no difference in terms of weight gain in an adolescent sample, but duration to obtain weight gain was significantly shorter for paroxetine (72 versus 97 days) [45,60]. In addition, because of the lethal risk with overdose in suicide attempts and the potential for fatal arrhythmia at low body weight, particularly among young subjects, this type of medication is no longer studied and is not recommended today for AN [6,37,40,45,48].

Selective Serotonin Reuptake Inhibitors (SSRIs)

There is today no clear evidence supporting the use of SSRIs in AN [48].

The three RCTs [56,57,61] on fluoxetine versus placebo provided controversial results (respectively 60 mg for the first and for the others 20 to 60mg, for seven weeks, one year, and 52 weeks, placebo 16, 44, and 16 subjects AD 15, 49, and 19 subjects). Most RCTs with placebo (2/3) reported negative results concerning the effect on eating psychopathology and weight gain [56] and on weight maintenance on a large sample at 12 months [45,48,57]. The only one that had positive results for the maintenance of weight at 12 months and for anxiety [61] had only 13 completers for the treatment and no associated psychological treatment [48]. Some authors hypothesised that fluoxetine inefficacy could be linked to malnutrition, and in particular, to a lack of dietary tryptophan. Tryptophan supplementation in addition to fluoxetine was evaluated in a double-blind controlled trial versus placebo (fluoxetine 20 to 60 mg, for six months, AD and placebo 11 subjects, AD with nutritional supplementation 15 subjects). Barbarich, et al. [62], did not show benefits from this supplementation on weight gain, anxiety or obsessive compulsive symptoms [45]. Three RCTs compared fluoxetine to nortriptyline, amineptine [63,64] (respectively for fluoxetine 60 mg, versus nortriptyline 75 mg, amineptine 300 mg for 16 weeks, 22 subjects and 13 subjects) or clomipramine / amisulpride [65] (respectively for fluoxetine 28 mg, clomipramine 58 mg/ amisulpride 50 mg for 12 weeks, 35 subjects), and failed to demonstrate any difference [40].

The effect of citalopram was only investigated in three open trials [66–68]. The authors of the third study with a control group (citalopram 20 mg, for 12 weeks, 19 subjects compared to 20 patients on a waiting list) found no improvement in terms of weight, but an improvement in depression, obsessive-compulsive symptoms, impulsiveness and trait-anger [48], and body dissatisfaction [45].

A small open-label study that compared sertraline with the placebo [69] reported that sertraline improved depressive symptoms, perceptions of ineffectiveness, a lack of interoceptive awareness, and perfectionism, but not weight gain [45]

Other Antidepressants

Monoamine oxydase inhibitors were evaluated in an open study among six patients for six weeks [70]. Mood and anxiety improved [45] but these drugs are no longer used, as a result of both their inefficacy on weight and their unfavourable side effect profile [48]. Venlaxine has only been studied in an open trial [71], in comparison with fluoxetine and in association with cognitive behavioural therapy, with no differences in weight or behaviour outcomes [45]. Mirtazapine and duloxetine used in AN have only been described in case reports on adults [48]. Concerning adolescents, mirtazapine was not found to be superior to other medications nor to no medication in AN [45].

In conclusion, antidepressants have no impact on weight gain [45,48], and their impact on eating symptoms or psychopathology is not clear. Tricyclics and monoamine oxydase inhibitors have adverse side effect profiles and should no longer be used in AN [45,48].

Antipsychotics

The rationale for treating AN with antipsychotics was initially linked to the hypothesis that obsessions regarding weight and body shape in AN (abnormal beliefs that are ego-syntonic and characterised by an acute lack of insight that persists even when the affected person's health status is endangered) could be viewed as delusional ideas and consequently could result from dopamine receptor hypersensitivity in AN [45]. Other arguments for their use in AN were based on the effect of these drugs on reward system regulation, their potential efficacy in controlling problematic frequency of physical activity (usually called hyperactivity in AN) and the weight gain side effects observed in other disorders [48]. Another recent argument is that second generation drugs also act on the salience network, known to be impaired in eating disorders, and that they could thus act by enhancing the reactivity of the anterior cingulate cortex and the salience network in the response to the reward value of food in AN. These drugs are mainly dopamine D2 and serotonin 5HT2A antagonists [71]. Finally, more recently, Frieling et al. [72] cited by Miniati et al. [48], have postulated the existence of an altered expression of the dopaminergic genes among patients exhibiting psychomotor hyperactivity. These drugs are dopamine D2 receptor antagonists with severe adverse effects. For second-generation drugs, the arguments also include positive effects on depression and anxiety symptoms arising from eating disorders [48]. First-generation antipsychotics (typical antipsychotics) and second-generation (atypical) antipsychotics have all been studied.

Four meta-analyses [27,38,41,43] and six reviews concerned each class of antipsychotic separately [6,37,40,45,48,51]. The reviews are considered for first-generation drugs, as they are mainly not included in meta-analyses, and also for second-generation drugs after 2012 (the most recent data in the meta-analyses). Since the end of the last review [48] five study reports have been published about antipsychotics in AN, two retrospective chart reviews on adults and adolescents with AN respectively [45] not reviewed here, one open-label study among adolescents [73] and one among adults [74] not reviewed here, and two RCTs [75,76]. Details concerning antipsychotic studies are presented in Table 4.

Table 4. Description of neuroleptics and antipsychotics studies [45,48].

Author	Study	Treatment Group	Daily Medication Dose	Length of Treatment	N	Mean Age ± SD (Years)	Results
Vandereycken and Pierloot, 1982	Double-blind placebo controlled crossover	pimozide placebo	4 to 6 mg	6 weeks	18	Non reported	Non-significant on weight gain
Vandereycken, [78] 1984	Double-blind placebo controlled crossover	sulpiride/placebo sequence placebo/sulpiride sequence	300 or 400 mg	2–3 weeks	99	23.2 ± 6.5 23.7 ± 9.6	Non-significant on weight gain
Ruggiero et al., [65] 2001	Open-label	clomipramine fluoxetine amisulpride	Mean= 57.7 ± 25.8 mg Mean = 26.0 ± 10.3 mg Mean = 50.0 ± 0.0 mg	3 months	10 13 12	23.7 ± 4.6 4.5 ± 5.1 24.3 ± 5.8	No significant difference between groups in term of weight gain significant increase for fluoxetine and amisulpride groups
Cassano et al., [79] 2003	Open label	haloperidol	Months 1–3 Mean = 1.2 ± 0.4 mg; Months 4–6 Mean = 1.1 ± 0.2 mg	6 months	13	22.8 ± 4.2	BMI increased significantly in chronic and treatment-resistant patients
Mondraty et al., [80] 2005	Double-blind placebo controlled	olanzapine chlorpromazine	10 mg 50 mg	Mean = 46 ± 31 days Mean = 53 ± 26 days	87 10	25.3 ± 7.42 5.3 ± 7.3	No significant difference in weight gain
Brambilla et al., [81] 2007a	Double-blind placebo controlled	olanzapine and cognitive behaviour therapy and nutritional rehabilitation placebo and cognitive behavioural therapy and nutritional rehabilitation	2.5 mg for 1 month; 5 mg for 2 months	3 months	10	23 ± 4.8	No difference for weight gain
Brambilla et al., [82] 2007b	Double-blind placebo controlled	olanzapine and cognitive behavioural therapy placebo and cognitive behavioural therapy	2.5 mg for 1 month; 5 mg for 2 months	3 months	15 15	23.7 ± 4.8 26.3 ± 8.5	No difference for weight gain between groups greater improvement on the Eating Disorder Inventory ineffectiveness and maturity fear scores in the olanzapine group
Bissada et al., [83] 2008	Double-blind placebo controlled	olanzapine placebo	Start : 2.5 mg; Max = 10 mg flexible dose regimen	10 weeks	16 18	23.6 ± 6.5 29.7 ± 11.6	Olanzapine: greater weight increase and faster achievement of weight goals
Attia et al., [84] 2011	Double-blind placebo controlled	olanzapine placebo	Start = 2.5 mg; Last 4 Weeks = 10 mg	8 weeks	11 12	27.7 ± 9.1	Olanzapine was associated with a small but significant increase in BMI compared to placebo
Kafantaris et al., [85] 2011	Double-blind placebo controlled	olanzapine and psychotherapy placebo and psychotherapy	Start = 2.5 mg; week 4 target = 10 mg	10 weeks	10 10	16.4 ± 2.2 18.1 ± 2.0	No significant difference in weight gain between groups
Hagman et al., [86] 2011	Double-blind placebo controlled	risperidone placebo	Mean = 2.5 ± 1.2 mg Mean = 3.0 ± 1.0 mg	17 weeks	18 2	16.2 ± 2.5 15.8 ± 2.3	No significant difference in weight gain between groups; the risperidone group showed greater reduction in drive for thinness over the first half of the study, but this was not sustained
Powers et al., [87] 2012	Double-blind placebo controlled	quetiapine placebo	Mean = 177.7 ± 90.8 mg	8 weeks	46	34 ± 14.5	No difference between quetiapine and placebo on weight, eating disorders, anxiety and depressive symptoms

BMI: Body Mass Index.

Meta-Analyses

The meta-analyses compared antipsychotics, mainly second-generation, to placebo in six to eight studies, but never exactly the same drugs, always with a majority of studies on olanzapine. 2/4 pooled first and second-generation antipsychotics [27,41], the two others only included second-generation drugs [38,43]. They concerned respectively:

- Eight RCTs (four on olanzapine [81,82], one on quetiapine [88], one on risperidone [86], one on pimoside [77] and one on sulpiride [78] versus placebo) with 102 subjects in the antipsychotic group and 114 in the comparator group (six placebo groups and one treatment-as-usual), one study [78] included one sample of adolescents, the last one [86] examined the effects on BMI, weight, glucose levels, depressive and anxiety symptoms, dropout rates from any cause, adverse effects, akathisia and drowsiness/sedation [27].

- Seven RCTs including five against placebo, four on olanzapine [81–84], one on risperidone [86], and two against chlorpromazine [80] or clomipramine or fluoxetine [65] with 72 subjects in the second-generation antipsychotic group and 75 in the comparator group, exploring weight gain and drive for thinness, body dissatisfaction, overall eating disorder symptoms and anxiety [38,43].

- Six RCTs (five on olanzapine [81,82,84,85] and one on sulpiride [78]), including one sample of adolescents [85], one with 73 subjects in the antipsychotic group and 72 in the placebo group, exploring weight post-treatment [41].

- Seven RCTs (four on olanzapine [81–84], two on quetiapine [87,88], and one on risperidone [86] with 91 subjects in the second-generation antipsychotic group and 99 in the placebo group, exploring BMI change, overall changes in anorectic symptoms, and number of dropouts [43].

No impact of antipsychotics was found in comparison to placebo on weight gain, whether antipsychotics were pooled or considered individually (evaluated in 4/4 meta-analyses), nor on eating disorder symptoms (evaluated in 3/4 meta-analyses [38]), nor was it found for akathisia [27], dropout [27], or glucose levels [27]. A recent paper by Attia et al. [76] reported an RCT on olanzapine increased to the maximum of 10 mg/day in four weeks compared to placebo. This study was conducted on a large sample of 152 adults AN (83 completers) with a long illness duration (mean age for placebo group 28 ± 10.9 and for olanzapine group 30.0 ± 11.0 years old and illness duration respectively 10.5 ± 9.5 and 12.6 ± 11.7). It showed a modest therapeutic effect of four months of olanzapine, compared with placebo on BMI (with an increase difference of 0.165 BMI points more per month). This study found no difference between groups in terms of clinical global impressions, obsessionality, anxiety and depressive symptoms, nor eating disorders symptoms (except an increase in shape concerns that was observed in the olanzapine group).

Drowsiness/sedation occurred significantly more often with antipsychotics than with placebo/usual care in the pooled analyses, and especially for olanzapine in an individual analysis [27]. Attia et al [76] found no significant differences in the frequency of the abnormal blood test to assess metabolic abnormalities between the olanzapine and placebo groups.

For the effect on anxiety and depressive symptoms, there was no apparent efficacy of antipsychotics according to the largest meta-analysis on the topic (pooling four studies) [27]. A recent small RCT study lasting three months among 30 adult outpatients with AN mentioned a superiority of Olanzapine (2.5 mg the first month and 5 mg the two following months) combined with cognitive behavioural therapy (CBT) versus placebo combined with CBT in improving obsessiveness-compulsivity, depression, anxiety and especially hostility (but not weight gain or specific aspects related to the AN eating pathology) without showing results [75].

Typical Antipsychotics other than those Explored in the Meta-Analyses

Haloperidol and chlorpromazine have generally not been evaluated in RCTs, and evidence levels for their efficacy and safety are poor [48]. Haloperidol as an adjunct to psychotherapy was found to be associated with weight over six months in one open study [45,48,79]. In an RCT, there was no difference in terms of weight gain between chlorpromazine and olanzapine [80] but olanzapine was superior for the reduction of anorexic ruminations [37].

Other Second-Generation Antipsychotics than those Explored in the Meta-Analyses

Amisulpride was studied in one study [45]. It was found to be superior to fluoxetine and clomipramine in a single blind RCT for weight gain (not for weight phobia, body image disturbance or amenorrhea) [65].

Aripiprazole was considered only in a case series of adults and young people [48].

In conclusion, according to the four meta-analyses considered here, antipsychotics had no impact on weight gain compared to placebo, and their impact on eating symptoms and psychopathology is not clear. Olanzapine had a modest effect on weight gain in one RCT including adults with a long duration of AN [76]. Typical antipsychotics have an adverse side effect profile and should not be used in AN, except perhaps haloperidol in severe AN [45]. Atypical antipsychotics could alleviate some symptoms, such anorexic ruminations, anxiety or depressive symptoms, but levels of evidence are low, and based only some small studies [75] and not supported by meta-analyses on the topic [27].

3.2.3. Lithium

The rationale for using lithium among patients with AN is mainly related to the fact that it induces weight gain in other disorders [37,48].

We found four reviews concerning lithium [6,37,48] all mentioning one RCT [89], but we found no other recent study.

This small RCT, involving lithium among adults (dose not mentioned, 16 patients and controls, evaluation criterion: weight gain at weeks three and four) showed a significant difference in terms of weight for the lithium-treated group, but not for other psychological dimensions [89]. However, the use of lithium is not recommended in AN, even for patients with severe and resistant forms. Sodium and fluid depletion are frequent in AN and could reduce lithium clearance, which could lead to lithium poisoning [45,48], as renal complications are frequent in AN [90].

3.2.4. Appetite Enhancers

Antihistamines

Four reviews [6,37,45,48] mentioned antihistamines but we did not find any more recent studies.

Cyproheptadine (CYP), a serotonin and histamine antagonist reputed to produce weight gain among children with asthma, was tested in two RCTs [37,48]. The first RCT in four arms compared Placebo and CPY both with and without cognitive behavioural therapy (12 mg to 32 mg maximum, duration not mentioned, 81 subjects in four groups: CYP and behavioural therapy or placebo, placebo and behavioural therapy, placebo; evaluation criterion: weight gain) [91]. The second compared placebo, CYP and amitriptyline (CPY 32 mg maximum, amitriptyline 160 mg maximum, duration: to 5% of target weight, 72 subjects in three groups, evaluation criterion: duration to 5% target weight) [92]. There was no clinically significant effect on weight gain with CYP in the first RCT. In the second, cyproheptadine marginally decreased the length of time to reach the weight gain objective for restricting AN patients, but it significantly impaired treatment efficacy for the binging/purging anorectic patients, compared to amitriptyline and placebo [45,48]. Thus antihistamines remain non-indicated in AN and should be avoided. No further study was found.

Opiates

One review [37] mentioned a study about cannabinoids and we did not find any more recent studies.

The opioid peptide system has been implicated in appetite and feeding regulation, linked to the hedonic value of food in both animals and humans. It has been hypothesised that both anorexia nervosa and bulimia nervosa could be opioid-mediated addictions [37]. In line with these hypotheses opiates and opiate antagonists have been used in order to stimulate eating in AN or to deactivate the suspected auto-addictive properties of food restriction. No study has been conducted in AN exclusively to test this hypothesis. Only one review by Aigner et al. [6] mentions one RCT that was conducted in a mixed sample of 19 AN binging/purging subtype and bulimia nervosa patients using naltrexone, 100 mg for 6 weeks [93]. Bingeing and purging behaviours decreased among both AN and bulimia nervosa patients. Naltrexone has no indication in AN.

Cannabinoids

Given the well-known impact of cannabis on appetite, cannabinoids have also been used and tested in AN. [45,51].

Two reviews mentioned cannabinoids, but we did not find any more recent studies [45,51].

Two RCTs evaluated cannabinoids. An earlier four-week double-blind crossover study [45] compared delta-9-terahydrocannabiol (delta-9-THC) to diazepam (delta-9-THC, 7.5 to 30 mg versus diazepam 1 to 15 mg, for four weeks, 11 subjects, evaluation criteria: weight gain, daily calorie intake), and showed no benefit of delta-9-THC [94]. In addition, three patients experienced severe dysphoric reactions under 9-Tetrahydrocannabinol administration. The second four-week crossover RCT (5 mg, 4 weeks, 24 subjects, evaluation criteria: weight gain, daily calorie intake), [95] compared low doses of dronabinol (a synthetic form of delta-9- tetrahydrocannabinol) to a placebo and observed a small significant gain of 0.73 kg for dronabinol. It had no impact on the total duration of physical activity but increased the average intensity of this physical activity [51].

In conclusion, cannabinoids have no proof of their efficacy nor of their safety in AN, they need further evaluation in AN, and should not be used in routine care practice.

Ghrelin

One review [45] mentioned ghrelin agonists, but we did not find any more recent studies.

In a small open trial, infusions of ghrelin over 14 days were delivered to five individuals with AN, and improved gastrointestinal discomfort and improved nutritional intake and weight gain were rapidly observed [96].

In conclusion, however, ghrelin has not proved its efficacy nor its safety in AN, and needs more evaluation in that setting.

3.2.5. Other Medications

Benzodiazepines

Only one review mentioned benzodiazepines [45], and we did not find any more recent studies.

Benzodiazepines are anxiolytic agonists of the gamma-aminobutyric acid (GABA) receptors. Although they are widely used in anorexia nervosa [7] studies that systematically investigated benzodiazepines in AN are scarce, and fairly recent [45]. An RCT on alprazolam in an AN inpatient setting comparing 75 mg of alprazolam prior to a laboratory test meal to placebo, did not find this drug beneficial in the treatment of AN [45]: alprazolam does not improve calorie intake and increases fatigue without reducing anxiety [97].

Clonidine

Clonidine is an alpha two adrenergic agonist used to treat hypertension. It was mentioned in only two reviews [6,48] reporting one placebo-controlled crossover study on four patients on 500–700 micrograms/day [98] and we did not find any more recent studies. No beneficial effect in AN was observed, but it was associated with hemodynamic side effects such as hypotension.

In conclusion, clonidine has not proved its efficacy in AN and should not be used in routine care practice.

N-Methyl-D-Aspartate Agonists and Antagonists

D-cycloserine is an N-methyl-D-aspartate (NMDA) receptor agonist known to facilitate extinction learning, a promising treatment for anxiety disorders. Only one review mentioned glutamatergic drugs [45], and they were reported in two RCTs. We did not find any more recent studies.

In one RCT [99], which used D-cycloserine versus placebo prior to meal exposure therapy, it was found that the D-cycloserin group was linked to a greater weight gain after four exposure sessions and at one-month follow-up [45].

The NMDA receptor antagonist amantadine was also used in a case series of 22 patients [100]. Amantadine administered 45 min before the main meal improved neuro-autonomic symptoms during the meal. Patients were able to eat all types of foods and their BMI increased over three months [45].

In conclusion, these drugs have no proof of their efficacy nor of their safety in AN and they need more evaluation in AN. They should not be used in routine care practice.

Oxytocin

Oxytocin is a neuropeptide hormone synthesised in the hypothalamus. It plays a role in pair bonding and in the regulation of broader social interactions, emotional reactivity and feeding behaviours. Some authors suggest that oxytocin could be a useful adjunct for the treatment for AN [51], but no review has published results. We found one recent RCT. The usefulness of oxytocin as a therapeutic agent in AN was tested in only one RCT in the course of hospital-based nutritional rehabilitation, comparing 16 AN patients under oxytocin 36 UI (intra-nasal) per day for four to six weeks and 17 patients receiving placebo. The weight gain was similar in the two groups, while eating concerns and cognitive rigidity lowered after oxytocin treatment [101].

3.3. Results: Somatic and Nutritional Treatments

Recent progress in understanding and progress in care provision for eating disorders has led to an overall consensus at the beginning of the 21st century on somatic and nutritional treatments in multidisciplinary approaches, and on evidence that weight restoration is a key aspect for the correction of many somatic functional disorders. Nevertheless, somatic medications or nutritional approaches for AN patients are more often used off-label, with no detailed guidelines for severe AN inpatient populations, nor for specific organic complications (osteoporosis, growth or puberty failure) treated by various highly specialized physicians.

Our literature review found various narrative reviews concerning somatic aspects of AN, but only a few recent systematic reviews concerning multi-organic somatic medications. In fact, most systematic reviews are concerned with the effects of weight gain or pharmacological treatments (hormone replacement, biphosphonates, teriparatide, and vitamin K) on bone mineral density and secondary osteoporosis [39,44,49,50] or they concerned nutritional therapeutic modalities and their impact on weight changes [42,46], or the efficacy of nasogastric enteral nutrition and adverse effects [47,52,53]. Most of the studies involved small samples, with heterogeneity within and among studies concerning evaluations, biomarkers and age range, with heterogeneous adolescent and adult populations, and various durations, often with an insufficient follow-up. There are very few studies only on child/adolescent populations, and more than 95% of the data mainly concerned female and Caucasian AN patients.

3.3.1. Nutritional Support and Refeeding

While weight gain and progressive weight restoration is an important first step in treating patients with AN, and is essential for medical stabilization before starting specific psychiatric care, it is clear that there is a lack of empirical evidence concerning initial refeeding strategies, and that heterogeneous medical practices are observed in everyday practice.

Approaches to Refeeding

One systematic review [42], including seven studies assessed and summarized nutritional treatments provided for 403 adolescent AN inpatients. Initial energy intake, regardless of refeeding protocols, ranged from 1000 kcal to >1900 kcal/day with a maximum energy intake during hospitalization ranging from 2000 to 4350 kcal/day. The maximum energy intake achieved was greater in the groups with additional enteral feeding (three comparative studies out of seven). The level of evidence for these results was not sufficient to propose any consensus on the most effective refeeding protocols, but it supported the need for future research on this topic.

One systematic review [46], including 27 studies and 2635 patients examined approaches to refeeding among adolescent and adult AN patients in various treatment settings, and 96% were observational/prospective or retrospective and conducted in hospital. This review focused on refeeding protocol analyses, patient clinical characteristics and somato-psychic outcomes. Thirteen studies described a meal-based approach to refeeding (calorie intake divided into meals and snacks), ten studies approached the topic with various combinations of nasogastric feeding and oral intake, one combined total parenteral nutrition and oral intake, three involved altered nutrient content (differing from current dietary recommendations). The main results of this systematic review concluded that the classic refeeding approach (starting the calorie level between 1000 and 1200 kcal/j) among mildly and moderately malnourished patients is too "conservative", and could be associated with lower weight gain and longer hospitalization. Higher calorie intake (calorie starting level between 1500 and 2400 kcal/j) with a meal-based approach, or a combination of nasogastric feeding and oral intake could be safe and well tolerated with appropriate monitoring. In the absence of sufficient evidence, a lower calorie approach in refeeding remains the rule for severely malnourished inpatients. Parenteral refeeding was associated with multiple adverse effects and is not recommended. The authors of the review suggested more research to evaluate the impact of different refeeding approaches on the duration of a hospital stay and long-term outcomes.

Enteral Feeding (EF)

Enteral feeding is indicated if under-nutrition is severe (BMI < 13) and/or associated with metabolic disorders, and/or if there is prolonged weight stagnation, despite adequate nutritional and psychiatric management [3]. EF is considered safe and well tolerated, and effectively enhances calorie intake and the rate of weight gain among patients with AN [102]. Enteral nutrition should always be performed using a small nasogastric tube. Although a few studies reported using percutaneous endoscopic gastrostomy [103], this route should not be used in the nutritional management of anorexia nervosa, because it can aggravate the distortion of body shape perception among patients. An isocaloric and isoprotidic solute should be used continuously (1 mL = 1 kcal) in the first days in case of severe undernutrition, in order to avoid post-stimulatory hypoglycaemia [104]; nocturnal refeeding can also be performed. Caloric progression should be cautious in the first days, beginning with 10–15 kcal/kg/d, and increasing slowly up to 30 to 40 kcal/kg/d at one week, in order to prevent refeeding syndrome [105], but some recent data also reported the potential risk of "underfeeding syndrome", supporting the interest of more aggressive refeeding therapies [106]. EF should be maintained only as needed, to ensure that patients retain normal eating behaviours. Progressive oral feeding should always be encouraged and accompanied by an experienced dietician [107].

One recent systematic review [53] including 10 studies, confirmed that EF is a safe therapeutic tool that is well tolerated for the management of AN patients, with an average weight gain > 1kg/week and enhanced calorie intake and weight gain in the four studies comparing EF to oral-only refeeding. Long-term effects associated with nasogastric enteral refeeding are only reported in the RCT study [108], with a higher mean body weight at 12 months in the EF group.

One systematic review [47] including 18 studies and 1427 adolescent and adult AN patients (1406 F/21 M), evaluated physiological and psychiatric outcomes and patient adherence to nasogastric feeding (NG). It can be noted that 95% of the studies were conducted in inpatient medical or psychiatric units and only one study concerned ambulatory patients [109]. Continuous NG was reported for 50% of the patients, and various tube refeeding methods (combined, overnight, bolus, not reported) for the others. Mean duration for NG use was 79.5 days. All studies reported a greater short-term weight gain for patients with NG than for patients fed per os, with 30% of non-adherent patients (interference with the tube or the feeding pump). NG could decrease bingeing/purging behaviours and improve cognitive functions and psychiatric comorbidities such as anxiety and depression symptoms. Results concerning the physiological tolerance of NG (digestive disorders), safety (partial symptoms of refeeding syndrome) and the psychiatric outcomes are confusing and should be taken with caution because of the many methodological limitations.

One systematic review [52], investigating the efficacy of enteral nutrition (EN) in the treatment of eating disorders included 22 studies and 1397 AN patients, 97.4 % of whom were females. One study concerned only hospitalized adolescent boys [110]. The nineteen studies evaluating the use of enteral nutrition in the treatment of anorexia nervosa, reported a significant short-term weight and/or BMI gain, but results were more uncertain in the long term. Five studies evaluated the characteristics and outcomes of the use of enteral nutrition in the treatment of binge-eating/purging behaviours, among which four studies were conducted in home settings [108,109,111,112]. The combined results of these studies confirmed that transient exclusive EN use decreased the frequency and severity of bingeing/purging behaviours. Three studies [113–115] on severe AN patients with BMI $\leq$ 11.5 reported that EN was initially better accepted than oral intake, and that EN is a safe and well-tolerated therapeutic strategy for high-risk patients. No major side effects in comparative studies were reported concerning transient hypophosphatemia, well controlled by biological monitoring, and transient and moderate digestive disturbances were resolved with treatment. Most studies reported various, transient EN interference strategies, without massive refusal for the reinstatement of tube feeding. Hale et al, discussed the limitations of the study, including various selection biases and ethical limitations for the conduct of blind randomized trials in the EN clinical context.

Oral Nutritional Supplementation

High-calorie liquid supplements can be prescribed to supplement oral food intake or to substitute for calories refused in meals, to increase energy intake and to promote weight gain [106]. Different types of oral supplements varying in flavour, volume, and nutritional composition exist, and need to be adapted to individual therapeutic purposes. Evidence is really scarce in the field of AN.

We found no systematic review on this topic, but benefits and adverse effects for high-energy liquid supplements among feeding methods are reported by Hart et al. [116] with the combined findings and conclusions of five descriptive studies [117–120]. Oral nutritional supplements can meet the high calorie requirements for weight gain in a smaller volume (125–300 mL) than food, and can thus be helpful for patients with digestive discomfort and/or for vulnerable patients in avoiding early satiety. This can lead to a better and faster nutritional recovery, and a reduction of hospital stays by shortening the duration of treatment. The main adverse effect is the risk of addiction to oral supplements creating an obstacle to food reintroduction, by reinforcing avoidance behaviours or by encouraging dependence on artificial food sources. These findings suggest that oral nutritional supplements can be considered as a part of dietary and medical care, and should be administered with precise and specific objectives explained to patients and integrated into a multidisciplinary approach.

Parenteral Feeding

Parenteral feeding is contraindicated in anorexia nervosa because of the major risk of metabolic and infectious complications [45].

Micronutrient Supplementation

No systematic review was found on this question. Several micronutrient deficiencies (including vitamins, minerals and trace elements) are described among patients with eating disorders [121]. These deficiencies are the consequence of restrictive food and low micronutrient intakes widely described among eating disorder patients [122]. Among malnourished patients, initial asymptomatic electrolyte, vitamin and trace element deficiencies can often worsen with re-feeding because of the increased needs, and lead to the occurrence of refeeding syndrome (RS) [45]. Prophylactic electrolyte and micronutrient supplementation is recommended for eating disorder patients with high risk of RS by the French and American guidelines on eating disorders [2,3], especially in long-lasting renutrition among adult AN patients with severe under-nutrition and a very low weight. This supplementation, in addition to unspecific vitamin and trace element supplementation, includes phosphorous (0.5–0.8 mmol/kg/d), and thiamin (200–300 mg/d) [105,123].

Zinc

Zinc deficiency is frequent in AN patients. Zinc is reported to be an appetite stimulator and to improve depression and anxiety. Zinc increases the expression of NPY and orexin m-RNA in experimental animals and plays a role in limiting the progression of cachexia and sarcopenia [124].

One RCT study [125] evidenced a BMI increase that was twice as rapid and an enhancement of brain neurotransmitters, including gamma-aminobutyric acid (GABA), in the group receiving zinc supplementation. No side effects are reported. Birmingham et al [125], suggest that daily oral supplementation should be considered for malnourished AN patients.

Vitamin B12 and Selenium

Other rare micronutrient deficiencies are reported, such as cases of sensory neuropathy resulting from vitamin B12 deficiency [126] and cases of cardiac involvement resulting from selenium deficiency [127]. There are no recommendations on specific supplementation with vitamin B12 or selenium. However, a plasma concentration assay should be performed, and supplementation should be administered if any specific clinical or biological symptoms are observed in severely malnourished AN patients.

Polyunsaturated Fatty Acids (PUFAs)

Polyunsaturated fatty acids (PUFAs) including essential fatty acids, linoleic (n-6) and alpha-linolenic n-3 (n-3) acids, and long-chain fatty acids (LC n-PUFAs), seem to provide different benefits for various neurological and psychic disorders by acting on the brain and the inflammatory system [128].

A recent comprehensive overview of the literature [129] reported that AN patients have modified PUFAs levels. Shih et al [129], reported on one case [130] and two cases series [131,132] concerning the effectiveness of polyunsaturated fatty acid supplementation and concluded that polyunsaturated fatty acids and particularly n-3 and n-6 PUFAs could be a novel adjunct medication for AN patients to treat food aversion, comorbid anxiety and depression and promote weight restoration.

3.3.2. Functional Digestive Disorders

Functional Digestive Disorders according to the Rome III criteria are common in anorexia nervosa [133–135]. Reported lesions are dysphagia and gastric burns, described respectively in 6% and 22% of patients, with no clear link to structural involvement of the oesophagus [136]. In a prospective cohort study including inpatients with eating disorders, 96% reported postprandial fullness, 90% reported abdominal distension and more than half complained of abdominal pain, gastric distension, early satiety and nausea [137]. Classic therapies are not very effective and there are few studies on the subject. Refeeding inducing a return to normal weight, remains the most effective therapeutic option; however no systematic review exists on this topic specifically in AN. We report here, empirical data concerning therapies provided in digestive disturbances associated with AN.

Drugs Acting on the Gastro-Oesophageal Cardia and Gastric Motility

According to the current guidelines of the American College of Gastroenterology [138], the prokinetic agents of choice are metoclopramide, erythromycin, azithromycin, and domperidone [139].

Metoclopramide is the first-line drug (moderate recommendation, moderate level of evidence [138]). It is a dopamine D-2 receptor antagonist that acts by stimulating the parasympathetic innervation of the stomach to increase the motility and contraction of the smooth muscles of the stomach. It should be started at a low dose, 2.5 mg 30 min before meals. This prescription should be monitored clinically because of the risk of acute dystonia and the cardiac risk with the prolongation of the QT interval.

Erythromycin is an antibiotic that also works at low doses, as a motilin agonist, which is a stimulant of gastric peristalsis. It has a prokinetic effect that improves the symptoms of gastroparesis. However, erythromycin has non-negligible adverse effects, and its effectiveness is limited to a few weeks because there is a saturation effect of the receptors. Long-term use can induce a decrease in the response to the drug (strong recommendation and a moderate level of evidence). Moshiree et al, have also shown that azithromycin has a similar motilin agonist effect to erythromycin and can be prescribed at a 250 mg daily dose [140].

Domperidone is a D-2 dopaminergic receptor agonist similar to metoclopramide with fewer central nervous system side effects (moderate recommendation and a moderate level of evidence) [138]. Due to the serious cardiac side effects, domperidone is subject to recent restrictions on use, particularly among underweight AN patients.

Other Drugs for the Gastro-Intestinal Tract

Trimebutine, a smooth muscle relaxant, can be useful in treating irritable bowel syndrome, particularly during the initial re-feeding period [141].

Proton pump inhibitors are often administered to AN patients in a context of gastroesophageal reflux or during tube re-feeding, and they are the first-line treatment because of their efficacy and supposed safety [142]. In fact, proton pump inhibitors have various potential side effects involving bone and renal and digestive functions, and they can interact with psychotropic medications in AN patients [143].

Laxatives

In the context of constipation in AN, the use of laxatives should be evaluated for the risk-benefit balance, and non-irritant osmotic laxatives should be proposed in priority in association with a gut muscle relaxant such as trimebutine. Indeed, they are not very effective, and there is a significant risk of abuse as a strategy for weight control. Their use should be cautious because they can lead to dehydration or hypokalaemia [144], and a progressive withdrawal is necessary to limit sub-occlusive risk.

Probiotics

The gut microflora contributes to the regulation of feeding behaviours and probably has a significant impact on the regulation of responses to stress [145]. Recent findings support the concept of altered host-microbe symbiosis in patients with AN, which could be one of the key factors in the pathophysiology of AN. Probiotic gut microflora modulation could be an interesting biotherapeutic strategy [146,147], but currently no data exists.

To sum up, digestive symptoms are common in patients with AN, they are a source of physical and psychic complaints, and can be a barrier to re-feeding. Functional digestive disorders should be appropriately managed using specific medications restricted in time to relieve patients and facilitate their adherence to the oral or enteral feeding program. Despite the lack of data on their efficacy in AN, these drugs should be considered as an adjunctive therapy on a case-by-case basis among patients with severe functional digestive symptoms, and their relevance should be regularly reassessed.

3.3.3. Endocrine Medications

Anorexia nervosa is associated with numerous neuroendocrine dysfunctions associated with modified plasma hormone levels and blunted, suppressed or paradoxical responses to dynamic tests, involving the hypothalamic-pituitary-gonadal growth hormone (GH)-insulin-like growth factor-I (IGF-I) and the hypothalamic-pituitary-adrenal axis, thyroid function, several adipokines, such as leptin, gut peptides such as ghrelin and YY peptide, and the posterior pituitary (oxytocin and anti-diuretic hormone). Endocrine disturbances can generate severe and irreversible complications involving osteoporosis, puberty, fertility or growth and can in addition perpetuate AN symptoms and psychiatric comorbidities [148,149].

Among AN patients, the majority of endocrine disturbances are attributable to weight reduction and to the low energy availability as a result of chronic starvation, but also due to neuro-psychic alterations, and consequently, the key treatment consists in weight restoration and in treating psychic disorders. Since hormone changes can also act as maintenance or aggravating factors on AN cognitive and behavioural symptoms, on psychiatric comorbidity (anxiety, depression) and on neuro-psychic function, it seems essential not to neglect endocrine comorbidities and to possess an adequate range of specific medications.

To date, no systematic review concerning endocrine medications exists, but we found a few recent, innovative studies on promising hormone treatments conducted among female AN patients: one study concerned recombinant human growth hormone (rhGH) replacement among adult AN women [150], one study concerned rhGH treatment among AN children [151], one study concerned oestrogen replacement among adolescent AN girls [152], one study concerned GnRH among weight-recovered AN [153] and one study concerned recombinant human leptin among underweight women [154]. We report these five studies on these innovative hormone medications in the following sections, and they are summarized in Table S1. All other studies about endocrine medications and bone health and osteoporosis were reported in previous systematic reviews and are summarized in Table 3.

Growth Hormone (GH)-Insulin-Like Growth Factor-I (IGF-I) Axis Medication

Nutritionally acquired resistance to GH, with high levels of this hormone and a disruption of the circadian dynamics of GH secretion, high levels of the GH secretagogue ghrelin, and low serum IGF-I levels have been reported among young AN patients [20]. The pathophysiological mechanisms underlying pubertal delay or arrest and low height velocity (HV) are complex during the critical window for the pubertal growth spurt. These mechanisms can affect adult height, but they are still incompletely understood. After the patients' nutritional and mental state has improved, catch-up growth is highly variable, from complete catch-up to a complete failure to gain height [155,156]. About one third of girls with severe early-onset AN are at risk for adult height deficit [157]. It remains unclear whether the high rates of associated psychiatric comorbidities, such as depression and anxiety, contribute to hypercortisolemia and persistent severe growth deficiency. It can also be noted that among children and adults, GH and IgF1 have various metabolic effects on body composition and trophic effects on bone formation and osteoblastic activity [150].

In a randomized placebo-controlled study, Fazeli et al [150], showed that suraphysiological rhGH administration for AN adult women for 12 weeks failed to increase IgF1 levels, but significantly decreased the total fat mass and fat mass percentage (rhGH, $-2.5 \pm 0.6\%$, vs. placebo, $2.2 \pm 1.1\%$; $p = 0.004$) and leptin levels in the rhGH group. Glucose, insulin, free fatty acid levels, bone markers (N-terminal propeptide of type 1 procollagen, type I collagen C-telopeptide), and weight did not differ between the two groups. These results support the independent metabolic roles of GH and IgF1 and the fact that suraphysiological rhGH is not a useful medication for adult AN women because of the negative effects on nutritional status via increased lipolysis, and on gonadal function via the effects of leptin.

In a proof-of-concept study reported by Léger et al [151], recombinant human growth hormone (rhGH) treatment has recently been shown to greatly increase HV among AN adolescents with delayed puberty and prolonged severe growth failure (HV < 2.5 cm/year for at least 18 months at the age of 13.3 ± 1.1 years) within one year of treatment instatement. Serum IGF-I levels increased to the mid-normal range for all patients; HV increased significantly, from a median of 1.0 (0.7–2.1) to 7.1 (6.0–9.5) cm/year after one year ($p < 0.002$). This increase in HV was also maintained in subsequent years and adult height (-0.1 ± 1.0 SD) was close to target height after 3.6 ± 1.4 years of rhGH. The treatment was well tolerated. Despite a substantial increase in body mass index (BMI) before the start of GH treatment, mean BMI SDS did not normalize entirely. These data indicate that the increase in HV observed in these patients was probably related to hGH therapy, with only a small potential contribution of the improvement in nutritional intake and BMI. To determine whether hGH therapy should be considered an appropriate option for AN adolescent patients, a randomized placebo-controlled study evaluating the effect of hGH treatment on growth, metabolic parameters, bone mineral density and overall course of the illness in this rare and severe condition in children is currently being conducted.

Hypothalamic-Pituitary-Gonadal Axis Medication

AN patients present functional hypogonadotropic hypogonadism including low levels of gonadal hormones (estradiol/testosterone), prepubertal patterns of gonadotropin hormones (Follicle Stimulating Hormone (FSH), Luteinizing Hormone (LH), reduced GnRH pulsatility with menstrual disorders in women, and fertility and sexuality disorders in both sexes [149]), although the literature on endocrinopathies among AN males is sparse [158]. Weight restoration is a crucial issue for gonadal function recovery, but individual BMI targets and time lapses to menstrual resumption are highly variable [159], and the indication for hormone replacement to restore menstrual function, and the efficacy of fertility-stimulating treatment among weight-recovered anorexic female patients, are frequently questioned. The potential impact of oestrogen on cognitive function among AN women following adolescent onset has recently been suggested [160].

One double-blind RCT reported by Misra et al [152] on 72 AN adolescent girls with an 18-month follow-up evaluated the impact of transdermal 17 ßestradiol (100 μg twice/week)/ 2.5 mg medroxyprogesterone acetate J1-J10/month) on anxiety, eating attitudes, and body image. Oestrogen replacement was linked to a decrease in anxiety trait scores evaluated on the Spielberger State-Trait Anxiety Inventory for Children (STAIC-trait scores) without impacting anxiety state scores (STAI-state). There was no effect of oestrogen replacement on eating disorder symptoms evaluated on the Eating Disorder Inventory (EDI II) or the Body Shape Questionnaire (BSQ-34 scores). BMI changes did not differ between groups. Oestrogen replacement leads to a reduction in trait anxiety among adolescent girls with AN that is independent from weight changes. However, oestrogen replacement did not directly impact eating attitudes and behaviours, body shape perception, or state anxiety. These results, to be confirmed, raise interesting questions and call for future research to confirm the impact of various oestrogen replacement therapies on cognitive functions, anxiety and depressive symptoms in AN.

One retrospective observational monocentric study reported by Germain et al [153], compared response to gonadotropin-releasing hormone therapy (GnRH) with 20 μg/90 min/four weeks induction cycles (repeated if there was no pregnancy) administered by a sub-cutaneous infusion pump to 19 weight-recovered AN patients (Rec-AN) (BMI > 18.5) and to patients with other causes of hypothalamic amenorrhea, including primary hypothalamic amenorrhea patients (PHA) and secondary hypothalamic amenorrhea patients (SHA). The study results reported higher estradiol and LH levels during induction cycles among Rec-AN patients than in the PHA and SHA groups; follicular recruitment and the ovulation rate were higher among Rec AN patients than among PHA patients, but similar to SHA patients; the cumulate pregnancy rate was 74 % for Rec-An (vs 73% for SHA et 14% for PHA). No adverse side effect and no excessive response to stimulation were reported. This study showed that pulsatile GnRH therapy could be a safe and efficient treatment in hypothalamic amenorrhea among weight-recovered AN patients.

Leptin

Previous animal model studies reported that leptin, an anorexigen adipokine regulating LH pulsatility, gonadal function, puberty development and fertility, could participate in starvation-induced amenorrhea among AN patients [161]. Leptin levels are decreased in malnourished AN patients, and recent research discussed the potential interest of recombinant human leptin treatment, which could normalize reproductive hormones and restore gonadal function among female AN patients, and the interest of combining recombinant human leptin with oestrogen therapy [162].

One prospective study, reported by Welt et al [154], concerned the use of recombinant human leptin (r-metHULeptin) for up to three months among eight secondary hypothalamic amenorrheic adult women (18–33 years) versus six amenorrheic control subjects. Amenorrhea among the treated patients was secondary to recently increased physical exercise or weight loss but without AN diagnosis. The study reported increased LH pulsatility after two weeks of treatment, and increased estradiol levels and ovarian activity, over a period of three months among treated subjects. Levels of thyroid hormones (free T3), IgF1 and IGF1-BP3 and osteoformation biomarkers also increased with leptin treatment. The safety and tolerance of leptin administration and the impact on eating behaviours among AN patients are in debate and require further research.

There are serious gaps in knowledge and no approved treatment for gonadal deficits or other endocrine dysfunctions in AN despite the various severe consequences on somatic, nutritional and psychiatric aspects of the low levels of reproductive hormones and other hormonal disturbances such as prolonged hypercortisolism. Recent studies suggest interesting new approach strategies, such as sexual hormone therapy to normalize oestrogen deficit, and restore puberty and fertility processes, with a potentially positive impact on cognitive functions, mood, anxiety, and bone health, and reduced spontaneous fracture risk. To date, there is no data concerning gonadal function treatments for male AN patients.

3.3.4. Bone and Osteoporosis Medication

Anorexia nervosa leads to a loss of bone mass, accompanied by low bone mineral density (BMD), secondary osteoporosis and increased fracture risk, as a result of malnutrition and hormonal imbalance [163]. Almost all adult AN patients (92%) have a BMD 1 SD below controls and 38% of patients have a BMD 2.5 SD below controls. For the same duration of amenorrhea, AN patients who develop AN during adolescence have lower BMD than those who present AN later in adult life. As suggested by Misra et al, long-term use of SSRIs could contribute to low bone mass in AN [164]. Given the impact of AN on bone metabolism, fracture risk should be assessed in AN patients using dual energy X-ray absorptiometry (DXA). The U.K. National Osteoporosis Society (NOS) recommends monitoring BMD by DXA every two years.

We found four systematic reviews concerning the treatment provided for bone health and osteoporosis [39,44,49,50]. One of them concerned the impact of weight gain/restoration on bone [44], one was about impact of oestrogen replacement on bone [39], and the two other studies concerned the impact of various somatic medications on bone health [49,50] We report these four systematic reviews in the following sections on the basis of the therapeutic strategies provided.

Weight Gain/Restoration

Restoring weight and normal function of the gonadal axis (with restoration of menses for women) is one of the goals of the treatment of AN and is essential for bone health.

In a systematic review [44] which included 18 studies with follow-up periods from 12 to 90 months of female adolescent AN patients, eight studies showed no significant change in BMD after weight gain/restoration (follow-up 12 months), one study showed decreased BMD after weight restoration (follow-up 12 months), and nine studies showed BMD improvements with weight gain (mean follow-up 30 months) without total catch-up with controls. Therefore, there is strong evidence for at least a stabilization of BMD with weight gain and/or weight restoration. Longer follow-up (more than 12 months) provides evidence of an increase in BMD with weight gain. Nonetheless low BMD and fracture risk persist after weight recovery. In an adult study [165] the patients whose menses were restored had an increase in spine BMD independently from weight restoration, and weight gain improved hip BMD, whereas the patients with no weight gain nor restoration of menses had an annual rate of BMD decrease of 2.5%. Weight gain and restoration of the gonadal axis can be difficult to obtain in clinical practice. In addition, BMD is persistently low a long time after recovery for AN patients without complete catch-up with weight and menses restoration [166]. The adjunction of complementary medications to treat low BMD and limit fracture risk among pre-menopausal AN women needs to be considered. Only one study [167] on male adolescents with AN was reported, evidencing a rapid and positive bone density evolution in case of weight restoration.

Oestrogen Replacement Therapy

Oestrogen inhibits bone resorption and hypogonadism resulting from food restriction in AN and contributes to increased bone resorption as a result of hypoestrogenia in women.

One cross-sectional study [168] has shown a higher spine BMD for AN subjects exposed to oral contraceptives (OC) combining oestrogen and progesterone compared to AN patients without OC, but Elkazaz et al. [169] reported that healthy premenopausal women with OC current use have a lower BMD compared to women with past OC use and/or non-use, and that this relationship seems in part mediated by IGF1 suppression by oestrogen and thus should not be recommended as a bone accrual medication for adult AN patients.

One systematic review [39] including 10 studies with eight placebo-controlled RCTs evaluated the influence of oestrogen therapies on bone mineral density (lumbar spine and femoral neck or hip BMD by DXA) among adolescent and premenopausal adult women with amenorrhea [39]. Five RCTs used oral contraceptives and three RCTs used hormone replacement therapy. The results were poor quality and generally disappointing regarding oral contraceptives with various ethinyl estradiol doses administered (20–35 µg/d) and various combined progestins, small samples and short follow-up. Of the five studies using oral contraceptives, only one reported increased BMD in the lumbar spine [170], while in the other studies bone loss was not modified or continued to progress. Lebow et al concluded that oral contraceptives were poorly effective in treating bone loss among adolescent or young adult amenorrheic AN patients [39]. Physiological hormone replacement therapy yielded more interesting results, particularly with one study reported by Misra et al, [171] on physiological transdermal oestrogen (17ß estradiol) replacement therapy among AN adolescent girls (with incremental doses of oestrogen mimicking oestrogen pubertal secretion for the youngest patients and 100 µg patches for bone-mature patients) combined with cyclic progesterone. This increased hip and spinal BMD, with an increment comparable to the healthy control group, in a well-designed randomized controlled 18-month trial, but it did not provide complete recovery at the end of the trial, as BMD was still lower in the AN group than in the control group [171]. Therefore, transdermal oestrogen replacement therapy, by bypassing the IgF1 suppressive effect of oral oestrogen, could be recommended for adolescent females suffering from AN.

Hormonal and Other Somatic Medications

One systematic review [49] concerning 20 studies (10/20 were double-blind RCTs) reported a synthetic assessment of the effectiveness of weight restoration and interventional studies exploring various somatic drugs (oestrogen replacement therapy, recombinant h-GH, recombinant h-IgF1, DHEA, biphosphonates, teriparatide) on bone health among adolescent and adult AN women.

The most recent systematic review [50] included 19 studies (10/19 were double-blind RCTs) and concerned adjuvant medications potentially active on bone, such as various oral contraceptives (OC) containing Ethinyl Estradiol (EE) (EE or EE/levonorgestrel or EE/progestin or EE/norgestimate), various oestrogen replacements (transdermal 17ßE/progesterone or oral EE/progesterone), teriparatide (TPt), alendronate, rhIgF1, menatetrenone (MED) (vitamin K2), risedronate and transdermal testosterone.

The results from these two systematic reviews concerning various medications and pharmacological interventions are summarized in the sections below.

Bisphosphonates

Biphosphonates inhibit osteoclast activity and bone resorption, they increase BMD and reduce fracture risk in post-menopausal women. Three trials have explored the impact of bisphosphonate treatment on BMD in AN (one RCT with alendronate [172], two with risedronate: one controlled trial [173] and one RCT [174]). After 1 year of alendronate in an adolescent AN group (baseline Zscore ≤ -1), weight was the main determinant of BMD. After controlling for body weight, alendronate increased femoral neck BMD. This does not provide sufficient proof to support the use of alendronate in adolescent osteoporosis in AN.

Among adult premenopausal AN patients with osteopenia (Tscore of -2.7 ± 2) [173] spine BMD had increased by 4.9±1% after nine months of treatment with risedronate compared to a decrease of $1 \pm 1.3\%$ in the control group. After one year of risedronate [174] (baseline Zscore -1.5 ± 0.7) spine BMD increased by 3.2%, whereas it was unchanged in the placebo group.

Oral bisphosphonates have been associated with upper gastrointestinal tract ulcerations. Nonetheless, in the three trials in AN no adverse effects on the gastrointestinal tract were reported. Intravenous bisphosphonates could be an option in AN, but they have yet to be tested in this population. The main question concerning the use of bisphosphonates in AN resides in its long half-life and its potential harm to the foetus in case of pregnancy. For the time being, for premenopausal adult AN women, the prescription of bisphosphonates cannot be widely recommended, and individual prescription should be discussed on a case-by-case basis.

Testosterone

In the studies using transdermal testosterone administration in women with AN there was no significant changes in markers of bone formation, and no increase in spinal BMD when transdermal testosterone was administered without risedronate [174,175].

DHEA

The sole significant effect of DHEA was observed when combined with oral contraceptive (20 μgEE/ 0.1 mg levonorgestrel) with a stabilisation of femoral neck BMD [176].

IgF1

RhIGF-1 replacement increased bone formation markers in both adolescents and adults AN patients [177–179]. Effectiveness of combined oral contraceptives or 17ß estradiol replacement and rhIgF1 are discussed [50].

Teriparatide

Teriparatide is a human recombinant parathyroid hormone, anabolic on bone and it is recommended for the treatment of post-menopausal osteoporosis. A six-month RCT [180] studied the impact of teriparatide among older AN patients (mean age 47, Tscore ≤ 2.5), and evidenced that teriparatide increased spine BMD by 6% (+ 0.2% in the control group). This result supports the use of teriparatide as anabolic agent for older AN patients.

Menatetrenone (MED) (Vitamin K2)

Administration of MED (vitamin K2) in AN among Japanese women over a nine-month period reduced bone loss, but there was no increase in BMD [181].

Evidence-based data from these recent comprehensive studies suggests that the safest and most effective strategy to protect and improve bone density in AN and prevent fractures among adolescent and premenopausal women is restoration of weight with the resumption of menses. The most promising available medications include 17 ß estradiol replacement (such as the transdermal estradiol patch) for adolescents and bisphosphonates for adults.

Vitamin D and Calcium Supplementation

Low levels of vitamin D and inadequate calcium intake are associated with increased fracture risk and low BMD. In addition, D3 hypovitaminosis could be responsible for the lack of inflammatory response and depressive symptoms among patients with long-term eating disorders. Calcium intake among adolescent AN patients has been described as comparable to that among controls, partly as a result of supplements [182]. While their intake and the bioavailability of oral ergocalciferol among young AN patients was similar to that of healthy controls, AN patients have lower serum levels of 25 and 1,25OH-Vitamin D [183]. In addition, patients who have lower serum levels of vitamin D (<20 ng/mL) have lower hip BMD [184]. After weight gain, the spine BMD increase was greater in the group of patients with higher serum vitamin D levels ($\geq$30 ng/mL) [185], supporting the use of oral vitamin D supplements to obtain sufficient serum levels during weight gain. No RCT prospective trial has been performed to evaluate the efficacy of calcium and vitamin D supplements alone on BMD among AN patients. Nevertheless, given the impact of calcium and vitamin D on bones, although the efficacy of calcium and vitamin D supplementation has been poorly evaluated in AN, we recommend a total intake of calcium of approximately 1000–1200 mg and vitamin D supplements if serum levels of vitamin D are insufficient or if there is a secondary hyperparathyroidism [186]. Since oral calcium supplements can be associated with an increased risk of incident coronary atherosclerosis, a calcium-rich diet should be privileged if possible among AN patients [187].

4. Discussion

The original aim of this multidisciplinary overview was to summarize all the literature published about the use of medication in the psychiatric, somatic and nutritional aspects in AN.

Evidence based on the efficacy of medication in anorexia nervosa is scarce whether for the psychological, somatic or nutritional sphere. The evidence base is sparse, as the literature reports mainly case reports, cases series, open studies and some RTCs. In addition, for the RCTs, methodologies have numerous failings such as the heterogeneity of study designs, research methods, population samples, and intervention modalities [6,37,44,45,50]. The aims of the published research were initially to find medication that would cure AN by overcoming the key resistant symptom, the need for weight gain. Many drugs have been tested in AN on the rationale of their side effect in terms of weight gain in other disorders (for example lithium, antihistamines, cannabinoids, etc.) or their action on clinical manifestations observed in AN (depression, anxiety, obsessions, hyperactivity). In parallel, some psychotropic drugs have been tested in connection with hypotheses of neurobiological etiopathogenic neuro-transmitter involvement in the development or maintenance of AN (for example noradrenalin and serotonin for antidepressants, dopamine for antipsychotics). Recently, new neuro-hormones involved in the regulation of dimensions altered in AN, such as appetite regulation (ghrelin) or social interactions (oxytocin) have been evaluated. However, oxytocin and ghrelin have not proved their efficacy nor their safety in AN. In relation to its anorexigen effect, oxytocin needs more evaluation in AN setting [188]. These neuro-hormones should not be used in routine care practice.

4.1. Somatic and Nutritional Aspects

Concerning somatic aspects, if weight gain is a crucial step to correct the majority of adaptive and functional changes resulting from undernutrition, somatic drugs have been explored from the late 1990s. The evidence of a higher risk of osteoporosis and spontaneous fracture among AN subjects with amenorrhea [17,19] raised the question of the use of bisphosphonate or oestrogen replacement to treat low bone density [39,49,50]. Other hormone replacement therapies for the endocrine consequences of AN, such as growth or pubertal delay, appeared in the 2000s in association with endocrine-paediatric management in the context of a multidisciplinary approach [151,157]. Two recent narrative update reviews on endocrine mechanisms and repercussions in AN report on available treatments and innovative therapeutic strategies in endocrinology [189,190]. Physicians' interest in refeeding modalities [191], relating to optimal daily calorie requirements [42], the risk of over-feeding and that of under-feeding, high calorie oral supplementation [116], vitamin supplementation and functional digestive disorder medications [139], is fairly recent and corresponds to the development of specific nutritional and dietary expertise, alongside the publication of international guidelines [2,3]. Finally, in the last 20 years, we have observed a paradigm shift concerning enteral tube feeding, considered initially as unethical and coercive, and now viewed as efficient, safe and well tolerated [53]. Promising somatic medications for new targets have developed recently, with micronutrients such as zinc, polyunsaturated fatty acids (PUFAs) used in refeeding, physiological oestrogen replacement or teriparatide to treat bone health, leptin to restore gonadic function, reproductive hormone for hormonal deficits and neuropsychic functions, and GH for severe growth retardation among prepubertal adolescents.

4.2. Psychotropic Drugs

Since the 1960s nearly all classes of psychotropic drugs have been tried in AN [45]. Psychotropic drugs were initially compared to placebo without psychotherapy, with very poor results, but the most recent studies now use psychotropic drugs as additional treatment to global treatment approaches including psychotherapy (individual and/or family therapy). This type of use stems from an international consensus, as attested by the NICE guidelines (the most recent international guidelines published) stipulating that medication cannot be considered as the sole treatment for Anorexia Nervosa (see Table 1).

Despite the evolution and improvement in study design, evidence-based data is scarce and possibly even less robust than it was in the WFSBP in 2011 [6] since atypical antipsychotics seem not to exhibit the efficacy they initially appeared to have.

The RCTs generally evidence negative results concerning weight, and contradictory results concerning eating disorder symptoms and psychiatric dimensions. This situation can be explained by discrepancies in study methodologies [45,48], including many limitations such as relatively short durations of treatment (weeks, or two to three months mainly) and the small sample sizes (fewer than 100 in RCTs, and generally fewer than 30). That said, one of the most important limitations to efficacy in AN is non-compliance with medication treatments: patients frequently do not take their medication.

This situation of a poor evidence base in the existing literature is discouraging [48]. It has led, in the more recent reviews published, to giving prominence to emergent or promising interventions and recommendations for research [24,40,45,51].

In this situation, if we refer only to the evidence-based elements, psychotropic drugs should not be prescribed in AN. However, the reality in the field is quite the reverse. All psychotropic drugs are widely prescribed to both adults and adolescents with AN, and this seems to be increasing [7]. In addition, more than half of the patients have more than one psychotropic drug prescribed simultaneously. Also, dangerous drugs such as bupropion or tricyclics, are still prescribed despite the conclusions of the literature [7]. The same observation has been made in other studies on adults and adolescents in different countries [7,8,192]. These papers highlight the disparity between research conclusions and clinical practice in the treatment of AN. This underlines the importance of consensual guidelines incorporating evidence-based data. We also need expert consensus and training for practitioners on this question, especially for ED specialists, who mostly base their practice on their experience and who seem more resistant to using guidelines than general practitioners [7]. Our "experience" is the result of a complex combination of elements. It is based on core beliefs derived from different sources, including, of course, evidence-based data. Evidence can be biased in favour of drug efficacy by the publication of positive results only [7]. In addition, some studies (or their coordinators) are sponsored by the industry and their results can be biased by conflicts of interest. This last point leads the latest NICE guidelines to exclude studies sponsored by the industry from the studies analysed to establish the evidence base retained for the guidelines [4]. In addition, our experience is also impacted by psychiatric theoretical orientations, [7] or good or bad experiences with one or several patients.

4.3. Use of Psychotropic Medication in AN

Once we have discussed these elements, the central question for this review is still unresolved: how should we use medication in AN?

As recommended by most guidelines, we need to evaluate the global situation of the patient, including psychiatric, medical, nutritional and social aspects, to propose the best-suited treatment. Medication should be prescribed on the basis of the clinical evaluation. This evaluation should include the patient's opinion about the treatment [4,24].

Concerning psychotropic medication, comorbidities (including mood disorders, anxiety disorders, obsessive disorders) should be evaluated and treated [18,45] if they are real disorders and not "artefacts" that will improve with re-feeding [193]. These disorders are usually treated by teams on the assumption that treating anxiety and depressive disorders facilitates AN treatment, or at least improves their quality of life [45]. These disorders are usually treated according to the specific recommendations for each, and taking into account the particular risks of side effects resulting from low weight and metabolic disturbances (possible depletion in potassium, phosphorus, magnesium, and zinc), and somatic complications concerning hematologic, renal, hepatic and heart functions that can interact with medication. Antidepressants and atypical antipsychotics are the most frequently evaluated drugs and the most widely used in practice.

Chlorpromazine is no longer used for AN because of its severe adverse effects, including seizures; low doses of haloperidol could be effective as an adjunct treatment for patients with severe, treatment-resistant conditions with marked self-image alteration [48]. Atypical antipsychotics can sometimes be useful to help patients with AN, in case of high levels of anxiety [75] or in adults with a long illness duration [76], but practitioners should be aware that they prolong the QT segment and can be dangerous in case of malnutrition by leading to cardiac death associated with ventricular arrhythmia. Their prescription should be monitored for safety, including regular electrocardiogram and ionogram assessments. In addition, because of the risk of metabolic syndrome, such as hyperglycaemia, dyslipidaemia or HTA, the usual guidelines for the monitoring of antipsychotics should be applied. Benzodiazepines are also widely used and their use is questionable, especially among young people, as they induce dependency and can lead to abuse or misuse [7].

A psychotropic drug can be useful to manage eating disorders or psychiatric symptoms. Himmerich et al. [194] in a recent survey among AN patients and carers and reported that people with anorexia nervosa want medication to help with anxiety and sleep problems [24]. However, the specific treatment of AN also requires re-feeding, and/or cessation of binging and purging, specific psychotherapy (individual or family therapy) and work on the social impact of the illness. Medications, and especially antidepressants, are less effective among those that are acutely ill and underweight [18].

Outside situations of emergency (suicidal ideas or risk, very severe anxiety or OCD), following the discussion with the patient, it is possible to wait a few weeks in order to later reassess the need for specific treatments for possible comorbidities [195]. In order to diagnose whether psychiatric symptoms are linked to a comorbid diagnosis or to malnutrition, it is useful to investigate the personal and family history of comorbid disorders and the chronology of appearance of AN and psychiatric symptoms. Diagnosis should be based on symptoms, their evolution, the chronology of onset and individual and familial history of comorbidities [18].

A general discussion with the patient (and the parents for a minor) is necessary to review side effects, risks, benefits, and alternatives. One important point to make is that psychotropic drugs do not induce weight gain in AN but can alleviate negative psychological symptoms. This will be important for the therapeutic alliance. Practitioners should always have in mind that to be efficient, a medication needs be taken, and AN patients are often not observant, especially for antipsychotics [37]. In addition, to be efficient, a medication needs be absorbed. When patients purge after they have taken their pills or have swallowing phobia or food orality disturbances, they cannot be efficient. Both points should be discussed with the patients.

As in other reviews, we will conclude on perspectives for future research on the topic of medication in AN.

4.4. Perspectives

Several perspectives suggest the need for the development of innovative treatments.

Part of the lack of evidence could be attributable to the heterogeneity of significant symptoms and the treatment responses encountered in AN. Very few studies thus far have stratified the subtypes or clinical features of the disorder. Anorexia nervosa is a heterogeneous disorder and a single "optimal" drug for all individuals is highly unlikely. Targeting more homogeneous subgroups could be helpful. Thus, growing evidence derived from various approaches supports a specific staging trajectory for anorexia nervosa, and there is preliminary evidence that interventions should be matched to the stage in the illness (for review see [196]). Interventions tailored according to the stage of the illness or the developmental trajectory could be valuable options. Certain other clinical features could be considered for more homogeneous subgroups of patients, since they could be associated with a specific form of the illness, or lower response to medication, for instance the AN subtype (AN-R, AN-BP, AN/B, AN/P), age (differentiating pre and post-pubertal adolescents and adults), gender, cultural environment, current and maximum pre-treatment BMI, associated personality traits, psychiatric comorbidities [45] or a history of childhood abuse [197,198]. A number of latent class and latent profile analyses have been performed on symptom and personality factors to stratify the endo-phenotypes spanning AN [197,199–201]. These sub-categorizations could be a starting point to homogenize samples.

Also, there is currently emphasis on using precision medicine to identify targets, which should lead to more effective treatments. Symptoms that maintain the disorder may differ across individuals and participate in the lack of evidence. A novel methodological perspective is thus to address the extreme heterogeneity within AN and to develop and adapt treatments to each individual, which could be of considerable interest in the near future [202].

Finally, beyond a categorical approach, treating one or several specific dimensions associated with the illness rather than the illness overall could be useful, since changing targets might change clinical outcomes. Some salient dimensions in AN, such as delay discounting or cognitive impulse control, could potentially be targeted by drugs or a neuromodulation approach [203].

Concerning non-psychotropic drugs used in AN, these are mainly used to treat medical conditions associated with AN. It is critical to underline that weight gain and restoration of normal weight is the first line of approach to the management of these conditions whenever possible. Therefore, refeeding modalities for weight gain or restoration, including the specific indications for enteral nutrition, oral nutritional supplementation, micronutrient supplementation and specific drugs for functional digestive disorders, seem absolutely essential, but to date no guidelines exist on nutritional therapeutic strategies for AN.

Among the drugs available, sex hormone treatments need to be discussed, as they are fairly widespread in use, but their effects are a source of considerable debate. Various arguments should be taken into account in the assessment of the risk-benefit balance of their prescription. As demonstrated by our results, oral contraceptives have failed to show any significant benefit in protecting bones among patients with AN. Although certain issues could explain this lack of effect, such as the heterogeneity of the patients included across studies, and variable treatment and follow-up durations, the suggestion is not to use oral contraception to protect bones in AN. On the other hand, transdermal estradiol has been found to be a more physiological form of oestrogen replacement and more promising than oral administration in managing osteopenia among adolescents with AN. This explains the position of the recent British national guidelines suggesting hormone replacement therapy with 17-β-estradiol (with cyclic progesterone) rather than oral contraception, and only for young AN women (13–17 years). Furthermore, the decision to prescribe oral contraception is not without drawbacks. For example, the return of menstrual function, which indicates adequate weight restoration, is masked by the cessation of bleeding induced by contraceptives. Also, its use can provide a sense of reassurance that patients are protected against osteopenia, which can reduce efforts for weight rehabilitation. On the other hand, it is important to keep in mind that amenorrhea, occurring in 66 to 84% of women suffering from anorexia nervosa, favours the absence of contraceptive measures, explaining a particularly high rate (up to 50%) of unwanted pregnancies in this population. Finally, somato-psychic tolerance and compliance with hormonal replacement are very limited due to fat phobia, menstruation and bleeding refusal in many adolescent AN patients. Recent studies evaluated the interest of testosterone replacement therapy in AN women based on the fact that hypothalamic amenorrhea is associated with a profound androgen deficit. Transdermal testosterone replacement increases spinal BMD when administered with risedronate and can stimulate bone formation [174]. In addition, this could be an effective medication in women with treatment-resistant depression by improving depression and cognitions [175]. Otherwise, as mentioned previously, SSRIs seems to be inefficient in conditions of undernutrition, and future studies should assess optimal renutrition and adapted hormone replacement to potentiate the effectiveness of psychotropic medications [49]. To date, testosterone replacement therapy is not recommended for female nor for male AN patients. Concerning the use of medications for bone health and BMD improvement, despite the promising results of studies on sexual hormone replacement, bisphosphonates and combined interventions among adolescent and premenopausal women, the safest and most effective strategy to protect and improve bone density and prevent spontaneous fractures risk is, for now, the restoration of weight and menstrual recovery. Further studies are needed to establish standards for the treatment of osteoporosis in AN.

There are no specific treatments taking into account particular aspects of adolescent or adult male AN patients and current proposed treatments are similar to those for AN women [158]. Specific research on the male AN population is insufficient and needs to be developed, particularly with regard to testosterone and other therapies, and the benefits of specific drugs on somatic, cognitive and psychiatric functions that can influence evolution and prognosis in AN boys and men.

4.5. Strengths and Limitations of This Overview

As stated by Pollock et al. (p16) [204] "overviews are a relatively new methodological innovation, and there are currently substantial variations in the methodological approaches used within different overviews". We defined a methodology for this overview on the basis of elements from the literature, but due to the characteristic of the literature concerning medication for AN we could not totally fulfil all the quality criteria previously defined [205].

Indeed, a good quality overview should include systematic reviews with four characteristics [205]: 1. They should not substantially overlap. 2. They should focus on the precise question asked by the overview. 3. They should be high quality. 4. They should be up-to-date.

There is considerable overlap between reviews and meta-analyses selected in our overview. In order not to bias our conclusions we focused on the more recent reviews or meta-analyses; when meta-analyses and reviews were available on the same studies we focused on the meta-analysis conclusions, and when two reviews were available we focused on the more recent one including the more recent research. We selected only systematic reviews with a well-defined methodology but methodological quality was not homogeneous.

The conclusions we have drawn are limited by the methodology of the systematic reviews included, which use different criteria and objectives, over different periods, possibly leading to different conclusions and possibly biased by their selection. In order to alleviate this limitation we developed a systematic overview using the PRISMA guidelines, mainly based on meta-analyses and systematic reviews of RCTs and open comparative studies, but not on narratives reviews, retrospective studies or case reports.

Our findings are also limited by the quality of the published literature on the topic of medication for AN, which also impacts the conclusions, since most of the studies published on the subject are open studies, retrospective studies or case series or case reports, and RCTs are rare. The reason for this situation is linked to both AN patient refusal to participate in RCTs and to the clinical context, and also to the relatively low frequency of AN. Otherwise, it is also linked to ethical reasons, particularly on the refeeding topic [52] or growth hormone replacement [151]. In addition, the existing RCTs are poor quality, as they were conducted with various methodological procedures, on heterogeneous, small samples, and over different durations of follow-up. Finally, these studies were mostly conducted over short treatment durations whereas AN is a chronic disorder.

5. Conclusions

Perspectives for future research on medication in AN should include more specific phenotyping for psychological dimensions and comorbidities, also taking into account more somatic and anthropometric data, such as premorbid weight, body composition, nutritional and hormonal markers of undernutrition, so as to optimize the assessment of the efficacy of medication.

There is a need to make progress and develop innovative therapeutic strategies, especially for severe, chronic forms of AN with resistant psychiatric comorbidities, and for pre-pubertal AN patients with severe somatic prognosis, by targeting medication more efficiently through improved understanding of their etiopathogenic mechanisms [189,190]. A future perspective is to address the extreme heterogeneity within AN and to develop psychotropic treatments for the various clinical dimensions observed. We should develop new, more sensitive and specific biomarkers, especially for bone microarchitecture, because evaluating BMD is not sufficient to predict fracture risk. In addition, we need better-adapted techniques to measure the benefits of weight gain and nutritional status, including body composition analyses [176].

There are exciting perspectives for the development of transdisciplinary studies, based on well-defined and phenotyped sub-groups, including psychotherapeutic approaches and evaluating the impact of optimized refeeding modalities, hormone replacement, other somatic medications, or psychotropic drugs.

Studies should evaluate synergistic benefits of these combined interventions on a global perspective, including renutrition, cognitive functions, somatic, and psychic outcomes over prolonged follow-up periods.

Supplementary Materials: The following are available online at http://www.mdpi.com/2077-0383/8/2/278/s1, Table S1: Selected studies concerning innovative hormonal medications for female patients with AN and/or hypothalamic amenorrhea.

Author Contributions: Conceptualization, C.B., S.G., F.B.-P. and N.G.; methodology, C.B., S.G., and N.G.; validation, C.B., N.G., C.S. and S.G.; investigation, C.B., S.G., F.B.-P., M.-E.C., J.C., V.D., P.D., P.G., M.H.-G., S.I., J.L., B.S. and N.G.; resources, C.B., S.G., F.B.-P., M.-E.C., J.C., V.D., P.D., P.G., M.H.-G., J.L., B.S. and N.G; writing—original draft preparation, C.B., S.G., M.-E.C., F.B.-P., J.C., V.D., P.D., P.G., M.H.-G., S.I., J.L., B.S., C.S. and N.G.; writing—review and editing, C.B., S.G., N.G.; project administration, C.B., N.G.; funding acquisition, C.B., S.G., F.B.-P., V.D., S.I., J.L., B.S. and N.G.

Funding: This research was funded by French Federation Anorexia Bulimia for translation and publication fees.

Acknowledgments: To Angela Verdier for reviewing the English of this paper, and to Wayne Hodgkinson for his friendly participation.

Conflicts of Interest: The authors have no conflict of interest to report. Except: S Guillaume reported that he received funding as a consultant by Janssen, Otsuka and Lundbeck Compagnies. J. Léger is currently investigator in a clinical trial using growth hormone (GH) from Novo-Nordisk, has received support for travel to international meetings from several GH manufacturers (Ipsen, Merck, Novo Nordisk, Lilly), fees for lectures from Ipsen Pharma and Merck, and consulting fees from Sanofi Genzyme.

References

1. Treasure, J.; Claudino, A.M.; Zucker, N. Eating disorders. *Lancet Lond. Engl.* **2010**, *375*, 583–593. [CrossRef]
2. American Psychiatric Association. *Practice Guideline for the Treatment of Patients with Eating Disorders*; American Psychiatric Association: Philadelphia, PA, USA, 2006.
3. Haute Autorité de Santé. *HAS Anorexia Nervosa Practice Guidelines*; HAS: Saint-Denis La Plaine, France, 2010.
4. National Institute for Health and Care Excellence. *NICE Eating Disorders Guidelines: Eating Disorders: Recognition and Treatment*; NICE: London, England, 2017.
5. Herpertz-Dahlmann, B.; van Elburg, A.; Castro-Fornieles, J.; Schmidt, U. ESCAP Expert Paper: New developments in the diagnosis and treatment of adolescent anorexia nervosa—A European perspective. *Eur. Child Adolesc. Psychiatry* **2015**, *24*, 1153–1167. [CrossRef] [PubMed]
6. Aigner, M.; Treasure, J.; Kaye, W.; Kasper, S. WFSBP Task Force on Eating Disorders World Federation of Societies of Biological Psychiatry (WFSBP) guidelines for the pharmacological treatment of eating disorders. *World J. Biol. Psychiatry Off. J. World Fed. Soc. Biol. Psychiatry* **2011**, *12*, 400–443. [CrossRef] [PubMed]
7. Garner, D.M.; Anderson, M.L.; Keiper, C.D.; Whynott, R.; Parker, L. Psychotropic medications in adult and adolescent eating disorders: Clinical practice versus evidence-based recommendations. *Eat. Weight Disord. EWD* **2016**, *21*, 395–402. [CrossRef] [PubMed]
8. Alañón Pardo, M.D.M.; Ferrit Martín, M.; Calleja Hernández, M.Á.; Morillas Márquez, F. Adherence of psychopharmacological prescriptions to clinical practice guidelines in patients with eating behavior disorders. *Eur. J. Clin. Pharm.* **2017**, *73*, 1305–1313. [CrossRef] [PubMed]
9. Marzola, E.; Nasser, J.A.; Hashim, S.A.; Shih, P.B.; Kaye, W.H. Nutritional rehabilitation in anorexia nervosa: Review of the literature and implications for treatment. *BMC Psychiatry* **2013**, *13*, 290. [CrossRef] [PubMed]
10. Sebaaly, J.C.; Cox, S.; Hughes, C.M.; Kennedy, M.L.H.; Garris, S.S. Use of fluoxetine in anorexia nervosa before and after weight restoration. *Ann. Pharm.* **2013**, *47*, 1201–1205. [CrossRef] [PubMed]
11. Mitchell, J.E.; Roerig, J.; Steffen, K. Biological therapies for eating disorders. *Int. J. Eat. Disord.* **2013**, *46*, 470–477. [CrossRef] [PubMed]
12. Campbell, K.; Peebles, R. Eating disorders in children and adolescents: State of the art review. *Pediatrics* **2014**, *134*, 582–592. [CrossRef] [PubMed]
13. Fazeli, P.K.; Klibanski, A. Anorexia nervosa and bone metabolism. *Bone* **2014**, *66*, 39–45. [CrossRef] [PubMed]
14. Van den Heuvel, L.L.; Jordaan, G.P. The psychopharmacological management of eating disorders in children and adolescents. *J. Child Adolesc. Ment. Health* **2014**, *26*, 125–137. [CrossRef] [PubMed]
15. Starr, T.B.; Kreipe, R.E. Anorexia nervosa and bulimia nervosa: Brains, bones and breeding. *Curr. Psychiatry Rep.* **2014**, *16*, 441. [CrossRef] [PubMed]
16. Brown, C.; Mehler, P.S. Medical complications of anorexia nervosa and their treatments: An update on some critical aspects. *Eat. Weight Disord. Stud. Anorex. Bulim. Obes.* **2015**, *20*, 419–425. [CrossRef] [PubMed]
17. Saraff, V.; Högler, W. Endocrinology and Adolescence: Osteoporosis in children: Diagnosis and management. *Eur. J. Endocrinol.* **2015**, *173*, R185–R197. [CrossRef] [PubMed]
18. Mairs, R.; Nicholls, D. Assessment and treatment of eating disorders in children and adolescents. *Arch. Dis. Child.* **2016**, *101*, 1168–1175. [CrossRef] [PubMed]
19. Jagielska, G.W.; Przedlacki, J.; Bartoszewicz, Z.; Racicka, E. Bone mineralization disorders as a complication of anorexia nervosa—Etiology, prevalence, course and treatment. *Psychiatr. Pol.* **2016**, *50*, 509–520. [CrossRef] [PubMed]
20. Misra, M.; Klibanski, A. Anorexia Nervosa and Its Associated Endocrinopathy in Young People. *Horm. Res. Paediatr.* **2016**, *85*, 147–157. [CrossRef] [PubMed]
21. Davis, H.; Attia, E. Pharmacotherapy of eating disorders. *Curr. Opin. Psychiatry* **2017**, *30*, 452–457. [CrossRef] [PubMed]
22. Drabkin, A.; Rothman, M.S.; Wassenaar, E.; Mascolo, M.; Mehler, P.S. Assessment and clinical management of bone disease in adults with eating disorders: A review. *J. Eat. Disord.* **2017**, *5*, 42. [CrossRef] [PubMed]
23. Robinson, L.; Micali, N.; Misra, M. Eating disorders and bone metabolism in women. *Curr. Opin. Pediatr.* **2017**, *29*, 488–496. [CrossRef] [PubMed]
24. Himmerich, H.; Treasure, J. Psychopharmacological advances in eating disorders. *Expert Rev. Clin. Pharm.* **2018**, *11*, 95–108. [CrossRef] [PubMed]

25. Hay, P.J.; Claudino, A.M. Clinical psychopharmacology of eating disorders: A research update. *Int. J. Neuropsychopharmacol.* **2012**, *15*, 209–222. [CrossRef] [PubMed]
26. Brewerton, T.D. Antipsychotic agents in the treatment of anorexia nervosa: Neuropsychopharmacologic rationale and evidence from controlled trials. *Curr. Psychiatry Rep.* **2012**, *14*, 398–405. [CrossRef] [PubMed]
27. Kishi, T.; Kafantaris, V.; Sunday, S.; Sheridan, E.M.; Correll, C.U. Are antipsychotics effective for the treatment of anorexia nervosa? Results from a systematic review and meta-analysis. *J. Clin. Psychiatry* **2012**, *73*, e757–e766. [CrossRef] [PubMed]
28. Misra, M.; Klibanski, A. Bone health in anorexia nervosa. *Curr. Opin. Endocrinol. Diabetes Obes.* **2011**, *18*, 376–382. [CrossRef] [PubMed]
29. Maguire, S.; O'Dell, A.; Touyz, L.; Russell, J. Oxytocin and anorexia nervosa: A review of the emerging literature. *Eur. Eat. Disord. Rev. J. Eat. Disord. Assoc.* **2013**, *21*, 475–478. [CrossRef] [PubMed]
30. Howgate, D.J.; Graham, S.M.; Leonidou, A.; Korres, N.; Tsiridis, E.; Tsapakis, E. Bone metabolism in anorexia nervosa: Molecular pathways and current treatment modalities. *Osteoporos. Int.* **2013**, *24*, 407–421. [CrossRef] [PubMed]
31. Balestrieri, M.; Oriani, M.G.; Simoncini, A.; Bellantuono, C. Psychotropic drug treatment in anorexia nervosa. Search for differences in efficacy/tolerability between adolescent and mixed-age population. *Eur. Eat. Disord. Rev. J. Eat. Disord. Assoc.* **2013**, *21*, 361–373. [CrossRef] [PubMed]
32. McElroy, S.L.; Guerdjikova, A.I.; Mori, N.; Keck, P.E. Psychopharmacologic treatment of eating disorders: Emerging findings. *Curr. Psychiatry Rep.* **2015**, *17*, 35. [CrossRef] [PubMed]
33. Lutter, M. Emerging Treatments in Eating Disorders. *Neurother. J. Am. Soc. Exp. Neurother.* **2017**, *14*, 614–622. [CrossRef] [PubMed]
34. Leppanen, J.; Ng, K.W.; Tchanturia, K.; Treasure, J. Meta-analysis of the effects of intranasal oxytocin on interpretation and expression of emotions. *Neurosci. Biobehav. Rev.* **2017**, *78*, 125–144. [CrossRef] [PubMed]
35. Leppanen, J.; Ng, K.W.; Kim, Y.-R.; Tchanturia, K.; Treasure, J. Meta-analytic review of the effects of a single dose of intranasal oxytocin on threat processing in humans. *J. Affect. Disord.* **2018**, *225*, 167–179. [CrossRef] [PubMed]
36. Moher, D.; Liberati, A.; Tetzlaff, J.; Altman, D.G. The PRISMA Group Preferred Reporting Items for Systematic Reviews and Meta-Analyses: The PRISMA Statement. *PLoS Med.* **2009**, *6*, e1000097. [CrossRef] [PubMed]
37. Flament, M.F.; Bissada, H.; Spettigue, W. Evidence-based pharmacotherapy of eating disorders. *Int. J. Neuropsychopharmacol.* **2012**, *15*, 189–207. [CrossRef] [PubMed]
38. Lebow, J.; Sim, L.A.; Erwin, P.J.; Murad, M.H. The effect of atypical antipsychotic medications in individuals with anorexia nervosa: A systematic review and meta-analysis. *Int. J. Eat. Disord.* **2013**, *46*, 332–339. [CrossRef] [PubMed]
39. Lebow, J.; Sim, L. The influence of estrogen therapies on bone mineral density in premenopausal women with anorexia nervosa and amenorrhea. *Vitam. Horm.* **2013**, *92*, 243–257. [PubMed]
40. Watson, H.J.; Bulik, C.M. Update on the treatment of anorexia nervosa: Review of clinical trials, practice guidelines and emerging interventions. *Psychol. Med.* **2013**, *43*, 2477–2500. [CrossRef] [PubMed]
41. De Vos, J.; Houtzager, L.; Katsaragaki, G.; van de Berg, E.; Cuijpers, P.; Dekker, J. Meta analysis on the efficacy of pharmacotherapy versus placebo on anorexia nervosa. *J. Eat. Disord.* **2014**, *2*, 27. [CrossRef] [PubMed]
42. Rocks, T.; Pelly, F.; Wilkinson, P. Nutrition Therapy during Initiation of Refeeding in Underweight Children and Adolescent Inpatients with Anorexia Nervosa: A Systematic Review of the Evidence. *J. Acad. Nutr. Diet.* **2014**, *114*, 897–907. [CrossRef] [PubMed]
43. Dold, M.; Aigner, M.; Klabunde, M.; Treasure, J.; Kasper, S. Second-Generation Antipsychotic Drugs in Anorexia Nervosa: A Meta-Analysis of Randomized Controlled Trials. *Psychother. Psychosom.* **2015**, *84*, 110–116. [CrossRef] [PubMed]
44. El Ghoch, M.; Gatti, D.; Calugi, S.; Viapiana, O.; Bazzani, P.V.; Dalle Grave, R. The Association between Weight Gain/Restoration and Bone Mineral Density in Adolescents with Anorexia Nervosa: A Systematic Review. *Nutrients* **2016**, *8*, 769. [CrossRef] [PubMed]
45. Frank, G.K.W.; Shott, M.E. The Role of Psychotropic Medications in the Management of Anorexia Nervosa: Rationale, Evidence and Future Prospects. *CNS Drugs* **2016**, *30*, 419–442. [CrossRef] [PubMed]
46. Garber, A.K.; Sawyer, S.M.; Golden, N.H.; Guarda, A.S.; Katzman, D.K.; Kohn, M.R.; Le Grange, D.; Madden, S.; Whitelaw, M.; Redgrave, G.W. A systematic review of approaches to refeeding in patients with anorexia nervosa: Refeeding in patients with anorexia nervosa. *Int. J. Eat. Disord.* **2016**, *49*, 293–310. [CrossRef] [PubMed]

47. Kells, M.; Kelly-Weeder, S. Nasogastric Tube Feeding for Individuals with Anorexia Nervosa: An Integrative Review. *J. Am. Psychiatr. Nurses Assoc.* **2016**, *22*, 449–468. [CrossRef] [PubMed]
48. Miniati, M.; Mauri, M.; Ciberti, A.; Mariani, M.G.; Marazziti, D.; Dell'Osso, L. Psychopharmacological options for adult patients with anorexia nervosa. *CNS Spectr.* **2016**, *21*, 134–142. [CrossRef] [PubMed]
49. Misra, M.; Golden, N.H.; Katzman, D.K. State of the Art Systematic Review of Bone Disease in Anorexia Nervosa. *Int. J. Eat. Disord.* **2016**, *49*, 276–292. [CrossRef] [PubMed]
50. Robinson, L.; Aldridge, V.; Clark, E.M.; Misra, M.; Micali, N. Pharmacological treatment options for low Bone Mineral Density and secondary osteoporosis in Anorexia Nervosa: A systematic review of the literature. *J. Psychosom. Res.* **2017**, *98*, 87–97. [CrossRef] [PubMed]
51. Brockmeyer, T.; Friederich, H.-C.; Schmidt, U. Advances in the treatment of anorexia nervosa: A review of established and emerging interventions. *Psychol. Med.* **2018**, *48*, 1228–1256. [CrossRef] [PubMed]
52. Hale, M.D.; Logomarsino, J.V. The use of enteral nutrition in the treatment of eating disorders: A systematic review. *Eat. Weight Disord. Stud. Anorex. Bulim. Obes.* **2018**, 1–20. [CrossRef] [PubMed]
53. Rizzo, S.M.; Douglas, J.W.; Lawrence, J.C. Enteral Nutrition via Nasogastric Tube for Refeeding Patients with Anorexia Nervosa: A Systematic Review. *Nutr. Clin. Pract.* **2018**. [CrossRef] [PubMed]
54. Lacey, J.H.; Crisp, A.H. Hunger, food intake and weight: The impact of clomipramine on a refeeding anorexia nervosa population. *Postgrad. Med. J.* **1980**, *56* (Suppl. 1), 79–85.
55. Halmi, K.A.; Eckert, E.; LaDu, T.J.; Cohen, J. Anorexia nervosa. Treatment efficacy of cyproheptadine and amitriptyline. *Arch. Gen. Psychiatry* **1986**, *43*, 177–181. [CrossRef] [PubMed]
56. Attia, E.; Haiman, C.; Walsh, B.T.; Flater, S.R. Does fluoxetine augment the inpatient treatment of anorexia nervosa? *Am. J. Psychiatry* **1998**, *155*, 548–551. [CrossRef] [PubMed]
57. Walsh, B.T.; Kaplan, A.S.; Attia, E.; Olmsted, M.; Parides, M.; Carter, J.C.; Pike, K.M.; Devlin, M.J.; Woodside, B.; Roberto, C.A.; et al. Fluoxetine after weight restoration in anorexia nervosa: A randomized controlled trial. *JAMA* **2006**, *295*, 2605–2612. [CrossRef] [PubMed]
58. Halmi, K.A. Perplexities of treatment resistance in eating disorders. *BMC Psychiatry* **2013**, *13*, 292. [CrossRef] [PubMed]
59. Crisp, A.H.; Lacey, J.H.; Crutchfield, M. Clomipramine and "drive" in people with anorexia nervosa: An in-patient study. *Br. J. Psychiatry J. Ment. Sci.* **1987**, *150*, 355–358. [CrossRef]
60. Strobel, M.; Warnke, A.; Roth, M.; Schulze, U. Paroxetine versus clomipramine in female adolescents suffering from anorexia nervosa and depressive episode—A retrospective study on tolerability, reasons for discontinuing the antidepressive treatment and different outcome measurements. *Z. Kinder. Jugendpsychiatr. Psychother.* **2004**, *32*, 279–289. [CrossRef] [PubMed]
61. Kaye, W.H.; Nagata, T.; Weltzin, T.E.; Hsu, L.K.; Sokol, M.S.; McConaha, C.; Plotnicov, K.H.; Weise, J.; Deep, D. Double-blind placebo-controlled administration of fluoxetine in restricting- and restricting-purging-type anorexia nervosa. *Biol. Psychiatry* **2001**, *49*, 644–652. [CrossRef]
62. Barbarich, N.C.; McConaha, C.W.; Halmi, K.A.; Gendall, K.; Sunday, S.R.; Gaskill, J.; La Via, M.; Frank, G.K.; Brooks, S.; Plotnicov, K.H.; et al. Use of nutritional supplements to increase the efficacy of fluoxetine in the treatment of anorexia nervosa. *Int. J. Eat. Disord.* **2004**, *35*, 10–15. [CrossRef] [PubMed]
63. Brambilla, F.; Draisci, A.; Peirone, A.; Brunetta, M. Combined cognitive-behavioral, psychopharmacological and nutritional therapy in eating disorders. 2. Anorexia nervosa—Binge-eating/purging type. *Neuropsychobiology* **1995**, *32*, 64–67. [CrossRef] [PubMed]
64. Brambilla, F.; Draisci, A.; Peirone, A.; Brunetta, M. Combined cognitive-behavioral, psychopharmacological and nutritional therapy in eating disorders. 1. Anorexia nervosa—Restricted type. *Neuropsychobiology* **1995**, *32*, 59–63. [CrossRef] [PubMed]
65. Ruggiero, G.M.; Laini, V.; Mauri, M.C.; Ferrari, V.M.; Clemente, A.; Lugo, F.; Mantero, M.; Redaelli, G.; Zappulli, D.; Cavagnini, F. A single blind comparison of amisulpride, fluoxetine and clomipramine in the treatment of restricting anorectics. *Prog. Neuropsychopharmacol. Biol. Psychiatry* **2001**, *25*, 1049–1059. [CrossRef]
66. Pallanti, S.; Quercioli, L.; Ramacciotti, A. Citalopram in anorexia nervosa. *Eat. Weight Disord. EWD* **1997**, *2*, 216–221. [CrossRef] [PubMed]
67. Calandra, C.; Gulino, V.; Inserra, L.; Giuffrida, A. The use of citalopram in an integrated approach to the treatment of eating disorders: An open study. *Eat. Weight Disord. EWD* **1999**, *4*, 207–210. [CrossRef] [PubMed]

68. Fassino, S.; Leombruni, P.; Daga, G.; Brustolin, A.; Migliaretti, G.; Cavallo, F.; Rovera, G. Efficacy of citalopram in anorexia nervosa: A pilot study. *Eur. Neuropsychopharmacol. J. Eur. Coll. Neuropsychopharmacol.* **2002**, *12*, 453–459. [CrossRef]
69. Santonastaso, P.; Friederici, S.; Favaro, A. Sertraline in the treatment of restricting anorexia nervosa: An open controlled trial. *J. Child Adolesc. Psychopharmacol.* **2001**, *11*, 143–150. [CrossRef] [PubMed]
70. Kennedy, S.H.; Piran, N.; Garfinkel, P.E. Monoamine oxidase inhibitor therapy for anorexia nervosa and bulimia: A preliminary trial of isocarboxazid. *J. Clin. Psychopharmacol.* **1985**, *5*, 279–285. [CrossRef] [PubMed]
71. Stip, E.; Lungu, O.V. Salience network and olanzapine in schizophrenia: Implications for treatment in anorexia nervosa. *Can. J. Psychiatry Rev. Can. Psychiatr.* **2015**, *60*, S35–S39.
72. Frieling, H.; Römer, K.D.; Scholz, S.; Mittelbach, F.; Wilhelm, J.; De Zwaan, M.; Jacoby, G.E.; Kornhuber, J.; Hillemacher, T.; Bleich, S. Epigenetic dysregulation of dopaminergic genes in eating disorders. *Int. J. Eat. Disord.* **2010**, *43*, 577–583. [CrossRef] [PubMed]
73. Spettigue, W.; Norris, M.L.; Maras, D.; Obeid, N.; Feder, S.; Harrison, M.E.; Gomez, R.; Fu, M.C.; Henderson, K.; Buchholz, A. Evaluation of the Effectiveness and Safety of Olanzapine as an Adjunctive Treatment for Anorexia Nervosa in Adolescents: An Open-Label Trial. *J. Can. Acad. Child Adolesc. Psychiatry J. Acad. Can. Psychiatr. Enfant Adolesc.* **2018**, *27*, 197–208.
74. Himmerich, H.; Au, K.; Dornik, J.; Bentley, J.; Schmidt, U.; Treasure, J. Olanzapine Treatment for Patients with Anorexia Nervosa. *Can. J. Psychiatry Rev. Can. Psychiatr.* **2017**, *62*, 506–507. [CrossRef] [PubMed]
75. Brambilla, F.; Amianto, F.; Dalle Grave, R.; Fassino, S. Lack of efficacy of psychological and pharmacological treatments of disorders of eating behavior: Neurobiological background. *BMC Psychiatry* **2014**, *14*, 376. [CrossRef] [PubMed]
76. Attia, E.; Steinglass, J.E.; Walsh, B.T.; Wang, Y.; Wu, P.; Schreyer, C.; Wildes, J.; Yilmaz, Z.; Guarda, A.S.; Kaplan, A.S.; et al. Olanzapine Versus Placebo in Adult Outpatients with Anorexia Nervosa: A Randomized Clinical Trial. *Am. J. Psychiatry* **2019**. [CrossRef] [PubMed]
77. Vandereycken, W.; Pierloot, R. Pimozide combined with behavior therapy in the short-term treatment of anorexia nervosa. A double-blind placebo-controlled cross-over study. *Acta Psychiatr. Scand.* **1982**, *66*, 445–450. [CrossRef] [PubMed]
78. Vandereycken, W. Neuroleptics in the short-term treatment of anorexia nervosa. A double-blind placebo-controlled study with sulpiride. *Br. J. Psychiatry J. Ment. Sci.* **1984**, *144*, 288–292. [CrossRef]
79. Cassano, G.B.; Miniati, M.; Pini, S.; Rotondo, A.; Banti, S.; Borri, C.; Camilleri, V.; Mauri, M. Six-month open trial of haloperidol as an adjunctive treatment for anorexia nervosa: A preliminary report. *Int. J. Eat. Disord.* **2003**, *33*, 172–177. [CrossRef] [PubMed]
80. Mondraty, N.; Birmingham, C.L.; Touyz, S.; Sundakov, V.; Chapman, L.; Beumont, P. Randomized controlled trial of olanzapine in the treatment of cognitions in anorexia nervosa. *Australas Psychiatry Bull. R. Aust. N. Z. Coll. Psychiatr.* **2005**, *13*, 72–75. [CrossRef] [PubMed]
81. Brambilla, F.; Monteleone, P.; Maj, M. Olanzapine-induced weight gain in anorexia nervosa: Involvement of leptin and ghrelin secretion? *Psychoneuroendocrinology* **2007**, *32*, 402–406. [CrossRef] [PubMed]
82. Brambilla, F.; Garcia, C.S.; Fassino, S.; Daga, G.A.; Favaro, A.; Santonastaso, P.; Ramaciotti, C.; Bondi, E.; Mellado, C.; Borriello, R.; et al. Olanzapine therapy in anorexia nervosa: Psychobiological effects. *Int. Clin. Psychopharmacol.* **2007**, *22*, 197–204. [CrossRef] [PubMed]
83. Bissada, H.; Tasca, G.A.; Barber, A.M.; Bradwejn, J. Olanzapine in the treatment of low body weight and obsessive thinking in women with anorexia nervosa: A randomized, double-blind, placebo-controlled trial. *Am. J. Psychiatry* **2008**, *165*, 1281–1288. [CrossRef] [PubMed]
84. Attia, E.; Kaplan, A.S.; Walsh, B.T.; Gershkovich, M.; Yilmaz, Z.; Musante, D.; Wang, Y. Olanzapine versus placebo for out-patients with anorexia nervosa. *Psychol. Med.* **2011**, *41*, 2177–2182. [CrossRef] [PubMed]
85. Kafantaris, V.; Leigh, E.; Hertz, S.; Berest, A.; Schebendach, J.; Sterling, W.M.; Saito, E.; Sunday, S.; Higdon, C.; Golden, N.H.; et al. A placebo-controlled pilot study of adjunctive olanzapine for adolescents with anorexia nervosa. *J. Child Adolesc. Psychopharmacol.* **2011**, *21*, 207–212. [CrossRef] [PubMed]
86. Hagman, J.; Gralla, J.; Sigel, E.; Ellert, S.; Dodge, M.; Gardner, R.; O'Lonergan, T.; Frank, G.; Wamboldt, M.Z. A double-blind, placebo-controlled study of risperidone for the treatment of adolescents and young adults with anorexia nervosa: A pilot study. *J. Am. Acad. Child Adolesc. Psychiatry* **2011**, *50*, 915–924. [CrossRef] [PubMed]

87. Powers, P.S.; Klabunde, M.; Kaye, W. Double-blind placebo-controlled trial of quetiapine in anorexia nervosa. *Eur. Eat. Disord. Rev. J. Eat. Disord. Assoc.* **2012**, *20*, 331–334. [CrossRef] [PubMed]
88. Court, A.; Mulder, C.; Kerr, M.; Yuen, H.P.; Boasman, M.; Goldstone, S.; Fleming, J.; Weigall, S.; Derham, H.; Huang, C.; et al. Investigating the effectiveness, safety and tolerability of quetiapine in the treatment of anorexia nervosa in young people: A pilot study. *J. Psychiatr. Res.* **2010**, *44*, 1027–1034. [CrossRef] [PubMed]
89. Gross, H.A.; Ebert, M.H.; Faden, V.B.; Goldberg, S.C.; Nee, L.E.; Kaye, W.H. A double-blind controlled trial of lithium carbonate primary anorexia nervosa. *J. Clin. Psychopharmacol.* **1981**, *1*, 376–381. [CrossRef] [PubMed]
90. Stheneur, C.; Bergeron, S.; Lapeyraque, A.-L. Renal complications in anorexia nervosa. *Eat. Weight Disord. EWD* **2014**, *19*, 455–460. [CrossRef] [PubMed]
91. Goldberg, S.C.; Eckert, E.D.; Halmi, K.A.; Casper, R.C.; Davis, J.M.; Roper, M. Effects of cyproheptadine on symptoms and attitudes in anorexia nervosa. *Arch. Gen. Psychiatry* **1980**, *37*, 1083. [PubMed]
92. Halmi, K.A.; Eckert, E.; Falk, J.R. Cyproheptadine for anorexia nervosa. *Lancet Lond. Engl.* **1982**, *1*, 1357–1358. [CrossRef]
93. Marrazzi, M.A.; Bacon, J.P.; Kinzie, J.; Luby, E.D. Naltrexone use in the treatment of anorexia nervosa and bulimia nervosa. *Int. Clin. Psychopharmacol.* **1995**, *10*, 163–172. [CrossRef] [PubMed]
94. Gross, H.; Ebert, M.H.; Faden, V.B.; Goldberg, S.C.; Kaye, W.H.; Caine, E.D.; Hawks, R.; Zinberg, N. A double-blind trial of delta 9-tetrahydrocannabinol in primary anorexia nervosa. *J. Clin. Psychopharmacol.* **1983**, *3*, 165–171. [CrossRef] [PubMed]
95. Andries, A.; Frystyk, J.; Flyvbjerg, A.; Støving, R.K. Dronabinol in severe, enduring anorexia nervosa: A randomized controlled trial. *Int. J. Eat. Disord.* **2014**, *47*, 18–23. [CrossRef] [PubMed]
96. Hotta, M.; Ohwada, R.; Akamizu, T.; Shibasaki, T.; Kangawa, K. Therapeutic potential of ghrelin in restricting-type anorexia nervosa. *Methods Enzym.* **2012**, *514*, 381–398.
97. Steinglass, J.E.; Kaplan, S.C.; Liu, Y.; Wang, Y.; Walsh, B.T. The (lack of) effect of alprazolam on eating behavior in anorexia nervosa: A preliminary report. *Int. J. Eat. Disord.* **2014**, *47*, 901–904. [CrossRef] [PubMed]
98. Casper, R.C.; Schlemmer, R.F.; Javaid, J.I. A placebo-controlled crossover study of oral clonidine in acute anorexia nervosa. *Psychiatry Res.* **1987**, *20*, 249–260. [CrossRef]
99. Levinson, C.A.; Rodebaugh, T.L.; Fewell, L.; Kass, A.E.; Riley, E.N.; Stark, L.; McCallum, K.; Lenze, E.J. D-Cycloserine facilitation of exposure therapy improves weight regain in patients with anorexia nervosa: A pilot randomized controlled trial. *J. Clin. Psychiatry* **2015**, *76*, e787–e793. [CrossRef] [PubMed]
100. Lechin, F.; van der Dijs, B.; Pardey-Maldonado, B.; Baez, S.; Lechin, M.E. Anorexia nervosa versus hyperinsulinism: Therapeutic effects of neuropharmacological manipulation. *Clin. Risk Manag.* **2011**, *7*, 53–58. [CrossRef] [PubMed]
101. Russell, J.; Maguire, S.; Hunt, G.E.; Kesby, A.; Suraev, A.; Stuart, J.; Booth, J.; McGregor, I.S. Intranasal oxytocin in the treatment of anorexia nervosa: Randomized controlled trial during re-feeding. *Psychoneuroendocrinology* **2018**, *87*, 83–92. [CrossRef] [PubMed]
102. Agostino, H.; Erdstein, J.; Di Meglio, G. Shifting Paradigms: Continuous Nasogastric Feeding with High Caloric Intakes in Anorexia Nervosa. *J. Adolesc. Health* **2013**, *53*, 590–594. [CrossRef] [PubMed]
103. Findlay, S.M.; Toews, H.; Grant, C. Use of Gastrostomy Tubes in Children and Adolescents with Eating Disorders and Related Illnesses. *J. Adolesc. Health* **2011**, *48*, 625–629. [CrossRef] [PubMed]
104. Heruc, G.A.; Little, T.J.; Kohn, M.R.; Madden, S.; Clarke, S.D.; Horowitz, M.; Feinle-Bisset, C. Effects of starvation and short-term refeeding on gastric emptying and postprandial blood glucose regulation in adolescent girls with anorexia nervosa. *Am. J. Physiol. Endocrinol. Metab.* **2018**, *315*, E565–E573. [CrossRef] [PubMed]
105. Hofer, M.; Pozzi, A.; Joray, M.; Ott, R.; Hähni, F.; Leuenberger, M.; von Känel, R.; Stanga, Z. Safe refeeding management of anorexia nervosa inpatients: An evidence-based protocol. *Nutrition* **2014**, *30*, 524–530. [CrossRef] [PubMed]
106. Garber, A.K.; Michihata, N.; Hetnal, K.; Shafer, M.-A.; Moscicki, A.-B. A Prospective Examination of Weight Gain in Hospitalized Adolescents with Anorexia Nervosa on a Recommended Refeeding Protocol. *J. Adolesc. Health* **2012**, *50*, 24–29. [CrossRef] [PubMed]
107. Ozier, A.D.; Henry, B.W. Position of the American Dietetic Association: Nutrition Intervention in the Treatment of Eating Disorders. *J. Am. Diet. Assoc.* **2011**, *111*, 1236–1241. [CrossRef] [PubMed]

108. Rigaud, D.; Brondel, L.; Poupard, A.T.; Talonneau, I.; Brun, J.M. A randomized trial on the efficacy of a 2-month tube feeding regimen in anorexia nervosa: A 1-year follow-up study. *Clin. Nutr.* **2007**, *26*, 421–429. [CrossRef] [PubMed]

109. Rigaud, D.J.; Brayer, V.; Roblot, A.; Brindisi, M.-C.; Vergès, B. Efficacy of Tube Feeding in Binge-Eating/Vomiting Patients: A 2-Month Randomized Trial with 1-Year Follow-Up. *J. Parenter. Enter. Nutr.* **2011**, *35*, 356–364. [CrossRef] [PubMed]

110. Silber, T.J.; Robb, A.S.; Orrell-Valente, J.K.; Ellis, N.; Valadez-Meltzer, A.; Dadson, M.J. Nocturnal nasogastric refeeding for hospitalized adolescent boys with anorexia nervosa. *J. Dev. Behav. Pediatr. JDBP* **2004**, *25*, 415–418. [CrossRef] [PubMed]

111. Rigaud, D.; Pennacchio, H.; Roblot, A.; Jacquet, M.; Tallonneau, I.; Verges, B. Efficacité de la nutrition entérale à domicile chez 60 malades ayant une anorexie mentale. *Presse Médicale* **2009**, *38*, 1739–1745. [CrossRef] [PubMed]

112. Daniel, R.; Didier, P.; Hélène, P. A 3-month at-home tube feeding in 118 bulimia nervosa patients: A one-year prospective survey in adult patients. *Clin. Nutr.* **2014**, *33*, 336–340. [CrossRef] [PubMed]

113. Gentile, M.G.; Pastorelli, P.; Ciceri, R.; Manna, G.M.; Collimedaglia, S. Specialized refeeding treatment for anorexia nervosa patients suffering from extreme undernutrition. *Clin. Nutr. Edinb. Scotl.* **2010**, *29*, 627–632. [CrossRef] [PubMed]

114. Gentile, M.G. Enteral Nutrition for Feeding Severely Underfed Patients with Anorexia Nervosa. *Nutrients* **2012**, *4*, 1293–1303. [CrossRef] [PubMed]

115. Rigaud, D.; Tallonneau, I.; Brindisi, M.-C.; Vergès, B. Prognosis in 41 severely malnourished anorexia nervosa patients. *Clin. Nutr.* **2012**, *31*, 693–698. [CrossRef] [PubMed]

116. Hart, S.; Franklin, R.C.; Russell, J.; Abraham, S. A review of feeding methods used in the treatment of anorexia nervosa. *J. Eat. Disord.* **2013**, *1*, 36. [CrossRef] [PubMed]

117. Arii, I.; Yamashita, T.; Kinoshita, M.; Shimizu, H.; Nakamura, M.; Nakajima, T. Treatment for inpatients with anorexia nervosa: Comparison of liquid formula with regular meals for improvement from emaciation. *Psychiatry Clin. Neurosci.* **1996**, *50*, 55–60. [CrossRef] [PubMed]

118. Hill, K.K.; Maloney, M.J.; Jellinek, M.S.; Biederman, J. Treating Anorexia Nervosa Patients in the Era of Manage Care. *J. Am. Acad. Child Adolesc. Psychiatry* **1997**, *36*, 1632–1633. [PubMed]

119. Imbierowicz, K.; Braks, K.; Jacoby, G.E.; Geiser, F.; Conrad, R.; Schilling, G.; Liedtke, R. High-caloric supplements in anorexia treatment. *Int. J. Eat. Disord.* **2002**, *32*, 135–145. [CrossRef] [PubMed]

120. Cockfield, A.; Philpot, U. Managing anorexia from a dietitian's perspective. *Proc. Nutr. Soc.* **2009**, *68*, 281. [CrossRef] [PubMed]

121. Achamrah, N.; Coëffier, M.; Rimbert, A.; Charles, J.; Folope, V.; Petit, A.; Déchelotte, P.; Grigioni, S. Micronutrient Status in 153 Patients with Anorexia Nervosa. *Nutrients* **2017**, *9*, 225. [CrossRef] [PubMed]

122. Chiurazzi, C.; Cioffi, I.; De Caprio, C.; De Filippo, E.; Marra, M.; Sammarco, R.; Di Guglielmo, M.L.; Contaldo, F.; Pasanisi, F. Adequacy of nutrient intake in women with restrictive anorexia nervosa. *Nutrition* **2017**, *38*, 80–84. [CrossRef] [PubMed]

123. Oudman, E.; Wijnia, J.W.; Oey, M.J.; van Dam, M.J.; Postma, A. Preventing Wernicke's encephalopathy in anorexia nervosa: A systematic review: Wernicke's and anorexia nervosa. *Psychiatry Clin. Neurosci.* **2018**, *72*, 774–779. [CrossRef] [PubMed]

124. Suzuki, H.; Asakawa, A.; Li, J.B.; Tsai, M.; Amitani, H.; Ohinata, K.; Komai, M.; Inui, A. Zinc as an appetite stimulator—The possible role of zinc in the progression of diseases such as cachexia and sarcopenia. *Recent Pat. Food Nutr. Agric.* **2011**, *3*, 226–231. [CrossRef] [PubMed]

125. Birmingham, C.L.; Gritzner, S. How does zinc supplementation benefit anorexia nervosa? *Eat. Weight Disord. EWD* **2006**, *11*, e109–e111. [CrossRef] [PubMed]

126. Franques, J.; Chiche, L.; Mathis, S. Sensory Neuronopathy Revealing Severe Vitamin B12 Deficiency in a Patient with Anorexia Nervosa: An Often-Forgotten Reversible Cause. *Nutrients* **2017**, *9*, 281. [CrossRef] [PubMed]

127. Birmingham, C.L.; Gritzner, S. Heart failure in anorexia nervosa: Case report and review of the literature. *Eat. Weight Disord. EWD* **2007**, *12*, e7–e10. [CrossRef] [PubMed]

128. Perica, M.M.; Delaš, I. Essential Fatty Acids and Psychiatric Disorders. *Nutr. Clin. Pract.* **2011**, *26*, 409–425. [CrossRef] [PubMed]

129. Shih, P.B.; Morisseau, C.; Le, T.; Woodside, B.; German, J.B. Personalized polyunsaturated fatty acids as a potential adjunctive treatment for anorexia nervosa. *Prostaglandins Other Lipid Mediat.* **2017**, *133*, 11–19. [CrossRef] [PubMed]

130. Ayton, A.K.; Azaz, A.; Horrobin, D.F. Rapid improvement of severe anorexia nervosa during treatment with ethyl-eicosapentaenoate and micronutrients. *Eur. Psychiatry* **2004**, *19*, 317–319. [CrossRef] [PubMed]

131. Ayton, A.K.; Azaz, A.; Horrobin, D.F. A pilot open case series of ethyl-epa supplementation in the treatment of anorexia nervosa. *Prostaglandins Leukot. Essent. Fatty Acids* **2004**, *71*, 205–209. [CrossRef] [PubMed]

132. Mauler, B.; Dubben, S.; Pawelzik, M.; Pawelzik, D.; Weigle, D.S.; Kratz, M. Hypercaloric diets differing in fat composition have similar effects on serum leptin and weight gain in female subjects with anorexia nervosa. *Nutr. Res.* **2009**, *29*, 1–7. [CrossRef] [PubMed]

133. Zipfel, S.; Sammet, I.; Rapps, N.; Herzog, W.; Herpertz, S.; Martens, U. Gastrointestinal disturbances in eating disorders: Clinical and neurobiological aspects. *Auton. Neurosci.* **2006**, *129*, 99–106. [CrossRef] [PubMed]

134. Malczyk, Ż.; Oświęcimska, J. Gastrointestinal complications and refeeding guidelines in patients with anorexia nervosa. *Psychiatr. Pol.* **2017**, *51*, 219–229. [CrossRef] [PubMed]

135. Hetterich, L.; Mack, I.; Giel, K.E.; Zipfel, S.; Stengel, A. An update on gastrointestinal disturbances in eating disorders. *Mol. Cell. Endocrinol.* **2018**. [CrossRef] [PubMed]

136. Wang, X.; Luscombe, G.M.; Boyd, C.; Kellow, J.; Abraham, S. Functional gastrointestinal disorders in eating disorder patients: Altered distribution and predictors using ROME III compared to ROME II criteria. *World J. Gastroenterol. WJG* **2014**, *20*, 16293–16299. [CrossRef] [PubMed]

137. Salvioli, B.; Pellicciari, A.; Iero, L.; Di Pietro, E.; Moscano, F.; Gualandi, S.; Stanghellini, V.; De Giorgio, R.; Ruggeri, E.; Franzoni, E. Audit of digestive complaints and psychopathological traits in patients with eating disorders: A prospective study. *Dig. Liver Dis.* **2013**, *45*, 639–644. [CrossRef] [PubMed]

138. Camilleri, M.; Parkman, H.P.; Shafi, M.A.; Abell, T.L.; Gerson, L. Clinical Guideline: Management of Gastroparesis. *Am. J. Gastroenterol.* **2013**, *108*, 18–37. [CrossRef] [PubMed]

139. Mascolo, M.; Geer, B.; Feuerstein, J.; Mehler, P.S. Gastrointestinal comorbidities which complicate the treatment of anorexia nervosa. *Eat. Disord.* **2017**, *25*, 122–133. [CrossRef] [PubMed]

140. Moshiree, B.; McDonald, R.; Hou, W.; Toskes, P.P. Comparison of the Effect of Azithromycin Versus Erythromycin on Antroduodenal Pressure Profiles of Patients with Chronic Functional Gastrointestinal Pain and Gastroparesis. *Dig. Dis. Sci.* **2010**, *55*, 675–683. [CrossRef] [PubMed]

141. Martínez-Vázquez, M.A.; Vázquez-Elizondo, G.; González-González, J.A.; Gutiérrez-Udave, R.; Maldonado-Garza, H.J.; Bosques-Padilla, F.J. Effect of antispasmodic agents, alone or in combination, in the treatment of Irritable Bowel Syndrome: Systematic review and meta-analysis. *Rev. Gastroenterol. México* **2012**, *77*, 82–90.

142. Mehler, P.S.; Linas, S. Use of a proton-pump inhibitor for metabolic disturbances associated with anorexia nervosa. *N. Engl. J. Med.* **2002**, *347*, 373–374. [PubMed]

143. Walder, A.; Baumann, P. Cardiac Left Bundle Branch Block and Pancytopenia in Anorexia Nervosa: Higher Risk with Mirtazapine and Pantoprazole? Case Report. *Pharmacopsychiatry* **2009**, *42*, 79–81. [CrossRef] [PubMed]

144. Sato, Y.; Fukudo, S. Gastrointestinal symptoms and disorders in patients with eating disorders. *Clin. J. Gastroenterol.* **2015**, *8*, 255–263. [CrossRef] [PubMed]

145. Mason, B.L. Feeding Systems and the Gut Microbiome: Gut-Brain Interactions with Relevance to Psychiatric Conditions. *Psychosomatics* **2017**, *58*, 574–580. [CrossRef] [PubMed]

146. Hanachi, M.; Manichanh, C.; Schoenenberger, A.; Pascal, V.; Levenez, F.; Cournède, N.; Doré, J.; Melchior, J.-C. Altered host-gut microbes symbiosis in severely malnourished anorexia nervosa (AN) patients undergoing enteral nutrition: An explicative factor of functional intestinal disorders? *Clin. Nutr.* **2018**. [CrossRef] [PubMed]

147. Schwensen, H.F.; Kan, C.; Treasure, J.; Høiby, N.; Sjögren, M. A systematic review of studies on the faecal microbiota in anorexia nervosa: Future research may need to include microbiota from the small intestine. *Eat. Weight Disord. Stud. Anorex. Bulim. Obes.* **2018**, *23*, 399–418. [CrossRef] [PubMed]

148. Misra, M.; Klibanski, A. Endocrine consequences of anorexia nervosa. *Lancet Diabetes Endocrinol.* **2014**, *2*, 581–592. [CrossRef]

149. Schorr, M.; Miller, K.K. The endocrine manifestations of anorexia nervosa: Mechanisms and management. *Nat. Rev. Endocrinol.* **2017**, *13*, 174–186. [CrossRef] [PubMed]

150. Fazeli, P.K.; Lawson, E.A.; Prabhakaran, R.; Miller, K.K.; Donoho, D.A.; Clemmons, D.R.; Herzog, D.B.; Misra, M.; Klibanski, A. Effects of Recombinant Human Growth Hormone in Anorexia Nervosa: A Randomized, Placebo-Controlled Study. *J. Clin. Endocrinol. Metab.* **2010**, *95*, 4889–4897. [CrossRef] [PubMed]
151. Léger, J.; Fjellestad-Paulsen, A.; Bargiacchi, A.; Doyen, C.; Ecosse, E.; Carel, J.-C.; Le Heuzey, M.-F. Can growth hormone treatment improve growth in children with severe growth failure due to anorexia nervosa? A preliminary pilot study. *Endocr. Connect.* **2017**, *6*, 839–846. [CrossRef] [PubMed]
152. Misra, M.; Katzman, D.K.; Estella, N.M.; Eddy, K.T.; Weigel, T.; Goldstein, M.A.; Miller, K.K.; Klibanski, A. Impact of Physiologic Estrogen Replacement on Anxiety Symptoms, Body Shape Perception, and Eating Attitudes in Adolescent Girls with Anorexia Nervosa: Data from a Randomized Controlled Trial. *J. Clin. Psychiatry* **2013**, *74*, e765–e771. [CrossRef] [PubMed]
153. Germain, N.; Fauconnier, A.; Klein, J.-P.; Wargny, A.; Khalfallah, Y.; Papastathi-Boureau, C.; Estour, B.; Galusca, B. Pulsatile gonadotropin-releasing hormone therapy in persistent amenorrheic weight-recovered anorexia nervosa patients. *Fertil. Steril.* **2017**, *107*, 502–509. [CrossRef] [PubMed]
154. Welt, C.K.; Smith, P.; Mantzoros, C.S. Recombinant Human Leptin in Women with Hypothalamic Amenorrhea. *N. Engl. J. Med.* **2004**, *351*, 987–997. [CrossRef] [PubMed]
155. Modan-Moses, D.; Yaroslavsky, A.; Kochavi, B.; Toledano, A.; Segev, S.; Balawi, F.; Mitrany, E.; Stein, D. Linear Growth and Final Height Characteristics in Adolescent Females with Anorexia Nervosa. *PLoS ONE* **2012**, *7*, e45504. [CrossRef] [PubMed]
156. Nehring, I.; Kewitz, K.; von Kries, R.; Thyen, U. Long-term effects of enteral feeding on growth and mental health in adolescents with anorexia nervosa—Results of a retrospective German cohort study. *Eur. J. Clin. Nutr.* **2014**, *68*, 171–177. [CrossRef] [PubMed]
157. Rozé, C.; Doyen, C.; Le Heuzey, M.-F.; Armoogum, P.; Mouren, M.-C.; Léger, J. Predictors of late menarche and adult height in children with anorexia nervosa. *Clin. Endocrinol.* **2007**, *67*, 462–467. [CrossRef] [PubMed]
158. Skolnick, A.; Schulman, R.C.; Galindo, R.J.; Mechanick, J.I. The endocrinopathies of male anorexia nervosa: Case series. *AACE Clin. Case Rep.* **2016**, *2*, e351–e357. [CrossRef] [PubMed]
159. Dempfle, A.; Herpertz-Dahlmann, B.; Timmesfeld, N.; Schwarte, R.; Egberts, K.M.; Pfeiffer, E.; Fleischhaker, C.; Wewetzer, C.; Bühren, K. Predictors of the resumption of menses in adolescent anorexia nervosa. *BMC Psychiatry* **2013**, *13*, 308. [CrossRef] [PubMed]
160. Chui, H.T.; Christensen, B.K.; Zipursky, R.B.; Richards, B.A.; Hanratty, M.K.; Kabani, N.J.; Mikulis, D.J.; Katzman, D.K. Cognitive Function and Brain Structure in Females with a History of Adolescent-Onset Anorexia Nervosa. *Pediatrics* **2008**, *122*, e426–e437. [CrossRef] [PubMed]
161. Chan, J.L.; Mantzoros, C.S. Role of leptin in energy-deprivation states: Normal human physiology and clinical implications for hypothalamic amenorrhoea and anorexia nervosa. *Lancet* **2005**, *366*, 74–85. [CrossRef]
162. Brown, L.M.; Clegg, D.J. Estrogen and Leptin Regulation of Endocrinological Features of Anorexia Nervosa. *Neuropsychopharmacology* **2013**, *38*, 237. [CrossRef] [PubMed]
163. Robinson, L.; Aldridge, V.; Clark, E.M.; Misra, M.; Micali, N. A systematic review and meta-analysis of the association between eating disorders and bone density. *Osteoporos. Int.* **2016**, *27*, 1953–1966. [CrossRef] [PubMed]
164. Misra, M.; Le Clair, M.; Mendes, N.; Miller, K.K.; Lawson, E.; Meenaghan, E.; Weigel, T.; Ebrahimi, S.; Herzog, D.B.; Klibanski, A. Use of SSRIs may Impact Bone Density in Adolescent and Young Women with Anorexia Nervosa. *CNS Spectr.* **2010**, *15*, 579–586. [CrossRef] [PubMed]
165. Miller, K.K.; Lee, E.E.; Lawson, E.A.; Misra, M.; Minihan, J.; Grinspoon, S.K.; Gleysteen, S.; Mickley, D.; Herzog, D.; Klibanski, A. Determinants of Skeletal Loss and Recovery in Anorexia Nervosa. *J. Clin. Endocrinol. Metab.* **2006**, *91*, 2931–2937. [CrossRef] [PubMed]
166. Hartman, D.; Crisp, A.; Rooney, B.; Rackow, C.; Atkinson, R.; Patel, S. Bone density of women who have recovered from anorexia nervosa. *Int. J. Eat. Disord.* **2000**, *28*, 107–112. [CrossRef]
167. Castro, J.; Toro, J.; Lázaro, L.; Pons, F.; Halperin, I. Bone Mineral Density in Male Adolescents with Anorexia Nervosa. *J. Am. Acad. Child Adolesc. Psychiatry* **2002**, *41*, 613–618. [CrossRef] [PubMed]
168. Seeman, E.; Szmukler, G.I.; Formica, C.; Tsalamandris, C.; Mestrovic, R. Osteoporosis in anorexia nervosa: The influence of peak bone density, bone loss, oral contraceptive use, and exercise. *J. Bone Min. Res.* **2009**, *7*, 1467–1474. [CrossRef] [PubMed]
169. Elkazaz, A.Y.; Salama, K. The effect of oral contraceptive different patterns of use on circulating IGF-1 and bone mineral density in healthy premenopausal women. *Endocrine* **2015**, *48*, 272–278. [CrossRef] [PubMed]

170. Hergenroeder, A.C.; Smith, E.O.; Shypailo, R.; Jones, L.A.; Klish, W.J.; Ellis, K. Bone mineral changes in young women with hypothalamic amenorrhea treated with oral contraceptives, medroxyprogesterone, or placebo over 12 months. *Am. J. Obs. Gynecol.* **1997**, *176*, 1017–1025. [CrossRef]
171. Misra, M.; Katzman, D.; Miller, K.K.; Mendes, N.; Snelgrove, D.; Russell, M.; Goldstein, M.A.; Ebrahimi, S.; Clauss, L.; Weigel, T.; et al. Physiologic estrogen replacement increases bone density in adolescent girls with anorexia nervosa. *J. Bone Min. Res.* **2011**, *26*, 2430–2438. [CrossRef] [PubMed]
172. Golden, N.H.; Iglesias, E.A.; Jacobson, M.S.; Carey, D.; Meyer, W.; Schebendach, J.; Hertz, S.; Shenker, I.R. Alendronate for the Treatment of Osteopenia in Anorexia Nervosa: A Randomized, Double-Blind, Placebo-Controlled Trial. *J. Clin. Endocrinol. Metab.* **2005**, *90*, 3179–3185. [CrossRef] [PubMed]
173. Miller, K.K.; Grieco, K.A.; Mulder, J.; Grinspoon, S.; Mickley, D.; Yehezkel, R.; Herzog, D.B.; Klibanski, A. Effects of Risedronate on Bone Density in Anorexia Nervosa. *J. Clin. Endocrinol. Metab.* **2004**, *89*, 3903–3906. [CrossRef] [PubMed]
174. Miller, K.K.; Meenaghan, E.; Lawson, E.A.; Misra, M.; Gleysteen, S.; Schoenfeld, D.; Herzog, D.; Klibanski, A. Effects of Risedronate and Low-Dose Transdermal Testosterone on Bone Mineral Density in Women with Anorexia Nervosa: A Randomized, Placebo-Controlled Study. *J. Clin. Endocrinol. Metab.* **2011**, *96*, 2081–2088. [CrossRef] [PubMed]
175. Miller, K.K.; Grieco, K.A.; Klibanski, A. Testosterone Administration in Women with Anorexia Nervosa. *J. Clin. Endocrinol. Metab.* **2005**, *90*, 1428–1433. [CrossRef] [PubMed]
176. DiVasta, A.D.; Feldman, H.A.; Beck, T.J.; LeBoff, M.S.; Gordon, C.M. Does Hormone Replacement Normalize Bone Geometry in Adolescents with Anorexia Nervosa? *J. Bone Min. Res. Off. J. Am. Soc. Bone Min. Res.* **2014**, *29*, 151–157. [CrossRef] [PubMed]
177. Grinspoon, S.; Baum, H.; Lee, K.; Anderson, E.; Herzog, D.; Klibanski, A. Effects of short-term recombinant human insulin-like growth factor I administration on bone turnover in osteopenic women with anorexia nervosa. *J. Clin. Endocrinol. Metab.* **1996**, *81*, 3864–3870. [PubMed]
178. Grinspoon, S.; Thomas, L.; Miller, K.; Herzog, D.; Klibanski, A. Effects of Recombinant Human IGF-I and Oral Contraceptive Administration on Bone Density in Anorexia Nervosa. *J. Clin. Endocrinol. Metab.* **2002**, *87*, 2883–2891. [CrossRef] [PubMed]
179. Miller, K.K.; Perlis, R.H.; Papakostas, G.I.; Mischoulon, D.; Iosifescu, D.V.; Brick, D.J.; Fava, M. Low-dose Transdermal Testosterone Augmentation Therapy Improves Depression Severity in Women. *CNS Spectr.* **2009**, *14*, 688–694. [CrossRef] [PubMed]
180. Fazeli, P.K.; Wang, I.S.; Miller, K.K.; Herzog, D.B.; Misra, M.; Lee, H.; Finkelstein, J.S.; Bouxsein, M.L.; Klibanski, A. Teriparatide Increases Bone Formation and Bone Mineral Density in Adult Women with Anorexia Nervosa. *J. Clin. Endocrinol. Metab.* **2014**, *99*, 1322–1329. [CrossRef] [PubMed]
181. Iketani, T.; Kiriike, N.; Stein, M.B.; Nagao, K.; Nagata, T.; Minamikawa, N.; Shidao, A.; Fukuhara, H. Effect of menatetrenone (vitamin K2) treatment on bone loss in patients with anorexia nervosa. *Psychiatry Res.* **2003**, *117*, 259–269. [CrossRef]
182. Misra, M.; Tsai, P.; Anderson, E.J.; Hubbard, J.L.; Gallagher, K.; Soyka, L.A.; Miller, K.K.; Herzog, D.B.; Klibanski, A. Nutrient intake in community-dwelling adolescent girls with anorexia nervosa and in healthy adolescents. *Am. J. Clin. Nutr.* **2006**, *84*, 698–706. [CrossRef] [PubMed]
183. Veronese, N.; Solmi, M.; Rizza, W.; Manzato, E.; Sergi, G.; Santonastaso, P.; Caregaro, L.; Favaro, A.; Correll, C.U. Vitamin D status in anorexia nervosa: A meta-analysis: Vitamin D in Anorexia Nervosa. *Int. J. Eat. Disord.* **2015**, *48*, 803–813. [CrossRef] [PubMed]
184. Gatti, D.; El Ghoch, M.; Viapiana, O.; Ruocco, A.; Chignola, E.; Rossini, M.; Giollo, A.; Idolazzi, L.; Adami, S.; Dalle Grave, R. Strong relationship between vitamin D status and bone mineral density in anorexia nervosa. *Bone* **2015**, *78*, 212–215. [CrossRef] [PubMed]
185. Giollo, A.; Idolazzi, L.; Caimmi, C.; Fassio, A.; Bertoldo, F.; Dalle Grave, R.; El Ghoch, M.; Calugi, S.; Bazzani, P.V.; Viapiana, O.; et al. Vitamin D levels strongly influence bone mineral density and bone turnover markers during weight gain in female patients with anorexia nervosa: GIOLLO et al. *Int. J. Eat. Disord.* **2017**, *50*, 1041–1049. [CrossRef] [PubMed]
186. Nakamura, Y.; Kamimura, M.; Koiwai, H.; Kato, H. Adequate nutrition status important for bone mineral density improvement in a patient with anorexia nervosa. *Clin. Risk Manag.* **2018**, *14*, 945–948. [CrossRef] [PubMed]

187. Anderson, J.J.B.; Kruszka, B.; Delaney, J.A.C.; He, K.; Burke, G.L.; Alonso, A.; Bild, D.E.; Budoff, M.; Michos, E.D. Calcium Intake from Diet and Supplements and the Risk of Coronary Artery Calcification and its Progression Among Older Adults: 10-Year Follow-up of the Multi-Ethnic Study of Atherosclerosis (MESA). *J. Am. Heart Assoc. Cardiovasc. Cereb. Dis.* **2016**, *5*, e003815. [CrossRef] [PubMed]
188. Giel, K.; Zipfel, S.; Hallschmid, M. Oxytocin and Eating Disorders: A Narrative Review on Emerging Findings and Perspectives. *Curr. Neuropharmacol.* **2018**, *16*, 1111–1121. [CrossRef] [PubMed]
189. Zipfel, S.; Giel, K.E.; Bulik, C.M.; Hay, P.; Schmidt, U. Anorexia nervosa: Aetiology, assessment, and treatment. *Lancet Psychiatry* **2015**, *2*, 1099–1111. [CrossRef]
190. Støving, R.K. Mechanisms in endocrinology: Anorexia nervosa and endocrinology: A clinical update. *Eur. J. Endocrinol.* **2019**, *180*, R9–R27. [CrossRef] [PubMed]
191. Bargiacchi, A.; Clarke, J.; Paulsen, A.; Leger, J. Refeeding in anorexia nervosa. *Eur. J. Pediatr.* **2018**, 1–10. [CrossRef] [PubMed]
192. Moore, J.K.; Watson, H.J.; Harper, E.; McCormack, J.; Nguyen, T. Psychotropic drug prescribing in an Australian specialist child and adolescent eating disorder service: A retrospective study. *J. Eat. Disord.* **2013**, *1*, 27. [CrossRef] [PubMed]
193. Mattar, L.; Huas, C.; Duclos, J.; Apfel, A.; Godart, N. Relationship between malnutrition and depression or anxiety in Anorexia Nervosa: A critical review of the literature. *J. Affect. Disord.* **2011**, *132*, 311–318. [CrossRef] [PubMed]
194. Himmerich, H.; Joaquim, M.; Bentley, J.; Kan, C.; Dornik, J.; Treasure, J.; Schmidt, U. Psychopharmacological options for adult patients with anorexia nervosa: The patients' and carers' perspectives. *CNS Spectr.* **2018**, *23*, 251–252. [CrossRef] [PubMed]
195. Woodside, B.D.; Staab, R. Management of psychiatric comorbidity in anorexia nervosa and bulimia nervosa. *CNS Drugs* **2006**, *20*, 655–663. [CrossRef] [PubMed]
196. Treasure, J.; Stein, D.; Maguire, S. Has the time come for a staging model to map the course of eating disorders from high risk to severe enduring illness? An examination of the evidence. *Early Interv. Psychiatry* **2015**, *9*, 173–184. [CrossRef] [PubMed]
197. Wildes, J.E.; Marcus, M.D.; Crosby, R.D.; Ringham, R.M.; Dapelo, M.M.; Gaskill, J.A.; Forbush, K.T. The clinical utility of personality subtypes in patients with anorexia nervosa. *J. Consult. Clin. Psychol.* **2011**, *79*, 665–674. [CrossRef] [PubMed]
198. Guillaume, S.; Jaussent, I.; Maimoun, L.; Ryst, A.; Seneque, M.; Villain, L.; Hamroun, D.; Lefebvre, P.; Renard, E.; Courtet, P. Associations between adverse childhood experiences and clinical characteristics of eating disorders. *Sci. Rep.* **2016**, *6*, 35761. [CrossRef] [PubMed]
199. Dechartres, A.; Huas, C.; Godart, N.; Pousset, M.; Pham, A.; Divac, S.M.; Rouillon, F.; Falissard, B. Outcomes of empirical eating disorder phenotypes in a clinical female sample: Results from a latent class analysis. *Psychopathology* **2011**, *44*, 12–20. [CrossRef] [PubMed]
200. Wildes, J.E.; Forbush, K.T.; Markon, K.E. Characteristics and stability of empirically derived anorexia nervosa subtypes: Towards the identification of homogeneous low-weight eating disorder phenotypes. *J. Abnorm. Psychol.* **2013**, *122*, 1031–1041. [CrossRef] [PubMed]
201. Goldschmidt, A.B.; Wonderlich, S.A.; Crosby, R.D.; Cao, L.; Engel, S.G.; Lavender, J.M.; Mitchell, J.E.; Crow, S.J.; Peterson, C.B.; Le Grange, D. Latent profile analysis of eating episodes in anorexia nervosa. *J. Psychiatr. Res.* **2014**, *53*, 193–199. [CrossRef] [PubMed]
202. Levinson, C.A.; Vanzhula, I.; Brosof, L.C. Longitudinal and personalized networks of eating disorder cognitions and behaviors: Targets for precision intervention a proof of concept study. *Int. J. Eat. Disord.* **2018**, *51*, 1233–1243. [CrossRef] [PubMed]
203. Dunlop, K.A.; Woodside, B.; Downar, J. Targeting Neural Endophenotypes of Eating Disorders with Non-invasive Brain Stimulation. *Front. Neurosci.* **2016**, *10*, 30. [CrossRef] [PubMed]

204. Pollock, A.; Campbell, P.; Brunton, G.; Hunt, H.; Estcourt, L. Selecting and implementing overview methods: Implications from five exemplar overviews. *Syst. Rev.* **2017**, *6*, 145. [CrossRef] [PubMed]
205. Ballard, M.; Montgomery, P. Risk of bias in overviews of reviews: A scoping review of methodological guidance and four-item checklist: Review of Methodological Guidance for Overviews of Reviews & Four-Item Checklist. *Res. Synth. Methods* **2017**, *8*, 92–108. [PubMed]

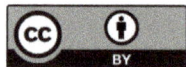 © 2019 by the authors. Licensee MDPI, Basel, Switzerland. This article is an open access article distributed under the terms and conditions of the Creative Commons Attribution (CC BY) license (http://creativecommons.org/licenses/by/4.0/).

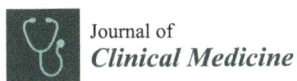
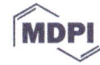

Review

Treatment of Anorexia Nervosa—New Evidence-Based Guidelines

Gaby Resmark [1,*], Stephan Herpertz [2], Beate Herpertz-Dahlmann [3] and Almut Zeeck [4]

1. Department of Psychosomatic Medicine and Psychotherapy, University Hospital Tuebingen, Osianderstr. 5, 72076 Tuebingen, Baden-Wuerttemberg, Germany
2. Department of Psychosomatic Medicine and Psychotherapy, LWL University Hospital, Ruhr-University Bochum, Alexandrinenstr. 1-3, 55791 Bochum, Nordrhein-Westfalen, Germany; stephan.herpertz@rub.de
3. Department of Child and Adolescent Psychiatry, Psychosomatics and Psychotherapy, University Hospital of the RWTH Aachen, Neuenhofer Weg 21, 52074 Aachen, Nordrhein-Westfalen, Germany; bherpertz@ukaachen.de
4. Department of Psychosomatic Medicine and Psychotherapy, University Hospital Freiburg, Hauptstr. 8, 79104 Freiburg, Baden-Wuerttemberg, Germany; almut.zeeck@uniklinik-freiburg.de
* Correspondence: gaby.resmark@med.uni-tuebingen.de; Tel.: +49-7071-29-86719

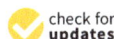

Received: 21 December 2018; Accepted: 28 January 2019; Published: 29 January 2019

Abstract: Anorexia nervosa is the most severe eating disorder; it has a protracted course of illness and the highest mortality rate among all psychiatric illnesses. It is characterised by a restriction of energy intake followed by substantial weight loss, which can culminate in cachexia and related medical consequences. Anorexia nervosa is associated with high personal and economic costs for sufferers, their relatives and society. Evidence-based practice guidelines aim to support all groups involved in the care of patients with anorexia nervosa by providing them with scientifically sound recommendations regarding diagnosis and treatment. The German S3-guideline for eating disorders has been recently revised. In this paper, the new guideline is presented and changes, in comparison with the original guideline published in 2011, are discussed. Further, the German guideline is compared to current international evidence-based guidelines for eating disorders. Many of the treatment recommendations made in the revised German guideline are consistent with existing international treatment guidelines. Although the available evidence has significantly improved in quality and amount since the original German guideline publication in 2011, further research investigating eating disorders in general, and specifically anorexia nervosa, is still needed.

Keywords: anorexia nervosa; guidelines; evidenced-based; treatment

1. Introduction

1.1. Anorexia Nervosa

Anorexia nervosa (AN) is a serious illness leading to high morbidity and mortality [1–4]. It is characterised by a restriction of energy intake, weight loss, fear of weight gain and distorted body image. According to the diagnostic criteria of the International Classification of Diseases, 11th Revision (ICD-11) [5] and the Diagnostic and Statistical Manual of Mental Disorders, 5th Edition (DSM-5) [6], the resulting malnutrition and low body weight may result in massive impairment to health. Often it takes years for patients with AN to achieve a first remission or to recover permanently. A quarter of adult patients go on to develop an enduring form of the disorder, and one-third of patients continue to suffer from residual symptoms in the long-term. The long-term outcome of adolescent-onset AN is more favourable [7]. Because of its severe and protracted course, AN represents a high emotional and economic burden for sufferers, carers and the society in general [8,9]. Age of onset peaks in middle to late adolescence, which affects educational and professional development. The consequences of starvation can have a negative impact on bone density, growth, and brain maturation, especially in children and adolescents. Many patients are affected by comorbid psychological diseases, such as depression, anxiety or obsessive–compulsive disorder. Additionally, the ego-syntonic nature of AN leads to a strong ambivalence regarding weight gain and recovery, which complicates and often slows down the recovery process. In light of these factors, treatment of AN remains challenging. To improve patients' chances of recovery, all individuals dealing with this illness should be well informed about the nature and challenges of treating AN.

1.2. Evidence-Based Treatment Guidelines for Eating Disorders

Evidence-based guidelines have been developed in several countries around the world to guide the treatment of different eating disorders, such as AN. These guidelines have the following aims [10]:

- To support all professionals involved in the diagnosis and treatment of eating disorders, as well as sufferers and their relatives, in deciding on adequate measures of care (prevention, diagnosis, therapy and aftercare);
- To improve health care outcomes;
- To minimise risks;
- To increase treatment safety and efficiency;
- To avoid non-indicated diagnostic and treatment methods.

Further, guidelines can reveal gaps in the health care system [11] and inspire new paths of research.

Treatment guidelines provide recommendations based on current scientific evidence. In cases where a lack of scientific evidence is available, recommendations are often provided based on expert opinion, influenced by years of clinical experience.

2. The German S3Guideline for the Diagnosis and Treatment of Eating Disorders

2.1. Historical Development of the S3-Guideline

In 2000, the German Society for Psychiatry, Psychotherapy and Psychosomatics (DGPPN) published a guideline for the diagnosis and treatment of eating disorders in Germany for the first time [12]. In the same year, a guideline of the German Society of Child and Adolescent Psychiatry, Psychosomatics and Psychotherapy (DGKJP) was also published [13]. Both guidelines were developed by expert groups using informal consensus (a representative group of experts from the relevant medical society prepares a recommendation which is adopted by the board of the society, development stage one) with the aim of developing recommendations for the diagnosis and treatment of eating disorders. In the autumn of 2003, a conference of members of the German Society for Psychosomatic Medicine and Medical Psychotherapy (DGPM) and the German College of Psychosomatic Medicine (DKPM) decided to develop an evidence-based guideline for eating disorders in Germany according to development stage three (S3, based on all elements of systematic development—logic, decision and outcome analysis, evaluation of the clinical relevance of scientific studies and periodic review).

One year later, in the spring of 2004, a group composed of psychiatrists, child and adolescent psychiatrists, medical specialists in psychosomatic medicine and psychologists with expertise in eating disorders, was formed. The group included representatives of the five professional societies (DGKJP, the German Psychological Society (DGPs), DGPM, DGPPN and DKPM) that are responsible for the care of patients with eating disorders within the German health care system. In 2010, the evidence-based guideline for the diagnosis and treatment of eating disorders was published online by the Association of the Scientific Medical Societies in Germany (AWMF) [14]. The AWMF advises on matters and tasks of fundamental and interdisciplinary interest in medicine and provides, among other things, a wide range of clinical practice guidelines on its website. The AWMF is the national member for Germany in the Council for International Organisations of Medical Sciences (CIOMS) at the World

Health Organisation, Geneva. In 2011, the guideline was made available in book format [15]. Based on the scientific guideline, a patient guideline was published in 2015 [16]; this guideline, supported by the German Society for Eating Disorders (DGESS), was designed to communicate the content of the scientific guideline to patients and relatives. The patient guideline, available both online [16] and in book format [17], addresses care structures and supports communication with professional health care providers, such as the family doctor, medical or psychological psychotherapists for adults or child and adolescent psychiatrists and psychotherapists.

Over the last two years, the scientific guideline has been revised, and a second edition will be available in German at the beginning of 2019, both online [14] and in book format. An English version of the guideline is currently in preparation and will be released at a later date. The scientific guideline addresses all age groups and is available in both a short and an extended version. The thematic structure of the recent guideline largely corresponds to the first edition and includes chapters covering epidemiology, diagnostics, the therapeutic relationship, AN, Bulimia nervosa (BN), Binge eating disorder (BED), physical sequelae and methodology. The chapter 'Diagnostics' is subdivided into sections on the diagnostics of psychological and somatic symptoms. In line with DSM-5 [6], two new categories of eating disorders have been added to the revised guideline: the 'Other Specified Feeding or Eating Disorders' (OSFED), which also include the 'Night Eating Syndrome', and the 'Avoidant Restrictive Food Intake Disorder' (ARFID), which replaces the old category of 'Eating Disorders Not Otherwise Specified' (EDNOS). With regard to the therapeutic studies on AN [18], BN [19] and BED [20], meta-analyses were performed based on a systematic literature search and assignment of pre-determined quality indicators (evidence level I).

2.2. Recommendation for AN—Differences between the First Version and the Revision

Changes in treatment recommendations were based on a systematic literature search (2008–2017), in which 26 new randomised controlled trials (RCTs) on psychotherapeutic treatments, 13 new RCTs on pharmacotherapy and 2 new RCTs on nutritional management were identified [14,18]. The evidence base has considerably improved since the first version, although studies still show a large heterogeneity in terms of samples (adolescents, adults, severe and enduring AN), setting (outpatient, day hospital, inpatient), treatment phase (acute, maintenance) and outcome measures used. It should be emphasised that an improvement in study quality can be seen. In recent years, for example, studies have been published with sample sizes that allow sufficient statistical power [21–26].

Treatment recommendations were based on a network-meta-analysis (see Section 2.3), newly published RCTs, systematic reviews, or lower levels of evidence (if RCTs or systematic reviews were not available). The guideline group discussed each recommendation in light of the available evidence, clinical relevance and suitability. The most relevant changes in the revised version concerning evidence levels and recommendations are summarised in Table 1. Evidence levels were assigned using the Oxford Centre of Evidence Based Medicine criteria [27]: An evidence level of I is given if there is evidence for a specific treatment based on a systematic review (or meta-analysis) of randomised controlled trials (Ia), or one randomised controlled trial with narrow confidence interval (Ib). An evidence level of II is based on cohort-studies (IIa: systematic review, or IIb: individual cohort study). Evidence level III refers to case-control studies and evidence level IV to case-control series.

Treatment recommendations in the German treatment guideline were graded according to levels 'A', 'B', '0' and 'KKP' [28]. 'A' is the strongest recommendation, which is usually based on evidence level I (something 'is to be done'). 'B' recommendations are less strong (something 'should be done'; evidence level II) and '0' recommendations are even less explicit (something 'may be done'). 'KKP' ('clinical consensus point') stands for recommendations, which are not based on empirical research and were derived from the experience of experts (good clinical practice). Grading of recommendations was based largely on the evidence level, but also took the following criteria into account: clinical relevance of effect sizes and end points, the balance of benefits and risks, ethical considerations, patient preferences and applicability. Grading of recommendations was discussed in several consensus meetings.

Table 1. German guideline—changes in treatment recommendations for AN.

Original guideline recommendations 2010 [15]	Guideline-revision recommendations 2019 [14]
General recommendations	
No recommendation concerning co-morbid conditions	(Evidence level IV; Clinical consensus point: good clinical practice): Co-morbid conditions should be systematically assessed and taken into consideration when treating patients with AN.
Treatment setting	
(Evidence level IV; 0): Inpatient treatment should take place in facilities able to offer a specialised multimodal treatment program.	(Evidence level IV; A): Same recommendation as original guideline, recommendation grading updated to A.
No recommendation concerning a stabilisation phase	(Evidence level IV; B): In order to reduce the probability of relapse, the final stage of inpatient therapy should aim to ensure that patients at least maintain their weight for a certain period and are prepared for the transition to an outpatient setting.
No specific recommendation concerning day hospital treatment for children and adolescents	(Evidence level Ib; A): A transfer to day hospital treatment after short-term inpatient treatment with sufficient physical stabilisation should be considered for children and adolescents, provided eating disorder-specific day hospital treatment can be carried out by the same treatment team, and close involvement of the relatives is ensured (evidence level Ib; A).
Psychotherapy	
(Evidence level II; B): Patients with AN are highly ambivalent towards change. Addressing ambivalence and motivation to change is a central task and should be maintained throughout the whole treatment process.	(Evidence level Ia; A): Same recommendation as original guideline, recommendation grading updated to A.
(Evidence level II; B): The outpatient treatment of first choice for AN should be evidence-based psychotherapy. (Clinical consensus point: good clinical practice): Patients with AN should be offered specialised therapy by a practitioner experienced with eating disorders. The choice of method should take into account the patient's preference and age.	(Evidence level Ib; B): Outpatient treatment of first choice for patients with AN should be evidence-based psychotherapy (FBT for children and adolescents; FPT, CBT-E, MANTRA or SSCM for adults), administered by practitioners experienced with eating disorders.
Nutritional management	
(Evidence level: not rated; statement): For orientation during the first days of treatment, the initial food intake (for enteral nutrition) of highly underweight patients can be quantified at approx. 30–40 kcal/kg.	(Evidence level IIa; statement): In patients with mild to moderate AN, an initial low caloric energy supply with gradual increase is not required for safe weight gain (avoidance of refeeding syndrome)—provided that medical monitoring is ensured.
No recommendation, but formulation of statements. For example, The basal metabolic rate is initially low and increases significantly with the onset of weight gain. The formulas for calculating basal metabolic rate obtained from normal and overweight people are not suitable for use with AN.	(Evidence level IV; Clinical consensus point: good clinical practice): The energy supply for the expected weight gain is highly variable and should be individually tailored to the patients as well as to the treatment phase and be continuously monitored.
Pharmacotherapy	
(Evidence level Ib; B): Neuroleptics are not suitable for achieving weight gain in AN. (Evidence level Ia; A): Antidepressants are not recommended for achieving weight gain in AN. This applies to both initial therapy and relapse prevention.	(Evidence level Ia; A): Same recommendations as original guideline, recommendation grading regarding neuroleptics updated to A.
(Evidence level IIa; B): If thinking is considerably restricted to weight phobia and eating and if hyperactivity is not controllable, an attempt to use low-dose neuroleptics (especially olanzapine) may be justified in individual cases. The indication for treatment should be limited to the duration of the symptoms mentioned above (no long-term treatment) and should only be applied within the framework of an overall treatment plan.	Same recommendation as original guideline, with altered recommendation levels: (Evidence level IIa; downgrading to 0): If thinking is considerably restricted to weight phobia and eating and if hyperactivity is not controllable, an attempt to use low-dose neuroleptics (especially olanzapine) may be justified in individual cases. (Clinical consensus point: good clinical practice): The indication for treatment should be limited to the duration of the symptoms mentioned above (no long-term treatment) and should only be applied within the framework of an overall treatment plan. The patient must be informed about the circumstances of the off-label use.

FBT, Family-Based Treatment; FPT, Focal Psychodynamic Therapy; CBT-E, Enhanced Cognitive Behaviour Therapy; MANTRA, Maudsley Model of Anorexia Nervosa Treatment for Adults; SSCM, Specialist Supportive Clinical Management.

Several key treatment recommendations did not change. They will be referred to in the comparison of evidence-based guidelines from other countries (see Section 3.2).

Up and down-grading of recommendations: Only one recommendation was downgraded. It is the recommendation for the use of low-dose neuroleptics in some cases of AN. The decision was based on the consideration that this recommendation should be followed only with caution and not as an overall clinical standard. In contrast, the recommendation not to use neuroleptics for the treatment of AN was upgraded due to an increase in evidence (systematic reviews). The same is true for the recommendation to continuously address motivation to change throughout treatment. Several studies show that motivation to change is a relevant predictor of treatment outcome. Recent high-quality trials made it possible to make specific recommendations regarding the use of specialised psychotherapeutic treatments. However, due to ethical reasons, no study compared an active treatment with untreated control groups. Therefore, it was decided that the recommendation should be classified as 'B' and not 'A'. A further recommendation was upgraded based on clinical relevance; Inpatient treatment should take place in facilities which are able to offer a specialised multimodal treatment programme. In Germany, some adult and child and adolescent psychiatric and psychosomatic hospitals are not specialised and have no experience with the treatment of patients with AN. Treatment in such facilities is, therefore, not recommended, due to high associated risks, not to mention high costs. The new guideline also includes the explicit recommendation to consider co-morbidity in patients with AN. Co-morbid conditions like borderline-personality disorder or post-traumatic stress disorder, for example, might require changes in treatment planning and prioritisation of therapy goals. Although empirical evidence is scarce, a recommendation for a stabilisation phase as a final phase in inpatient treatment was included, as relapse after discharge is common [29–31], and the transition from one service level to another service level (especially to a level with less supervision and support) is a major challenge for patients with AN. Finally, there was new empirical evidence suggesting that a short inpatient stay for weight stabilisation followed by day hospital treatment is as effective as long-term inpatient treatment for children and adolescents with AN, providing there is continuity in the therapists that are responsible and if there is sufficient support by family members [23].

2.3. Network-Meta-Analysis

Based on the systematic literature search (see Section 2.2), a network-meta-analysis was conducted to answer the following question: What is the comparable effectiveness of different psychotherapeutic treatments for AN? Additionally, two further questions were addressed using standardised mean change statistics: What is the amount of weight gain that can be expected in different treatment settings? And: What is the amount of weight gain that can be expected in adolescents vs. adults?

Predefined inclusion and exclusion criteria were used to select the studies. Each study was rated by two independent researchers and additionally assessed for quality [18]. For more details on data analysis see [18].

Network-meta-analysis: 18 randomised controlled studies met inclusion criteria for the data-analysis. Ten studies were on adolescents (625 patients), and 8 studies were on adults (622 patients). No treatment approach was found to be superior. However, there were several limitations to the analysis and interpretation of results. All studies compared active treatments with each other, with no study including an untreated control group. Only a few comparisons were replicated. Furthermore, the majority of studies on adolescents evaluated family-based treatment approaches mostly by the same group of researchers, while interventions in adults were almost exclusively on an individual basis. The manualised treatment approaches that were evaluated in high quality trials comprise the Maudsley Model of Anorexia Nervosa Treatment for Adults (MANTRA) [25], Focal Psychodynamic Therapy (FPT) [26,32,33], Enhanced Cognitive Behaviour Therapy (CBT-E) [26,34,35], Specialist Supportive Clinical Management (SSCM) for adults [25,35,36], and family-based treatment (FBT) for adolescents [21,22,24].

Standardised mean change statistics (SCM): Analyses were conducted with 38 studies (1164 patients). Seventeen of these studies were naturalistic studies, and four studies were on adolescents (350 patients). For a course of up to 27 weeks, significantly higher weight gains can be expected in inpatient treatment compared to outpatient treatment (for adults: mean weight gain of 537 g/week in inpatient treatment vs. 105 g/week in outpatient treatment; for adolescents: mean weight gain of 615 g/week in inpatient treatment vs. 192 g/week in outpatient treatment). The estimated effect sizes for weight gain in adolescents were significantly higher compared to adults (in RCTs: SMC = 1.97 vs. 1.02, in naturalistic studies SMC = 1.84 vs. 1.42, respectively).

In sum, there are several existing manualised psychotherapeutic treatments for AN, which can be considered evidence-based and effective. However, there is a need for replication studies. There are differences regarding treatment response and most suitable treatment approach in adult versus adolescent patients.

3. Comparison of the German S3-Guideline with International Evidence-Based Clinical Treatment Guidelines

3.1. International Evidenced-Based Eating Disorders Guidelines

There are currently several additional evidence-based guidelines available, which provide recommendations regarding the diagnosis and treatment of eating disorders. Most of the guidelines were written by multidisciplinary groups (comprising health care professionals and researchers), and most were designed solely for use by health specialists involved in the treatment of eating disorders. The most recent of these guidelines are the Dutch [37] and the revised British guidelines [38], both published in 2017. The British guideline [38], published by the National Institute for Health and Care Excellence (NICE), addresses all age groups (children, adolescents and adults), and all eating disorder categories (AN, BN, BED and Other Specified Feeding or Eating Disorders (OSFED)). Several lay members of the community were involved in the development of this guideline. The Dutch guideline addresses AN, BN and BED [39]. This guideline, designed to be used by both specialists and population members, is only available in Dutch [39]. Healthcare professionals collaborated with patients and relatives, as well as health insurance representatives, during the developmental stages of the guideline [39].

The next most recent guideline, published in 2016, is the Danish guideline [40]. This 'quick guide', provides a brief overview, designed solely for the treatment of AN. The guideline is available in English, and it addresses all age groups. The full-length version of this guideline is only available in Danish. The Australian and New Zealand guideline [41] was published in 2014 by the Royal Australian and New Zealand College of Psychiatrists. Community members and stakeholders collaborated with healthcare professionals and academics in the development of the guideline. This guideline contains two sections separately addressing AN in children and adolescents, and in adults. BN and BED, as well as avoidant/restrictive food intake disorder, are also addressed.

In 2012, the American Psychiatric Association (APA) released a guideline watch [42], reviewing new evidence published since the last APA guideline in 2006, but gives no explicit recommendations [43]. This guideline addresses AN, BN and BED, and also makes reference to EDNOS. The guideline is designed primarily for the treatment of adults, but also briefly addresses the treatment of children and adolescents. The French guideline [44], published in 2010, is written specifically for AN. It addresses all age groups and is available in English. In 2009, the Spanish guideline [45] for eating disorders was published. This guideline, which concerns eating disorder patients over 8 years of age, is written not only for healthcare specialists, but also for the population and educational professionals. It addresses AN, BN, BED and EDNOS.

In addition to these national guidelines, several more specific evidence-based guidelines also exist. A guideline, developed specifically for the Canadian province of British Columbia, was released in 2010 [46]. This guideline addresses AN, BN and EDNOS (except BED), and advisesthe on treatment of all age groups. In 2011, the World Federation of Societies of Biological Psychiatry (WFSBP) released a guideline specifically addressing the pharmacological treatment of eating disorders [47]. This guideline, written in English, addresses the pharmacological treatment of AN, BN and BED. In 2014, the Management of Really Sick Patients with Anorexia Nervosa (MARSIPAN and Junior

MARSIPAN) guideline [48] was published, a guideline which specifically addresses the treatment of children, adolescents and adult patients with 'severe' AN.

In line with an evidence-based approach, most of the guidelines explicitly state that the development of the guideline involved a systematic literature review, a rating of the identified literature, and a complex consensus process, involving collaboration and review by numerous experts [14,38,41,43–48]. Only the MARSIPAN [48] and WFSBP guidelines [47] do not explicitly refer to a complex consensus process, and the British Columbia guideline [46] does not mention a rating system. The Danish 'quick guide' [40] has a complete absence of information on the methodological process. However, the inclusion of evidence levels in the guide implies that the developmental process was rigorous. A detailed review of the evidence upon which the recommendations are based is only available in the British guideline and the Danish full-length guideline. A more detailed comparison of the methods employed in developing the guidelines goes beyond the scope of this review article. All of the guidelines are available online. The Australian and New Zealand, MARSIPAN, WFSBP and APA guidelines are published in online scientific journals and partly in print versions, and the remainder of the guidelines are available on the relevant publishing society's website.

3.2. Commonalities and Differences

3.2.1. Treatment Setting

For adults: Similar to the German guideline [14], all remaining guidelines (excluding the Danish [40] and WFSBP guidelines [47]) recommend outpatient treatment as a first treatment option, suggesting day patient or inpatient treatment as a more intensive treatment option if outpatient treatment proves ineffective [38,39,41,43,44,46,48]. The German guideline states, however, that in some cases this 'stepped-care' approach may not be appropriate.

Inpatient treatment is recommended in cases with a BMI <15 kg/m^2, rapid or continuing weight loss (>20% over 6 months), high physical risk, severe co-morbid conditions or denial of illness. If these criteria are met, an inpatient setting may be necessary for initial treatment. Likewise, all remaining guidelines (excluding the Danish and WFSBP guidelines) also suggest more intense treatment settings from the outset in cases of severe medical instability. All of these guidelines provide information regarding hospital admission criteria with varying degrees of detail, but agree on the necessity to judge the need for hospitalisation on an individual and multifactorial basis. Further, they state that compulsory treatment is possible in the case of extreme medical complications. The Danish and WFSBP guidelines do not make reference to treatment setting. For an overview of indicators of high medical risk and the handling of medical complications see the review of Zipfel and colleagues [4].

For children and adolescents: Corresponding to the treatment recommendations for adults, outpatient treatment is proposed as the first line treatment for children and young people by the German [14] and most other guidelines [38,41,43,44] if the patient is in a stable medical state. If more intensive care is needed, several guidelines suggest a graduated procedure from inpatient to partial and finally to outpatient treatment programs [40,44,45]. Only the German guideline [14] gives a special recommendation for a referral to day patient treatment. Interestingly, the British and accordingly the Spanish guidelines advise admitting children and young people to a setting with age-appropriate facilities, which are near to their home and have the capacity to provide appropriate educational activities [38,45].

Regarding medical risk and necessity for inpatient treatment, the Australian and New Zealand, British Columbia, British, APA and French guidelines [38,41,44,46,49] provide exact criteria, such as a BMI below the 3rd percentile or an expected body weight (EBW) below 75%, an abnormally low heart rate or blood pressure, electrolyte disturbances, etc. However, the exact values vary between countries. As for adults, these guidelines also indicate psychiatric risk factors, such as suicidality or severe self-injurious behaviour. The German and Spanish guidelines [14,45] are more unspecific to indicate hospitalisation (see above). The German and French guidelines [14,44] also refer to psychosocial risks, such as social isolation and family crisis, to consider inpatient treatment.

3.2.2. Psychotherapy

For adults: All guidelines except for the Danish [40] and WFSBP [47] address the efficacy of specific psychological interventions. No guideline recommends one single superior treatment option. The German [14], British [38] and Dutch guidelines [39] conclude that cognitive-behavioural therapy (CBT or CBT-E respectively), MANTRA, and SSCM are equally effective treatment options, and so, all treatments are recommended as first-line options. Additionally, the German guideline recommends FPT as another first-line treatment option. The remaining guidelines all review evidence for CBT, as well as a variety of other treatments including SSCM [41], psychodynamic therapy [43–46], interpersonal therapy [43,45,46], behaviour therapy [45] and 'systematic and strategic therapies' [44]. These guidelines all conclude that psychological interventions are effective, however, state that there is insufficient evidence to identify which is the most efficacious. The French [44], Dutch [39] and APA guidelines [43] also suggest that psychological interventions may not be as effective in severely malnourished patients.

The Danish guideline [40] also recommends the use of psychotherapeutic treatments, however, does not make any recommendations regarding specific interventions. This guideline provides a 'weak recommendation' that both group and individual psychotherapeutic treatment be considered as first-line treatment options, based on 'very low evidence' which suggests the approaches are equally effective. Recommendations for the inclusion of alternative elements, such as meal support and supervised physical activity, during the treatment phase are mentioned. Other guidelines make specific recommendations against alternative treatments; for example, the German [14] and the Australian and New Zealand guidelines [41] state that nutritional counselling alone should not be used as the sole treatment, and the British guideline [38] recommends against the use of alternative physical therapies, such as yoga, warming therapy, transcranial magnetic stimulation and acupuncture. The Spanish guideline [45] also advises against the use of excessively rigid behavioural programs for inpatients.

Some guidelines make recommendations regarding the required duration of treatment. The Australian and New Zealand guideline [41] states that a longer-term follow-up is necessary as relapse is common, and the Spanish guideline [45] states that duration of treatment should span at least six months for outpatients and twelve months for inpatients. The APA guideline [43] states that due to the enduring nature of the illness, psychotherapeutic treatment is usually required for at least one year, and the British guideline [38] makes specific recommendations regarding the time span of treatments, for example suggesting that CBT treatment for eating disorders should consist of 40 sessions over 40 weeks. The French guideline [44] recommends that treatment should last at least one year after significant clinical improvement, and the German guideline [14] states that after outpatient treatment, patients should regularly meet with their general practitioner (GP), or other care coordinator, for at least one year. The German guideline also recommends that the last phase of inpatient treatment before transfer to an outpatient setting should include a stabilisation period where patients demonstrate that they can maintain the achieved weight gain for a specified amount of time.

Some treatment guidelines make additional specific recommendations. The German [14], French [44], MARSIPAN [48] and Australian and New Zealand guidelines [41] all emphasise the importance of adopting a multi-disciplinary, collaborative approach to treatment. In a similar vein, the German [14], British Columbia [46] and APA guidelines [43] highlight the importance of effective communication between all involved health workers, and recommend identifying someone to act as the primary care coordinator, such as the patient's GP.

The MARSIPAN guideline [48] is specifically written regarding the treatment of patients who have a severe or enduring form of AN. The Australian and New Zealand [41] and British Columbia guidelines [46] also include comprehensive sections which address the treatment of such patients and suggest taking an alternative approach, focused on enhancing quality of life. The French [44], German [14] and APA guidelines [43] also briefly mention the treatment of patients with enduring AN. Other guidelines provide information regarding other additional elements related to AN. For example, both the Spanish [45] and French guidelines provide information regarding the care required for pregnant patients. Additionally, the APA and British Columbia guidelines include recommendations for therapists and specialists regarding communicating with patients (for example addressing the therapeutic relationship, boundaries). The German guideline does not entail any recommendations, but devotes a separate chapter to this topic.

For children and adolescents: All guidelines strongly recommend the involvement of parents or near caregivers in all treatment settings. The Australian and New Zealand, Spanish, APA and German guidelines explicitly mention family-based treatment or therapy (FBT) [14,41,43,45]. However, the Australian and British guidelines also propose alternatives if FBT is not appropriate, such as other forms of family therapy [41], as well as individual treatment, such as adolescent-focused therapy (AFT) or CBT, in older adolescents [38,41]. No guideline gives an explicit advice whether conjoint or separate FBT should be conducted. The French guideline does not refer to FBT, but to family therapy in general [44]. The British guideline also does not specifically use the term FBT, but has its own terminology instead (anorexia nervosa-focused family therapy, FT-AN) [38]. Although many key features of this treatment resemble FBT, FT-AN also includes other approaches, such as multi-family therapy, conjoint or separate family therapy and exclusion or inclusion of a family meal, which is a core feature of FBT. The British guideline also requests therapists and staff to be aware of or address carers' needs [38].

A summary of guidelines' essential key recommendations regarding psychotherapy for AN is shown in Table 2.

Table 2. International guidelines' key recommendations regarding psychotherapy for AN.

Recommendation	AUS [41]	BC [46]	DEN [40]	FR [44]	GER [14]	NETH [39]	SP [45]	UK [38]	US [43]
For adults:									
Psychotherapy in general	+	+	+	+	+	+	+	+	+
Not as efficient in severely malnourished patients	N.R.	N.R.	N.R.	✓	N.R.	✓	N.R.	+	+
Specific psychological interventions	✓	✓	N.R.	✓	✓	✓	✓	✓	✓
CBT/CBT-E	+	+	N.R.	+	+	+	+	+	+
Psychodynamic Therapy	N.R.	+	N.R.	+	+	N.R.	+	N.R.	+
FPT	N.R.	N.R.	N.R.	N.R.	+	N.R.	N.R.	N.R.	N.R.
MANTRA	N.R.	N.R.	N.R.	N.R.	+	+	N.R.	+	N.R.
SSCM	+	N.R.	N.R.	N.R.	+	+	N.R.	+	N.R.
IPT	N.R.	+	N.R.	N.R.	N.R.	N.R.	+	N.R.	+
For children and adolescents:									
Involvement of parents/near caregivers	+	+	+	+	+	+	+¹	+	+
Family therapy	FBT or other forms of family therapy	FBT	FBT or other forms of family therapy	Family therapy	FBT or other forms of family therapy	FBT?	Family therapy (systemic or not)	FT-AN	FBT or other forms of family therapy

✓ recommendation given; + explicit recommendation in favour; N.R., no recommendation reported; AUS, Australia and New Zealand; BC, British Columbia; DEN, Denmark; FR, France; GER, Germany; NETH, The Netherlands; SP, Spain; UK, United Kingdom; US, United States; CBT(-E), (Enhanced) Cognitive Behaviour Therapy; FPT, Focal Psychodynamic Therapy; MANTRA, Maudsley Model of Anorexia Nervosa Treatment for Adults; SSCM, Specialist Supportive Clinical Management; IPT, Interpersonal Therapy; FBT, Family-Based Treatment/Therapy; FT-AN, AN-focused Family Therapy; ¹ and siblings; ?, ambiguous evidence.

3.2.3. Nutritional Management

For adults: The WFSBP guideline [47] suggests that nasogastric feeding is effective for malnourished patients, however, does not address risks associated with refeeding, or provide any specific nutritional or weight gain recommendations. All remaining guidelines, (excluding the Danish guideline [40]), recommend nasogastric feeding for severely malnourished patients, when oral feeding is not an option [14,38,39,41,43,44,46,48]. These guidelines address the risk of refeeding syndrome, recommending that treatment is administered by experienced staff. The APA guideline [43] recommends nasogastric feeding over parenteral feeding, and the British guideline [38] explicitly recommends against parenteral nutrition. The German guideline also discusses the use of percutaneous endoscopic gastronomy feeding as a potential alternative, when patients will not tolerate nasogastric feeding [14]. The Danish guideline does not provide any recommendations regarding refeeding, nutritional intake or weight restoration.

In the original German guideline [15], an initial food intake of approximately 30 to 40 kcal/kg per day was recommended for highly underweight patients (see Table 1), which, upon revision, was considered too strict. The revised German guideline [14], as well as the Danish [40], French [44] and WFSBP guidelines [47], do not give specific recommendations regarding energy intake during refeeding. Both the British [38] and MARSIPAN guidelines [48] recommend commencing refeeding at 5 to 10 kcal/kg/day for severely underweight patients, and gradually increasing to 20 kcal/kg/day within 2 days. The British Columbia guideline [46] also recommends beginning refeeding at 5 to 10 kcal/kg/day if severity factors (e.g., nasogastric feeding) are involved. In the absence of severity factors, intake of 20 to 25 kcal/kg/day is recommended, and intake should not exceed 70 to 80 kcal/kg/day. The Spanish guideline [45] recommends a slightly higher caloric intake of 25 to 30 kcal/kg/day for severely malnourished patients, and they also provide a recommended upper limit of 1000 kcal/day. The APA guideline [43] recommends initiating refeeding at 30 to 40 kcal/kg/day, and also suggests that males may require a significantly higher energy intake to gain weight. The Dutch guideline has an even higher recommended refeeding starting point of 40 to 60 kcal/kg/day for severely underweight patients [39]. The Australian and New Zealand guideline [41] does not provide a recommended nutritional intake based on weight, but instead recommends a specific starting intake of 1433 kcal/day, with increases of 478kcal every 2 to 3 days.

Several guidelines also provide recommendations regarding appropriate weekly weight gain goals in inpatient and outpatient settings. Five guidelines recommend a minimum weight gain of 0.5 kg/week in an inpatient setting; the German [14], French [44] and Spanish guidelines [45] recommend weight gain ranging between 0.5 and 1 kg/week, the Australian and New Zealand guideline [41] recommends weight gain between 0.5 and 1.4 kg/week, and the Dutch guideline suggests weight gain ranging between 0.5 and 1.5 kg/week [39]. In contrast, the British Columbia guideline [46] suggests a higher minimum weight gain ranging from 0.8 to 1.4 kg/week, and the APA guideline [43] suggests a minimum weight gain ranging from 0.9 to 1.4 kg/week. The remaining guidelines [38,40,47,48] do not provide specific weight gain recommendations. Only four of the guidelines provide recommendations regarding weight gain per week in an outpatient setting. The French guideline recommends a weight gain of 0.25 kg/week, while the German, APA guidelines and Dutch recommend a weekly gain of between 0.2 to 0.5 kg [39].

For children and adolescents: The British guideline for the management of severely ill young people with AN (Junior MARSIPAN) [48,50] advocates to commence refeeding at about 40 kcal/kg/day and increase the meal plan by 200 kcal/day, while the others do not explicitly give calorie specifications for children and adolescents. Almost all guidelines recommend nasogastric tube feeding, if a meal plan and supplement drink tops are not managed [14,41,43,45,50].

The French, Danish and German guidelines emphasise the necessity of achieving a target weight at which menstruation can reoccur [14,40,44]. While the French guideline does not give any threshold criteria, the German guideline defines the 25th age-adapted BMI-percentile (with the 10th percentile as a minimum) in contrast to the Danish guideline with the 50th weight-for height percentile as target weight.

Supplementary nutritional counselling is advised by the British, Spanish and German guidelines for children and adolescents and their carers to help young people meet their dietary needs for pubertal development and growth [14,38,45]. According to these guidelines, growth and pubertal development should be regularly monitored in this age group.

3.2.4. Psychopharmacology

For adults: Use of pharmacotherapy is addressed in all treatment guidelines excluding the Danish guideline [40]. All of these guidelines emphasise the lack of evidence surrounding medication use for AN, and most guidelines emphasise that caution must be taken when administering medication, due to the physical complications associated with AN (e.g., cardiac problems). The Spanish [45], APA [43] and British guidelines [38] explicitly state that medication should not be used as the sole treatment. The British guideline also states that there is no proven benefit of combined treatment over psychotherapy alone in treating patients without comorbidities. All guidelines excluding the MARSIPAN [48], Danish and British guidelines give cautious recommendations for the use of antipsychotic medications. The French guideline [44] provides a cautionary recommendation, without addressing specific medications or effects. The remaining guidelines all make specific reference to the antipsychotic olanzapine; the German [14], WFSBP [47], Dutch [39], Australian and New Zealand [41], and APA guidelines recommended it to assist with anxious and obsessional thoughts, the WFSBP and Spanish guidelines suggest that it may be useful for improving general psychological symptoms, and the British Columbian [46], Spanish and APA guideline cautiously recommended it for improvements in weight gain. In contrast, the German guideline recommends against the use of antipsychotics for weight gain. The German guideline states there is no conclusive evidence to recommend the use of antidepressants for the core symptoms of AN, and the Dutch guideline also explicitly recommends against the use of selective serotonin reuptake inhibitors (SSRIs) [39]. In contrast, antidepressants are cautiously recommended by the French, WFSBP and APA guidelines, to assist with co-occurring symptoms of depression, obsessive–compulsive or anxiety disorder. Specifically, the APA guideline discusses the advantages of using selective serotonin reuptake inhibitors in combination with psychotherapy to address persistent depressive or anxiety symptoms, but recommends against the use of monoamine oxidase inhibitors and bupropion, due to adverse reactions and health risks. The APA guideline cautiously recommends the use of pro-motility agents for use against bloating, and use of antianxiety agents before eating for some patients. Similarly, the MARSIPAN guideline [48] discusses the use of benzodiazepines for particularly anxious patients. The WFSBP and APA guidelines discuss potential weight gain benefits of taking zinc supplements, while the German guideline suggests restricting zinc supplementation to cases with proven zinc deficiency.

For children and adolescents: With the exception of hormone replacement therapy the German and most other international guidelines do not give any specific recommendations for this age group. The Junior MARSIPAN guideline concludes that it 'may be necessary to prescribe regular sedative antipsychotic medication, such as olanzapine', if the patients are extremely agitated and resist refeeding [48]. It also gives clear recommendations for ECG monitoring if antipsychotics are applied. Hormone replacement therapy: In several guidelines including the German guideline the prescription of an oral contraceptive is not recommended [38,41,43]. The British guideline suggests considering a bone mineral density scan after one year of underweight in children and adolescents. Moreover—in correspondence to the German guideline—the British guideline suggests to consider transdermal estrogen replacement in combination with cyclic progesterone application in girls with a bone age over 15 years and long-term underweight as well as incremental physiological doses of estrogen in those below 15 years [14,38]. Similar indications are mentioned in the APA and the Australian and New Zealand guidelines [41,43].

4. Discussion

This review provides an overview of the newly revised and published German S3-guideline for eating disorders [14]. In particular, it highlights the changes in recommendations regarding the treatment of AN since the publication of the original guideline in 2011 [15]. In summary, family-based therapy approaches are recommended for adolescents, whereas individual approaches are suggested for adults. There is no evidence indicating the superiority of one specialised approach over another. In more intensive settings, as well as in adolescents, higher weight gains can be expected. To date, there is no convincing evidence for the positive effect of pharmacotherapy regarding the core symptoms of AN.

The revised German guideline is currently the most recent eating disorder treatment guideline internationally. Recommendations are, therefore, based on the most up to date research findings and evidence available. The development of this guideline involved a rigorous process, including a comprehensive literature review and analysis, and consultation and contribution by many experts in the eating disorder field. The findings of the literature review and network analysis are also available in English [18].

The German guideline also includes an easily comprehensible guide for sufferers with eating disorders and their relatives [17], which has been developed with the help of patient representatives. The German guideline, hereby, stresses the necessity of providing information and support to significant others, who often bear a high emotional burden, but also play an important role in helping patients to overcome the eating disorder. The guideline has been published in two different formats—as a scientific book (only the original version so far) and on the website of the Association of the Scientific Medical Societies in Germany (AWMF, awmf.org [14]), where it is freely available.

Similar to the Dutch guideline, the original version of the German guideline has been published in German only, which limits its distribution and implementation to Germany, Austria and Switzerland. An English translation of the revised version, which is currently in preparation, is, therefore, an invaluable step towards increasing the utility of this guideline.

The review also explores the similarities and differences between the German guideline and other existing international guidelines. There is significant homogeneity among the international guidelines in the recommendations derived from the existing evidence. All agree that there is no superior treatment for AN, if specialised approaches are compared. There are, however, some inconsistencies regarding aspects, such as medication and nutritional management. Most guidelines implemented a thorough methodology. We think there is a need for European research initiatives which aim to enhance the evidence base and clinical guidance regarding AN across the different participating countries. Recommendations must, however, take into account the specificities of the national health care systems.

Overall, evidence for treatment of AN has increased, yet even in the latest German guideline, many of the recommendations are still based on expert opinion. Guidelines do not only mirror the current state of research but also point out gaps that need to be bridged. There is still a need for more research in the field of eating disorders, particularly in AN. In view of the so-called 'research-practice gap', it needs to be mentioned that guidelines are not designed to propagate conformist standard therapy, or to restrict clinicians' individual willingness to learn and innovate. They should not be seen as directives, but as advice.

5. Conclusions

The German S3-guideline is, at present, the most recently revised evidence-based treatment guideline for AN. Based on newly available evidence, several amendments have been made regarding treatment recommendations, since the original guideline publication in 2011. Overall, the recommendations provided in the German guideline are fairly consistent with those provided in other international evidence-based eating disorder guidelines. Adult and adolescent patients should be distinguished in terms of treatment response and the most suitable treatment approach. Although the existing guidelines provide a sound base of information, which can be used by healthcare professionals to guide diagnosis and treatment decisions, further research regarding the treatment of AN is still urgently needed.

Author Contributions: Conceptualisation, G.R. and A.Z.; methodology, A.Z.; investigation, G.R.; writing—original draft preparation, G.R., S.H., B.H.-D. and A.Z.; writing–review and editing, G.R.

Funding: The S3-guideline was funded by the Christina Barz-Stiftung in the Association of German Academic Foundations.

Acknowledgments: The support of the publication fund of the University Hospital Tuebingen was greatly appreciated. We would also like to thank all contributors to the German S3-guideline and the Arbeitsgemeinschaft der Wissenschaftlichen Medizinischen Fachgesellschaften (AWMF). The authors would like to thank Brigid Kennedy for her help in preparing this manuscript.

Conflicts of Interest: The authors declare no conflict of interest.

References

1. Teufel, M.; Friederich, H.-C.; Groß, G.; Schauenburg, H.; Herzog, W.; Zipfel, S. Anorexia nervosa – Diagnostik und Therapie. *PPmP* **2009**, *59*, 454–466. [CrossRef] [PubMed]
2. Treasure, J.; Zipfel, S.; Micali, N.; Wade, T.; Stice, E.; Claudino, A.; Schmidt, U.; Frank, G.K.; Bulik, C.M.; Wentz, E. Anorexia nervosa. *Nat. Rev. Dis. Primers* **2015**, *1*, 15074. [CrossRef] [PubMed]
3. Zipfel, S.; Löwe, B.; Reas, D.L.; Deter, H.C.; Herzog, W. Long-term prognosis in anorexia nervosa: Lessons from a 21-year follow-up study. *Lancet* **2000**, *355*, 721–722. [CrossRef]
4. Zipfel, S.; Giel, K.E.; Bulik, C.M.; Hay, P.; Schmidt, U. Anorexia nervosa: Aetiology, assessment, and treatment. *Lancet Psychiat.* **2015**, *2*, 1099–1111. [CrossRef]
5. World Health Organization (WHO) ICD 11 International Classification of Diseases 11th Revision. Available online: https://icd.who.int/ (accessed on 17 December 2018).
6. American Psychiatric Association. *Diagnostic and Statistical Manual of Mental Disorders*, 5th ed.; American Psychiatric Publishing: Washington, DC, USA, 2013.
7. Wentz, E.; Gillberg, I.C.; Anckarsäter, H.; Gillberg, C.; Råstam, M. Adolescent-onset anorexia nervosa: 18-year outcome. *Br. J. Psychiatry* **2009**, *194*, 168–174. [CrossRef] [PubMed]
8. Egger, N.; Wild, B.; Zipfel, S.; Junne, F.; Konnopka, A.; Schmidt, U.; de Zwaan, M.; Herpertz, S.; Zeeck, A.; Löwe, B.; et al. Cost-effectiveness of focal psychodynamic therapy and enhanced cognitive-behavioural therapy in out-patients with anorexia nervosa. *Psychol. Med.* **2016**, *46*, 3291–3301. [CrossRef] [PubMed]
9. Stuhldreher, N.; Konnopka, A.; Wild, B.; Herzog, W.; Zipfel, S.; Löwe, B.; König, H.-H. Cost-of-illness studies and cost-effectiveness analyses in eating disorders: A systematic review. *Int. J. Eat. Disord.* **2012**, *45*, 476–491. [CrossRef] [PubMed]
10. Jäger, B.; Herpertz, S. S3-Leitlinie Diagnostik und Therapie der Essstörungen. *PiD* **2013**, *14*, 16–21. [CrossRef]
11. Giel, K.; Groß, G.; Zipfel, S. Neue S3-Leitlinie zur Behandlung von Essstörungen. *Psychother. Psychosom. Med. Psychol.* **2011**, *61*, 293–294. [CrossRef] [PubMed]
12. Fichter, M.; Schweiger, U.; Krieg, C.; Pirke, K.; Ploog, D.; Remschmidt, H. *Behandlungsleitlinie Eßstörungen, Praxisleitlinien in Psychiatrie und Psychotherapie*, 4th ed.; Steinkopff-Verlag: Darmstadt, Germany, 2000.
13. Herpertz-Dahlmann, B.; Hebebrand, J.; Remschmidt, H. *Leitlinien zur Diagnostik und Therapie von psychischen Störungen im Säuglings-, Kindes- und Jugendalter: Hrsg. d. Dtsch. Ges. für Kinder- u. für Kinder-& Jugendpsychiatrie u. Psycho*, 3rd ed.; Deutscher Ärzteverlag: Köln, Germany, 2000.
14. Herpertz, S.; Herpertz-Dahlmann, B.; Fichter, M.; Tuschen-Caffier, B.; Zeek, A. S3-Leitlinie Diagnostik und Behandlung der Essstörungen (Online). Available online: https://www.awmf.org/leitlinien/detail/ll/051-026.html (accessed on 29 January 2019).
15. Herpertz, S.; Herpertz-Dahlmann, B.; Fichter, M.; Tuschen-Caffier, B.; Zeeck, A. *S3-Leitlinie Diagnostik und Behandlung der Essstörungen*; Springer: Berlin, Germany, 2011.
16. Zeeck, A.; Herpertz, S. Diagnostik und Behandlung von Essstörungen - Ratgeber für Patienten und Angehörige: Patientenleitlinie der Deutschen Gesellschaft für Essstörungen (Online). Available online: https://www.dgppn.de/_Resources/Persistent/4c462ba248a0ce039579c678d467c33092a283a0/Patientenleitlinie%20Essst%C3%B6rungen%202015.pdf (accessed on 29 January 2019).

17. Zeeck, A.; Herpertz, S. *Diagnostik und Behandlung von Essstörungen - Ratgeber für Patienten und Angehörige: Patientenleitlinie der Deutschen Gesellschaft für Essstörungen*; Springer: Berlin, Germany, 2015.
18. Zeeck, A.; Herpertz-Dahlmann, B.; Friederich, H.-C.; Brockmeyer, T.; Resmark, G.; Hagenah, U.; Ehrlich, S.; Cuntz, U.; Zipfel, S.; Hartmann, A. Psychotherapeutic treatment for anorexia nervosa: A systematic review and network meta-analysis. *Front. Psychiatry* **2018**, *9*. [CrossRef]
19. Svaldi, J.; Schmitz, F.; Baur, J.; Hartmann, A.S.; Legenbauer, T.; Thaler, C.; von Wietersheim, J.; de Zwaan, M.; Tuschen-Caffier, B. Efficacy of psychotherapies and pharmacotherapies for bulimia nervosa. *Psychol. Med.* **2018**, 1–13. [CrossRef] [PubMed]
20. Hilbert, A.; Petroff, D.; Herpertz, S.; Pietrowsky, R.; Tuschen-Caffier, B.; Vocks, S.; Schmidt, R. Meta-analysis of the efficacy of psychological and medical treatments for binge-eating disorder. *J. Consult. Clin. Psychol.* **2019**, *87*, 91–105. [CrossRef] [PubMed]
21. Agras, W.S.; Lock, J.; Brandt, H.; Bryson, S.W.; Dodge, E.; Halmi, K.A.; Jo, B.; Johnson, C.; Kaye, W.; Wilfley, D.; et al. Comparison of 2 family therapies for adolescent anorexia nervosa: a randomized parallel trial. *JAMA Psychiatry* **2014**, *71*, 1279–1286. [CrossRef]
22. Eisler, I.; Simic, M.; Hodsoll, J.; Asen, E.; Berelowitz, M.; Connan, F.; Ellis, G.; Hugo, P.; Schmidt, U.; Treasure, J.; et al. A pragmatic randomised multi-centre trial of multifamily and single family therapy for adolescent anorexia nervosa. *BMC Psychiatry* **2016**, *16*, 422. [CrossRef] [PubMed]
23. Herpertz-Dahlmann, B.; Schwarte, R.; Krei, M.; Egberts, K.; Warnke, A.; Wewetzer, C.; Pfeiffer, E.; Fleischhaker, C.; Scherag, A.; Holtkamp, K.; et al. Day-patient treatment after short inpatient care versus continued inpatient treatment in adolescents with anorexia nervosa (ANDI): A multicentre, randomised, open-label, non-inferiority trial. *Lancet* **2014**, *383*, 1222–1229. [CrossRef]
24. Le Grange, D.; Hughes, E.K.; Court, A.; Yeo, M.; Crosby, R.D.; Sawyer, S.M. Randomized clinical trial of parent-focused treatment and family-based treatment for adolescent anorexia nervosa. *J. Am. Acad. Child. Adolesc. Psychiatry* **2016**, *55*, 683–692. [CrossRef]
25. Schmidt, U.; Magill, N.; Renwick, B.; Keyes, A.; Kenyon, M.; Dejong, H.; Lose, A.; Broadbent, H.; Loomes, R.; Yasin, H.; et al. The Maudsley outpatient study of treatments for anorexia nervosa and related conditions (MOSAIC): Comparison of the Maudsley model of anorexia nervosa treatment for adults (MANTRA) with specialist supportive clinical management (SSCM) in outpatients with broadly defined anorexia nervosa: A randomized controlled trial. *J. Consult. Clin. Psychol.* **2015**, *83*, 796–807.
26. Zipfel, S.; Wild, B.; Groß, G.; Friederich, H.-C.; Teufel, M.; Schellberg, D.; Giel, K.E.; de Zwaan, M.; Dinkel, A.; Herpertz, S.; et al. Focal psychodynamic therapy, cognitive behaviour therapy, and optimised treatment as usual in outpatients with anorexia nervosa (ANTOP study): Randomised controlled trial. *Lancet* **2014**, *383*, 127–137. [CrossRef]
27. Phillips, B.; Ball, C.; Sackett, D.; Badenoch, D.; Straus, S.; Haynes, B.; Dawes, M. Oxford Centre for Evidence-based Medicine - Levels of Evidence (March 2009). Available online: https://www.cebm.net/2009/06/oxford-centre-evidence-based-medicine-levels-evidence-march-2009/ (accessed on 19 November 2018).
28. Kopp, I.B.; Selbmann, H.-K.; Koller, M. Consensus development in evidence-based guidelines: From myths to rational strategies. *Z. Arztl. Fortbild. Qualitatssich.* **2007**, *101*, 89–95.
29. Carter, J.C.; Mercer-Lynn, K.B.; Norwood, S.J.; Bewell-Weiss, C.V.; Crosby, R.D.; Woodside, D.B.; Olmsted, M.P. A prospective study of predictors of relapse in anorexia nervosa: Implications for relapse prevention. *Psychiatry Res.* **2012**, *200*, 518–523. [CrossRef] [PubMed]
30. Eckert, E.D.; Halmi, K.A.; Marchi, P.; Grove, W.; Crosby, R. Ten-year follow-up of anorexia nervosa: Clinical course and outcome. *Psychol. Med.* **1995**, *25*, 143–156. [CrossRef] [PubMed]
31. Strober, M.; Freeman, R.; Morrell, W. The long-term course of severe anorexia nervosa in adolescents: Survival analysis of recovery, relapse, and outcome predictors over 10-15 years in a prospective study. *Int. J. Eat. Disord.* **1997**, *22*, 339–360. [CrossRef]
32. Friederich, H.-C.; Herzog, W.; Wild, B.; Zipfel, S.; Schauenburg, H. *Anorexia Nervosa: Fokale Psychodynamische Psychotherapie*, 1st ed.; Hogrefe Verlag: Göttingen, Germany, 2014.
33. Friederich, H.-C.; Wild, B.; Zipfel, S.; Schauenburg, H.; Herzog, W. *Anorexia Nervosa: Focal Psychodynamic Psychotherapy*, 2019th ed.; Hogrefe Publishing: Boston, MA, USA, 2019.
34. Fairburn, C. *Cognitive Behavior Therapy and Eating Disorders*, 1st ed.; Guilford Press: New York, NY, USA, 2008.
35. Touyz, S.; Le Grange, D.; Lacey, H.; Hay, P.; Smith, R.; Maguire, S.; Bamford, B.; Pike, K.; Crosby, R. Treating severe and enduring anorexia nervosa: a randomized control trial. *Eur. Psychiatry* **2015**, *30*, 357. [CrossRef]

36. McIntosh, V.V.W.; Jordan, J.; Carter, F.A.; Luty, S.E.; McKenzie, J.M.; Bulik, C.M.; Frampton, C.M.A.; Joyce, P.R. Three psychotherapies for anorexia nervosa: A randomized, controlled trial. *Am. J. Psychiatry* **2005**, *162*, 741–747. [CrossRef] [PubMed]
37. Dutch Foundation for Quality Development in Mental Healthcare. Practice Guideline for the Treatment of Eating Disorders [Zorgstandard Eetstoornissen]. Available online: https://www.ggzstandaarden.nl/zorgstandaarden/eetstoornissen (accessed on 8 November 2018).
38. National Guideline Alliance (UK). Eating Disorders: Recognition and Treatment. Available online: https://www.nice.org.uk/guidance/ng69/ (accessed on 1 October 2018).
39. Hilbert, A.; Hoek, H.W.; Schmidt, R. Evidence-based clinical guidelines for eating disorders: International comparison. *Curr. Opin. Psychiatry* **2017**, *30*, 423–437. [CrossRef] [PubMed]
40. Danish Health Authority. National Clinical Guideline for the Treatment of Anorexia Nervosa; Quick Guide. Available online: https://www.google.com/url?sa=t&rct=j&q=&esrc=s&source=web&cd=1&ved=2ahUKEwi0ws31keDeAhXIzKQKHWGUBAUQFjAAegQICRAC&url=https%3A%2F%2Fwww.sst.dk%2Fda%2Fudgivelser%2F2016%2F~{}%2Fmedia%2F36D31B378C164922BCD96573749AA206.ashx&usg=AOvVaw2q2_ZWBhf6MqnHgZp8vfxR (accessed on 1 October 2018).
41. Royal Australian and New Zealand College of Psychiatrists Clinical Practice Guidelines Team for Anorexia Nervosa. Australian and New Zealand clinical practice guidelines for the treatment of anorexia nervosa. *Aust. N. Z. J. Psychiatry* **2004**, *38*, 659–670. [CrossRef] [PubMed]
42. Yager, J.; Devlin, M.J.; Halmi, K.A.; Herzog, D.B.; Mitchell, J.E.; Powers, P.; Zerbe, K.J. Guideline Watch (August 2012): Practice guideline for the treatment of patients with eating disorders, 3rd ed. *FOCUS* **2012**, *12*, 416–431. [CrossRef]
43. Yager, J.; Devlin, M.J.; Halmi, K.A.; Herzog, D.B.; Mitchell, J.E.; Powers, P.; Yerbe, K.J. Practice Guideline for the Treatment of Patients with Eating Disorders, 3rd ed. Available online: https://www.google.com/url?sa=t&rct=j&q=&esrc=s&source=web&cd=1&cad=rja&uact=8&ved=2ahUKEwiajvSW0djeAhXNposKHUmuB8QQFjAAegQICBAC&url=https%3A%2F%2Fpsychiatryonline.org%2Fpb%2Fassets%2Fraw%2Fsitewide%2Fpractice_guidelines%2Fguidelines%2Featingdisorders.pdf&usg=AOvVaw1mmGEBSYOQgyC9FX4fGjBs (accessed on 1 October 2018).
44. Haute Autorité de Santé. Clinical Practice Guidelines: Anorexia Nervosa: Management. Available online: https://www.has-sante.fr/portail/upload/docs/application/pdf/2013-05/anorexia_nervosa_guidelines_2013-05-15_16-34-42_589.pdf (accessed on 1 October 2018).
45. Working Group of the Clinical Practice Guideline for Eating Disorders. Clinical Practice Guideline for Eating Disorders. Available online: http://www.guiasalud.es/GPC/GPC_440_Eat_Disorders_compl_en.pdf (accessed on 1 October 2018).
46. Ministry of Health. Clinical Practice Guidelines for the BC Eating Disorders Continuum of Services. Available online: http://mh.providencehealthcare.org/sites/default/files/BC%20Eating%20Disorders%20Clinical%20Practice%20Guidelines.pdf (accessed on 1 October 2018).
47. Aigner, M.; Treasure, J.; Kaye, W.; Kasper, S.; The WFSBP task force on eating disorders. World Federation of Societies of Biological Psychiatry (WFSBP) guidelines for the pharmacological treatment of eating disorders. *World J. Biol. Psychiatry* **2011**, *12*, 400–443. [CrossRef] [PubMed]
48. Robinson, P.; Rhys Jones, W. MARSIPAN: Management of really sick patients with anorexia nervosa. *BJPsych Adv.* **2014**, *24*, 20–32. [CrossRef]
49. Treatment of Patients with Eating Disorders. In *APA Practice Guidelines for the Treatment of Psychiatric Disorders: Comprehensive Guidelines and Guideline Watches*, 3rd ed.; American Psychiatric Association: Arlington, VA, USA, 2006.
50. Robinson, P.H.; Kukucska, R.; Guidetti, G.; Leavey, G. Severe and enduring anorexia nervosa (SEED-AN): A qualitative study of patients with 20+ years of anorexia nervosa. *Eur. Eat. Disord. Rev.* **2015**, *23*, 318–326. [CrossRef]

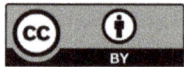

© 2019 by the authors. Licensee MDPI, Basel, Switzerland. This article is an open access article distributed under the terms and conditions of the Creative Commons Attribution (CC BY) license (http://creativecommons.org/licenses/by/4.0/).

MDPI
St. Alban-Anlage 66
4052 Basel
Switzerland
Tel. +41 61 683 77 34
Fax +41 61 302 89 18
www.mdpi.com

Actuators Editorial Office
E-mail: actuators@mdpi.com
www.mdpi.com/journal/JCM

www.ingramcontent.com/pod-product-compliance
Lightning Source LLC
LaVergne TN
LVHW070618100526
838202LV00012B/677